RUSSIAN DOCTOR

RUSSIAN DOCTOR

Vladimir Golyakhovsky

Translated from the Russian by
Michael Sylwester and
Eugene Ostrovsky

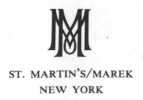

ST. MARTIN'S/MAREK
NEW YORK

Design by Manuela Paul

Library of Congress Cataloging in Publication Data

Golyakhovsky, Vladimir.
    Russian doctor.

    1. Golyakhovsky, Vladimir.   2. Orthopedists—Soviet
Union—Biography.   3. Jews—Soviet Union—Biography.
4. Soviet Union—Social life and customs.   I. Title.
RD728.G64A37 1984   617.3'0092'4 [B]   83-21204
ISBN 0-312-69609-4

First Edition
10 9 8 7 6 5 4 3 2 1

To my son—a future American doctor.

FOREWORD

Americans believe that all Russians are communists, while Russians think that all Americans are millionaires. Neither know much about each other.

I left Russia five years ago as a forty-eight-year-old successful orthopedic surgeon, capable of providing a comfortable living for my family, as comfort goes in Russia. I enjoyed my life, but I was not a communist. That is precisely the reason why I had finally come, after a long and tortuous mental journey, to the decision to emigrate. Leaving the country meant the loss of everything: social and professional status; orderly life; comforts to which I had grown accustomed. The reasons why I did it are disclosed in this book. In America I wrote the history of my life interspersed with my observations of people and events amassed over the quarter-century of my medical career. All information is factual except for a few names, changed to protect those who still live in Russia.

From beyond the ocean my former country looks like a giant iceberg. From afar, outsiders cannot see more than a fraction of reality. But I knew only too well its hidden underwater parts because I was both a physician and a writer; as a doctor, I came in close contact with thousands of patients—from the country's leader Nikita Khrushchev to a poor suicidal girl; as a writer, I trained myself to observe characters and circumstances.

It was difficult to select a suitable format for this book. It is not really a personal memoir, nor a compendium of real-life stories. Willy-nilly, I had to be its main protagonist, for all the events and facts described in the book are only pasted together with the glue of my participation. It was an enormous task to persuade literary agents and publishers that my manuscript merited attention. If not for the invaluable assistance of Michael Sylwester, the book may not have appeared. Mike believed in the book even more fervently than its author did. He commenced translating the manuscript into English at his own peril, sacrificing a whole year of nights and days off. With his aid I managed to breach the wall of indifference. For these reasons I am infinitely grateful to Mike. Unfortunately, he could not finish the translation. I am grateful to his successor, Eugene Ostrovsky, for his labors. Several fragments from the initial part of the book were translated by Leo Stern, to whom I also owe a debt of gratitude.

Since the time my family and I left Russia we have gone through many emigration hardships. For five years now we have been gradually adapting to a new, American way of life in New York City. In this city, nothing can surprise: it has everything, all kinds of people and all kinds of things. Still, several curious New Yorkers, having learned the highlights of my life, asked me two typical questions: Am I glad to have left Russia? and Do I like it here in America?

Not all of them were patient enough to bear with my explanations, though I tried to be concise and clear (who of us is not forever in a hurry?!). If the reader has more time and patience, enough to read the book to the end, he will have no difficulty guessing my reply to the former question.

As for the latter, all I can say is that I did not become a millionaire when I became an American.

However . . . that is an entirely different story.

Dr. Vladimir Golyakhovsky
New York City, 1983

1

I was sitting at a long wooden table in the Marble Hall of the Second Moscow Joseph Stalin Medical School taking my fourth and last entrance exam, on chemistry, one day in August 1947. I was a seventeen-year-old high school graduate. The competition was intense, because there were four applicants for each position. Each applicant had chosen randomly a card with three questions from a table and had then sat down for a few minutes to think about how he would answer.

About a fifth of the applicants and several of the teachers giving the exam were war veterans. Almost all of them were wearing their military uniforms with all their ribbons, but without their rank insignia. Most of them simply did not have the money to buy a civilian suit; the ribbons showed how well they had fought in the war.

The applicant sitting next to me was a young but gray-haired veteran with eight awards and medals on his chest. He was obviously having a hard time trying to think of the answers. After years of war, the veterans had forgotten the formulas and theorems that were still fresh to me. I felt sorry for him, so I began to whisper his answers to him, and he mouthed them word for word, trying to memorize them.

Our examiner sat across the table and pretended not to notice our cheating. He was wearing the same kind of uniform and medals, but looked twice as old. He suddenly asked: "Where did you finish the war?"

"In Prague," my young neighbor answered proudly. "I was a senior lieutenant in the tank troops."

"Which unit?"

"The Third Guards Tank Army under General Rybalko."

"Why didn't you say so earlier? I was in the same army. I was a major in a brigade under General Yakubovskiy."

"My platoon was in the very next brigade," the young veteran said enthusiastically. "We were fighting right next to each other."

"Side by side!" the older veteran exclaimed. He jumped up to embrace his comrade across the table. Everybody in the room stopped what they were doing and looked at the two veterans, so they lowered their voices.

"Look," said the examiner to his young comrade, "I'll just give you a five [the highest score]. Let's go out now and have a drink together."

He closed his examination book and they prepared to leave. I realized that if the examiner left I would have to pick another card and prepare another answer for another examiner.

"What about me?" I asked.

"You?" He then seemed to understand my predicament. He opened his book again and wrote something next to my name and then reached out with a smile to shake my hand. "You already passed. I'll give you a five too—for providing the correct answers to a combat veteran who had fallen into a difficult peacetime situation. As your reward, you will become a doctor."

They both walked out, their boots thumping across the floor. They would drink vodka and reminisce about army buddies who had died and who had survived. And I would become a medical student.

When I was accepted into the medical school, I expected big changes in my personal life. In those first few years after the war, all Soviet people expected things to get better. The war, which had caused millions to die and untold injuries, marked the absolute depth of suffering. The government and the media encouraged the universal expectation that better times would now come.

World War Two became a watershed in our family history: my parents' younger years were over and their maturity and my coming of age lay ahead. We all rejoiced when my father, Yuly Zak, came home after the war after serving as chief surgeon general with several armies for four years. He retired from the military service as a colonel with fourteen decorations. He was forty-seven at the time, and the first doctor and university graduate in a large and poor Jewish family. Several generations of Zaks had lived in Russia, with all the bitter experience of life under the czars, and had been exposed to the horrors of Russian anti-Semitism. In their predicament, the family had to roam from one place to another within the Pale of settlement reserved for Russian Jews. My father's grandfather, Rabbi Blumshtein, became the first rabbi in the city of Nizhny Novgorod, present-day Gorki; a permit for residence there was issued to him by the special decree of the czar. For a time, the family settled down, but then, when the Revolution erupted, the family fortunes declined again and several Zaks fled to begin new lives in Europe and in America. Those who stayed behind tried to make amends with the new regime.

My father had dreamed of becoming a doctor ever since he was a baby. Jews were enrolled into universities without discrimination after the Revolution, and in 1926, he graduated from the University of Kazan. He vacationed in Sukhumi, on the Black Sea Coast, where he became infatuated with Augusta Golyakhovsky, a beautiful twenty-six-year-old nurse in a trade union sanatorium. My mother-to-be was a descendant of an ancient noble family with an exquisite coat of arms and long military history. Several generations of her ancestors were Cossack generals, but her father, Vladimir, was a railroad official. Although none of my maternal relatives had any formal education they had had good tutors, and several were talented musicians and painters. Count Leo Tolstoy was their distant relative, and several of his works, including *War and Peace,* made reference to the Golyakhovsky family.

My mother was educated at a special institution for the daughters of the nobility. Together with other girls from the aristocratic families she was selected to greet Czar Nicholas II on the three-hundredth anniversary of the Romanov dynasty. All her relatives fought against the communists during the Revolution. Many of them died, and many fled to Europe, leaving behind their mansions and real estate. Those few who stayed in Russia adjusted to the new regime. My mother became a nurse, living on a miserable paycheck. My father went mad about her and proposed in a month. When he had returned to Kazan, he sent her money for railroad fare, and soon she came to him, carrying a small valise containing her second dress and wearing fancy felt boots. It still puzzles me how she could have abandoned her milieu to marry into a poor Jewish family. Their marriage defies all logic, yet they lived happily for over fifty years.

When my mother moved in, there was no private bedroom for the newlyweds in the house and it often happened that the family of seven living there had only herring for dinner. My dad had a lot of the entrepreneur in him; he was a hard worker but very unsure of himself. He would waver in many situations, lose his nerve and become overcome by doubts. "Weh, what will happen to us?" he would say. He was not a skinflint, but he loved money and did not part with it easily. He was uninhibited, nervous, and a babbler, thus epitomizing many features of the Russian Jew.

My mom, his antipode, was serenity itself, always preserving her sense of humor and confident there was no difficult situation without a resolution. She was impractical, spent a lot of money, and never cared. These features betrayed her former aristocracy. Different circumstances shaped their vastly different characters. Well, it was the Cossacks, on my maternal side, who for over one hundred years had been staging the pogroms of the Jews!

Their one common feature was sociability. As far back as I can remember, they were surrounded by people from all walks of life, highly intellectual types as well as commoners. They were all attracted by my parents' geniality, high spirits, and hospitality. My mother had a quick sense of humor; my dad was "a regular fellow" and could play the piano well. My mother had a deep interest in literature, history, and the arts, while my father barely knew anything outside his profession but adored dispensing medical advice. His counsel was always to the point; he was a good doctor.

My young mother liked it that her husband was an educated person, a doctor with a future, whereas my father worshiped his Russian beauty wife and was fond of showing her off to his friends and colleagues. My birth on December 24, 1929, in Kazan, exactly nine months to the day after my mother had moved in, was a merry event for all the Jewish kith and kin on my father's side. My Russian relatives, on my mother's side, lived very far from us then. All father's aunts and cousins would come and help the young inexperienced mother to coddle me. One wintry day, when I was only ten days old, she took me and headed for the University of Kazan. On entering the ancient building with the white marble pillars she drew back the warm wrapper from my face.

"When you grow up, my son, be a learned man," she said.

I, of course, do not remember the occasion, but I did as she wished. My parents had no other children: life was too difficult for them as it was.

My father made a very good start as a doctor but he failed to win admission to fellowship because of his religion. The Jews were allowed to get an education, but all kinds of obstacles were put in their way when they tried to advance themselves. In search of a new job, my parents relocated to the city of Gorki, where my father was appointed head doctor of a hospital and was assigned a comfortable two-bedroom apartment with a spacious parlor. However, we had to vacate the apartment in a few months when we were evicted by the chief of the local secret police, who had an eye for it. My infuriated father intended to go to the courts. His wise friends talked him out of it, pointing out that the best thing for him to do was to flee the town. Their line of reasoning was that the chief of the secret police could have him arrested and even executed on the pretext of his political unsoundness. My father was not a Communist Party member, and this could be interpreted as silent opposition to the regime.

"Since we're not lucky in the provinces, let's move to Moscow," my mother suggested.

My father had been raised in a provincial community and, in his heart, was scared of life in the capital. My mother, an aristocrat, was sold on the throbbing cultural life of a metropolitan center.

"You needn't think that we shall have it harder in Moscow," she reasoned. "I think that you will have better opportunities there and you will find a medical job faster. And our son, when he grows up, will be better off there, too."

My mother was being unrealistic because we had no place to live in Moscow. However, my father's elder brother Michael Zak had ceded him a small bedroom in his two-bedroom apartment in a wooden two-story house on the outskirts of the city. We lived in it for twenty-five years.

I remember a few episodes of those hard times whose meaning I could not grasp as a child. My mother tried to protect me, seeing that I was well fed and clothed while my parents were not— they only began buying good things for themselves in their late thirties. So I grew up pampered, and thus my first encounter with the outside world was painful. On September 1, 1937, my mother brought me to the gates of the grammar school and I was enrolled into the first grade under my father's name as Vladimir Zak. On that day our schoolmistress addressed the class of forty boys and girls with these words: "Kids, do you know what a nationality is?"

We answered in the affirmative.

"I will call out different nationalities that make up our nation and, please, raise your hands when I name yours," she suggested.

It looked like a game and we liked it.

"Russian," she said; most of the children raised their hands.

I was puzzled because I knew that my mother was Russian and my father was Jewish. "Ukrainian," the school mistress called out. Several hands went up. "Jewish," she said and I, happy that my turn had come at last, raised my lonely hand. I remember how the atmosphere in class changed. There was silence, and then general laughter broke out. The children pointed their fingers at me. "Zak is a Jew, Zak is a Jew!" they cried out. I could hardly understand what was wrong. Didn't I raise my hand like the others?

"Children, you should not laugh at Zak. Jewish is a nationality like any other," the schoolmistress tried to calm the class in a none-too-confident voice. The children did not seem to agree with her. But at last they quieted down, and I sat there stunned by the revelation: it hurts to be a Jew.

Back home, I told my story. My father was visibly distressed and buried his head in his hands. My mother acted firmly and with calm, taking a step that was to change my life: she went with me to a new grammar school and had me enrolled under her Russian name as Vladimir Golyakhovsky. My father did not object; he felt it was necessary.

No one has teased me as Jew since then, but the scar remained. All my life I had to hide my Jewish origins in order to conform to the norms of the Soviet society. I suffered and the people who knew my story continued to consider me Jewish.

I do not know whether I am Russian or Jewish to this day. I rather think I am both.

In our small room, my parents slept on a bed behind a curtain; grandmother slept on a fold-out couch; and I slept on several suitcases in one of the corners. We shared a common kitchen, toilet, and bathroom not only with my father's brother's family but also with a third family who lived in the third room. We kept potatoes in the bathtub, and there was barely enough wood for the wood furnace, much less to heat water. Each of the families had a separate table with a hot plate in the kitchen, and all of the families shared a single sink. In all, there were nine adults. Most Soviets lived this way.

Despite these difficult conditions, our life seemed easy and happy. My father earned a relatively high salary, and my parents had a lot of well-educated friends—doctors, lawyers, actors, writers, scientists, and so on. My parents liked to invite as many as ten people to parties in our apartment. They would move the furniture out into the corridor so that they could dance. During these parties, I would often study in the quiet bathroom with the potatoes.

Many of my parents' friends were Jews, and they felt that their condition was hardly better than it had been before the war. Many of them had prospered during the war, because the communists had needed their skills and talents so badly that they allowed them to occupy many of the middle-level positions in government and industry.

Jewish families were starting to advance their children up through society. In general, Jews felt that the Nazi atrocities had finally discredited anti-Semitism for all time.

2

The first lecture on the first day of classes in medical school on Marxism-Leninism-Stalinism was held in an auditorium decorated with big portraits of Lenin and Stalin. The instructor, Professor N. Dubinin, recited quotations and slogans without sense and axioms without proof. Nobody paid any attention to this gobbledygook, of course, and I remember that I gazed at one of my classmates, Lena

Kozak, a beautiful blonde, during the whole lecture. Nevertheless, these lectures subconsciously taught us that ideological submission was more important than professional accomplishment.

These political lectures took up about a third of my class time during my six years at the medical school. I studied the history of the Communist Party, the basics of Marxism-Leninism, political economy, dialectical materialism, and Marxist-Leninist philosophy. All of this instruction was completely dogmatic. The professors followed a strictly established schedule of instruction based on the textbooks and allowed no deviations or even rational explanations to interfere with the program. The holiest of all Marxist scripture at that time was the fourth chapter of *A Short History of the Bolshevik Party,* because supposedly Stalin Himself had written it.

The official awe toward this chapter went far beyond the awe felt for the Ten Commandments; students were asked to memorize it. Naturally, no one did so, but no one could refuse pretending to do so. As a result all the students murmured the text under their breath, exactly as a hasty parishioner drones a familiar, wearisome prayer. We uttered the words of the text without a thought, and I never discovered what the chapter contained.

If a student failed to do an assignment for any of these classes —for example, if he didn't write a summary of *Lenin's Materialism and Empirocriticism*— the Komsomol (Communist Youth League) called a meeting to threaten the student with expulsion from the school if he missed a second assignment. No such measures were ever taken if a student missed an assignment in any medical courses.

In Russia, medical students do not have to study at a college first and so are unprepared to study medicine. To compensate, we had to study theory in the classroom for the entire first two years. We studied general medicine during the third, fourth, and fifth years and a specialty such as surgery or pediatrics during the sixth.

The professors of the Moscow Medical School surpassed those in staffs of other medical schools. The equipment, although not in adequate supply, was still the best. And in the capital we felt the pulse of the public life of the country more sharply than in the provinces. News was spread in Moscow within minutes by means of rumors. It was published in the newspapers several weeks later. Soviet people privately discussing public or political news asked each other: "Have you heard?" and not: "Have you read?"

I began to hear about the campaign against cosmopolitans in 1948. It began with the art critic Yuzovskiy, a Jew. Although he had only been known to a small circle of intellectuals, he suddenly became the target of widely publicized accusations that he lacked patriotism and worshiped the West. In the following months, hundreds of writers, scientists, actors, and artists were accused of the same crimes, which were generally labeled "cosmopolitanism." The communists called meetings at factories, institutes, universities, theaters, publishing houses, and other organizations, and made these accusations. The victims were fired, arrested, and often sent to Siberian labor camps. Most of the people the communists accused of "cosmopolitanism" were Jews.

The first victim at our school was a very popular professor, Dr. Anatoly Geselevich, a fifty-year-old Jew, a member of the Communist Party. He headed the department of topographic anatomy and operative surgery and had written the best textbook on his specialty. All of us students loved to attend his articulate and thoughtful lectures. He was a pleasant and witty man with a Vandyke beard. He joked easily and laughed loudly. He wore a military uniform with the rank of colonel and the Lenin Medal.

The accusation against him was made one day in 1948 at a meeting of the Party members. The Party secretary, Dr. V. Dobrynina (a relative of the Soviet ambassador to the United States Anatoly Dobrynin), a biochemist, began to read a speech about Dr. Geselevich's cosmopolitanism. She said that his articles, lectures, and textbooks had propagandized Western scientists more than Russian and Soviet scientists. Specifically, she accused him of not citing the works of the great Russian anatomist and surgeon of the nineteenth century, Dr. Nikolay Pirogov.

The news of this accusation instantly spread throughout the school and among all medical professionals in Moscow. The people who heard the news divided into two camps. One group, which consisted of communists and Russians, openly discussed the accusations with interest and approval. The other, smaller group, mainly Jews, whispered about the accusations with alarm. Everybody noted that Dr. Dobrynina had read the speech, which meant that it had been written by someone above her.

In the following days, Dr. Geselevich's appearance changed dramatically. His back and shoulders drooped, and his face was full of worry. He continued to give his lectures and referred to Russian physicians more often, but his lectures lost their originality. His son Viktor was a student in the class with me, and I once noticed tears in his eyes.

At the next Party meeting, the communists heard the conclusions of a commission that had investigated the accusations against Dr. Geselevich. The commission, which consisted of professors who belonged to the Party, accused Dr. Geselevich of worshiping Western science and culture, of lacking patriotism, and of failing to teach his students pride in Russian and Soviet science. The commission referred to Dr. Geselevich without his title of "professor" and openly called him a "rootless cosmopolitan."

Two of Dr. Geselevich's graduate students, Yury Lopukhin, a Russian, and Ilya Movshovich, a Jew, both of them friends of mine, defended him, although both were communists. The debate became loud and angry. Finally, Dr. Geselevich asked permission to speak for himself. The participants argued about this for a while and then allowed him five minutes.

"I thank this whole collective and especially the secretary of the Party Committee," he said, "for this profound and principled criticism. As you know, I place the interests of the Party and nation above everything else. For this reason, I have carefully studied and followed the works of the great Stalin for my whole life. I will use his techniques and your criticisms to guide all of my future work."

The communists at the meeting received his speech with mixed reactions. Most of the people whispered among themselves. Some were suspicious, some relieved. One of the students, Boris Yelenin, got up to speak. During the war, he had served as a captain in the brutal counterintelligence organization "Smersh."

"We students," he said, "don't need any professors who worship the West and who want to inspire that worship in us. The Party and that great genius of Humanity, Comrade Stalin, have taught us that the ideological education of our future specialists is the most important task of any institute of higher education. We must therefore purify our collective of such homeless cosmopolitans. We must and we will. Comrades, we have earned this right with our blood on the Front."

At first, everybody remained silent. Then, Yekaterina Furtseva, the regional Party secretary, whom many believed was the source of the accusations, began to applaud. Dr. Valentina Dobrynina applauded too, and then the others began. Even Lopukhin and Movshovich pretended to applaud. Dr. Geselevich looked around at his applauding colleagues and comrades and then even he started to applaud.

This submission did not save him, though; several days later he was expelled from the Party and fired. We, the students, skipped his replacement's class as much as possible.

Dr. Geselevich could not find another job for a year. Finally he was hired to work in a small medical library at a salary one-sixth of his previous one. Ironically, he remained the Soviet Union's best expert on the historical accomplishments of Russian medicine, and his textbook was considered to be the most authoritative one in his field for many years.

The student Boris Yelinin was promoted to second secretary of the Party committee. He was the first student to hold this position, and he used it to tell the medical teachers what and how to teach. The teachers were so intimidated by him that they always gave him the highest grades. From then on, he also received a special "Stalin stipend," which was much higher than the stipend that the other students received.

The constant accusations about worship of the West led to the practice of replacing the names of famous Western scientists with the names of Russian scientists. Thousands of books and hundreds of dissertations were written to prove the leading role of Russian science. For example, the electric light was supposedly invented by the great Yablochkin (and not by Edison), the radio was invented by the great Popov (and not by Guglielmo Marconi), and the airplane was invented by the great Mozhaysky (and not by the Wright brothers). In medicine, it turned out that the great Russian doctors M. Mudrov, N. Pirogov, G. Zakharin, S. Botkin, I. Pavlov, and N. Filatov had developed all of the basic theories about medical pathology and had invented all the modern methods of treatment. Various symptoms, syndromes, and illnesses that had been named after Western medical scientists were renamed after Russian scientists. We students were assigned to study the biographies of these Russian scientists in more detail than we were to study the diseases themselves.

Dr. Joseph Tager, a fifty-year-old Jew, was an X-ray specialist and the author of many important articles and books. He was such a good lecturer that doctors and students came from distant cities to hear him speak. He orated like an actor, with wonderful voice and dramatic gestures, and he illustrated his explanations with vivid examples.

One day he was lecturing on bone transplants, a new method of treatment that promised hope to thousands of war invalids. He illustrated his lecture with fascinating X rays that showed the process by which transplanted bones take root in the body. At one point in this lecture, he joked that the first case of a successful bone transplant was when God created Eve out of Adam's rib. I remember that almost everybody laughed.

The next day, the Party Committee called him in and showed him an unsigned letter that a group of students had written. The essence of the letter was that: "The Jewish Professor Tager is propagandizing religion in his lectures and in particular is telling the students unscientific and anti-Marxist myths from the Bible. We Soviet students do not want to listen to this religious propaganda and demand that this pseudo-scientist be removed from his position as an instructor."

In the following meeting, Dr. Tager was accused of "rootless cosmopolitanism" because of this incident. He was fired from his job.

Of course, many of us saw the foolishness of this practice, but we were too afraid to say anything. We submissively recited the facts of Russian scientific priority in class but often told jokes about it among ourselves.

At about this time, it became impossible to check out of the library any scientific book or journal from a Western country without written permission. In order to obtain this permission, the scientist had to explain in writing why he needed to read this material. Many of the scientists who submitted these explanations were subsequently accused of "homeless cosmopolitanism."

3

Many students, especially those who didn't live with their parents, lived in very poor and difficult conditions. About half of the seven hundred students in the class suffered from chronic hunger and exhaustion. During the first years after the war, thousands of Soviets died of dystrophy caused by malnutrition. In fact, the anatomy department had hundreds of dystrophic corpses in formaldehyde baths in the cellar.

Medical students received a stipend of 22 rubles ($33) a month, out of which they had to pay tuition of 20 rubles a semester. Even after the government ended tuition payments in 1949, students could only live on their stipends if they ate only bread and water. Fortunately, my mother made several sandwiches for me every day. I would eat only one of them and give the others to my classmates.

Many of the students worked at various physical jobs during the nights to earn extra money. They may have earned an extra four rubles per night, but they sometimes fell asleep during classes the next day as a result. During the first semester about 5 percent of the student body had to drop out of the school for some reason. The young veteran whom I helped during the entrance exam left to take a job as the director of the university club for 85 rubles ($127) a month.

"I felt bad," he told me, "that I didn't become a doctor, because I had dreamed about that career during the whole war. If only I survive, I thought, I'll become a doctor. I have a wife, though, and a new baby, and I have to support them."

Indeed, it was generally more difficult for veterans. They were too old for their parents to support, and they had often become parents themselves.

Women were in a clear majority in my class, accounting for some 70 percent of the student body. Naturally, like all other male students, I was intrigued by them. From the very first days we all fell victim to the love fever that for many of us later culminated in marriage.

Our coeds fell into two uneven groups: innocent young girls constituted the larger group, while experienced women schooled in the ways of the world were the minority. My ideal fell midway between the two categories: a girl not exactly of the touch-me-not variety, but not overexperienced either.

Some of the girls in our class were World War Two veterans pushing thirty. To us, eighteen- or nineteen-year-old youths, they looked like old women.

One of them stood apart from the other veterans. It was rumored that she had served in the war as a marksman with thirty-four kills to her credit, that she had the rank of captain and seven combat medals. But she never wore her military uniform or decorations, always appearing at school in the same dark-blue old but tidy costume. And she rarely if ever joined a conversation. There was an element of mystery in her looks and behavior and she attracted me —but as a symbol of longing, not a woman of flesh and blood. I have always been a romantic, and her halo of mystery aroused my interest.

She usually stood alone in a corner and chain-smoked the little cigarettes, Gvozdyky, during breaks. She was painfully thin. She had beautiful black hair and a typically Jewish long nose and large eyes. She might have been beautiful, but she never smiled; her expression was always impassive. She never went to Komsomol meetings.

I had never talked with her, but I felt sorry for her. One day, I told my father about her and asked him to help her. He told me to give her his telephone number; if she called, he would try to do something for her.

During the following days, I tried to get her attention so that I could introduce myself. I would stand next to her during the breaks, but she just smoked and looked into space.

I explained this to my father, and he called the dean and had him call Marina to the telephone. My father then told her that he had a job to offer and that the dean had recommended her to fill it. The pay was 50 rubles a month for answering the phone evenings at the duty desk of the Institute of Surgery, where my father was the deputy director. She accepted the offer.

I avoided her after that, because I didn't want her to suspect that I had gotten her the job. I noticed, however, that she bought a new blue suit a couple of months later and some new shoes a few months after that. She remained a loner, but at least she looked better.

She evidently told my father about herself, though. One night as we were eating borscht he asked me: "Do you know what a background this young protegé Marina has?"

And he told me that her whole family—parents, younger sisters, brother, grandmother, grandfathers, aunts, nephews—had died in Nazi concentration camps. In addition, her fiancé and his family had also perished. The Nazis had taken them all away from Riga, Latvia, in 1941. Marina alone had escaped. She joined the Red Army and became a sniper with the rank of captain.

"She personally killed thirty-four Nazi soldiers," my father added, "but she thought that she should have killed three more, because thirty-seven of her own loved ones had been killed."

On another evening, my father talked about her again: "She is truly courageous. No wonder she won five medals. She has been sending letters all over the world and to all kinds of Jewish organizations in an effort to find any survivors from her family. I told her that this was dangerous, but she answered that she hadn't been afraid on the front and wasn't going to start being afraid during peacetime. That was very well put, but there is a lot of danger during peacetime too." I understood that he meant the secret police.

One day in 1949, my father mentioned her again: "Mr. Zuskin, the head director of the Jewish theater, is a new patient in our institute. He has a wide circle of Jewish contacts, so I asked him to help Marina find her relatives abroad."

Zuskin's help apparently gave Marina new hope, because she looked much happier when I saw her in the following days.

Suddenly, though, she stopped coming to class. At about the same time, my father starting coming home very depressed every night. I finally asked him if he had seen Marina.

"She's been arrested."

"Arrested! What for?"

"You remember that I told you that the Jewish director Zuskin was a patient in our institute? Well, the police came and arrested him right from his bed, where he was lying with a fever. At the same time, some other people came to the office where Marina was working and arrested her too. They would have arrested me too, for admitting Zuskin for treatment, but luckily I had had the director of the institute sign the papers to admit him. The director is Russian, Dr. A. Vishnevsky, so they couldn't accuse him of participating in a Jewish conspiracy. The director vouched for me, so the police didn't arrest me with Zuskin and Marina . . . yet. They asked her who helped her to get a job, but she didn't say about me. She truly is a courageous woman."

Zuskin and Marina never returned. We learned later that they died in prison. Marina, the Soviet war hero, was the thirty-eighth and last member of a Jewish family that was totally destroyed.

4

Since my father was a surgeon, I heard stories and comments about surgery throughout childhood. When I became a medical student, I decided that I wanted to become a surgeon, and therefore learned everything I could about what went on in operating rooms. In all that I heard, I was most struck by two things.

The first was that the quality and availability of the surgical instruments was very low. These included even simple items like scalpels, thread, pincers, clamps, hypodermic needles, cotton, and alcohol. Surgeons and nurses always had to expend a lot of effort, time, and worry to make sure that they had the things they needed to operate.

The second was the behavior of most surgeons in the operating room. They fidgeted, cursed, yelled, threw their instruments, and brought their assistants to hysterics. The higher the position of the surgeon, the more this tended to be true. And since most patients were only given local anesthetics, they watched all of this wild behavior in horror.

Once my father told me, "I like to go to two places to receive esthetic pleasure—to the plays at the Artistic Theater and to the operating room of Dr. Sergey Yudin."

The shows at the Artistic Theater really were beautiful, and I too liked them, but I had never seen any of Dr. Yudin's operations.

He was the most popular surgeon in Moscow, possibly even in the Soviet Union. My father was well acquainted with him, so I asked my father to arrange for me to observe one of Dr. Yudin's operations.

Dr. Yudin was about fifty-five years old. He came from a family of noble Russian intellectuals and could speak several European languages. He founded the Sklifasovskiy Surgical Institute of Emergency Medicine in Moscow, the first of its kind in the Soviet Union, invented many surgical techniques, and wrote textbooks that educated several generations of Soviet surgeons. Dr. Yudin was a Russian patriot who constantly promoted the authority of Russian surgery in his books and lectures, especially during World War Two. He traveled to the United States and he was the only Soviet doctor who belonged to the Royal Society of England, which made him a baronet.

Dr. Yudin gave me permission to attend one of his operations, in which he intended to make an esophagoplasty from the small intestine—a new and rare technique at that time. The amphitheater was full of invited professors of surgery, and I humbly sat behind them.

Dr. Yudin was a very tall man, and the operating table seemed somewhat too low for him. He operated calmly and quietly, without the usual nervousness and yelling that I had seen in other surgeons. The only time he spoke was to explain his procedures to his audience, wittily and subtly drawing parallels with other methods and with the work of other world-famous surgeons.

I was enchanted as I watched his hands. Dr. Yudin operated with his long fingers in the same way that a pianist played a keyboard. He often handled several instruments—scalpels, scissors, clamps, and pincers—at the same time. All of his tools were imported from America, England, and other foreign countries that he had visited. I had never seen such instruments before. The patient's tissues separated and joined like piano keys under Dr. Yudin's fingers. It was an esthetic pleasure for the audience to watch his performance.

His surgical nurse was a short woman of about forty-five years named Marina. Although Dr. Yudin officially had a family, Marina was his *de facto* wife, a situation that everybody knew about. They worked very well together. She stood on a stool and crisply handed Dr. Yudin his instruments.

After the operation, we all went to Dr. Yudin's office, where he gave us a lecture on the operation, pronouncing all of the foreign words perfectly. I very much admired his technique, his instruments, and his whole manner of behavior.

After the lecture, he walked over to a sink and urinated into it, with absolutely no embarrassment in front of his male colleagues. It turned out that in his nature he was still a Russian *muzhik* (peasant) at heart.

On one occasion in 1949, he operated on a high-ranking British diplomat in Moscow. The operation was very difficult, but the patient was saved from death. In gratitude, the British ambassador organized a reception for the famous surgeon and Marina. Two weeks later, both of them were arrested as a result of reports to the police by some of Dr. Yudin's students and assistants. They were convicted at a secret trial, but rumors about what had happened had quickly spread. They were sentenced to ten years in prison camps, allegedly for contacts with foreigners for the purpose of espionage.

Dr. Yudin and Marina were exiled to a remote corner of Siberia, where they were allowed to work in a small hospital for prisoners. He was, however, only allowed to work as a housekeeper —to clean an operating room, or assist his surgical nurse, Marina.

5

My parents had no religion. My father never observed Judaic traditions and the Jewish holidays, nor went to the synagogue. Judaism was never discussed in our house. While Orthodox Christianity was denounced by the authorities, practicing Judaism was considered a crime. People who dared to visit the one and only synagogue in Moscow were believed to be active Zionists. Of course, nobody had any clear idea about what Zionism was; popular feeling equated it with fascism.

One day, my parents took me, a small boy, to a seder at the

house of an elderly aunt of my father's whose husband was a believer. For the first time in my life I saw the Judaic rites observed and Judaic garments: men who wore yermulkas on their heads and tephillins. I heard lengthy prayers muttered in Yiddish, which I could not understand. To my surprise, my father knew these rituals and participated in them with pleasure. When the guests started dancing, my parents joined them. Then my father explained that in his day he had attended classes in Heder, the Jewish school where he learned all these rituals.

"I have come tonight to please my aunt and her husband, since they are believers," he caressed my hair, "I am not."

Confronted with the state-instigated, all-pervading atheistic propaganda at school, and outside my house in general, and comparing it to the attitudes of my kin, I had been in two minds about religion for quite some time.

In June 1941, when the war against Hitler's Germany broke out, I was eleven. On the very first day of the hostilities my father was called up and had to go to the front. Before his departure, he bid farewell to all of us, in turn, and my maternal grandmother, an Orthodox Christian, blessed him with the sign of the cross. I was surprised. My father stood very somber while my grandmother was whispering, then he said: "Pray for me, so that I may stay alive."

My mother also made the sign of the cross—she had never done this in front of me. Then I realized two things: first, people concealed their religion out of fear of reprisals by the authorities preaching atheism; second, when the fear of death overpowered the fear of the authorities, their hidden religious beliefs broke through and they turned to God. I later met many people whose predicament made them conceal or manifest their religion, depending upon the circumstances. About one-half of the population were believers. Although I was not one, I felt respect for the religious beliefs of other people. I always wanted to read the Bible and the Scriptures but could not do so—it was virtually impossible to get them.

University students ran the risk of being expelled if they chose to manifest openly their devotion to religion.

"Are you a believer?" the doctor asked one Russian lad wearing a cross around his neck as he stood naked before the members of the medical board, who examined all applicants who had passed the entrance examinations.

"Yes, I believe in the Lord," he said and lowered his eyes.

"So you do," the doctor drawled.

The young man was refused admission on the pretext of poor health although he was as fit as he could be. Upset but not dislodged, the youth turned up at the medical school on September 1, the day the classes began, and pressed for explanations. They brought out his file and showed him the entry: "Psychic abnormalcy of religious nature."

In the medical school, we never discussed religion. Many of my fellow students were superstitious, particularly at the end of the semester, on the eve of examinations. Nobody was reprimanded for that, nobody cared. However, a fellow student, a Russian girl, was reported to the Komsomol by somebody who saw her attending services at the Yelokhovsky Cathedral, one of the few functioning churches in Moscow. The Party Committee then instructed several active Komsomol members to follow her and they found that the report was true. A Komsomol meeting was then convened to discuss the subject "A moral image of the Soviet student." At the meeting, the girl was reproached for her religious habits. She did not balk, however, and challenged her detractors, the dean of the faculty and the Party secretary.

"My religious beliefs are my private affair. I do not try to convert anyone and do not think it is right to interfere with my personal feelings. I have good grades, am capable, and will become a good doctor. The rest does not concern anyone except myself. Squealing on me is much worse abuse compared to religion, anyway," she asserted.

The students now had to vote for her expulsion from the Komsomol by raising their hands, as was customary. About two-thirds raised their hands immediately; the others hesitated for half a minute, and then raised their hands, too. I voted with the latter group. Although I barely knew the girl I had no doubt that she was right. However, to vote against her expulsion meant to be expelled next. I felt revulsion and disgust at being coerced into committing an outrage. The others who were hesitant must have felt likewise. Yet no one dared to vote for her. After the meeting was over, we walked away feeling degraded. I tried not to look at my fellow students and especially at the hapless coed, not to show how humiliated I felt. I had had a similar experience in grammar school, when the other children had teased me because of my Jewishness. I was a child then, and the wounds healed faster in those days. This time it took me many weeks before I regained my composure, but I garnered forever a feeling of resentment and despair.

Due to our youth and ignorance we could not have our own opinions about the complex problems of the sciences. Everything that occurred in front of our eyes divided us into two groups: the majority unquestioningly believed the official versions of the accusations made against our teachers; the minority was profoundly suspicious of the correctness of the repressive measures. All of us were oppressed by the unstable situation; the professors' nervousness was conveyed to us.

Youth knows little, but it feels sharply. We were bombarded with various unpleasant changes: the programs for studying were changed in the departments, the books with which we studied were banned, teachers changed, our fellow students disappeared. We were questioned more dogmatically in the political sciences. We suspected a KGB informer in each of our neighbors, and we tried to be extremely cautious in our conversations. But we were young and could not always control ourselves; we wanted to be joyful, calm, brave. It was impossible!

On the second floor, to the side of auditorium No. 2, there was an inconspicuous narrow door. There was no sign on the door, but all the students knew the office as "the first department" or "the special department." The head of this department was Captain Matveyev, a representative of the secret police, who kept a file on everybody at the school. He wore an ordinary gray suit and frequently slithered out of his office to mingle silently among the students and teachers in the halls. At night, he invited students into his office to ask them about their classmates and teachers. Most students played dumb to evade these questions, but at least 20 percent did inform Matveyev regularly. Some informed out of conviction, some for passing grades. Captain Matveyev could force any professor to pass any bad student and flunk any good student. One of my classmates was especially vulnerable, because he lived on his stipend only and had failed a physics exam four times. Before this student attempted the test for a fifth time, Captain Matveyev called him into his office and promised him that if he would become an informer, the next exam would consist of a single question about the formula for a hanging drop of fluid. The next day, Professor Nikolay Sokolov indeed gave only that question and the student passed. A few of us realized what had happened, because one of my friends had seen the student leave Matveyev's office late that night.

Usually, we didn't know who the informers were, but they were everywhere. Any student who made indiscreet comments or jokes inevitably disappeared from the school.

On New Year's Eve, 1950, a real crime took place at the medical school. A miser, Dr. Ignatov, a seventy-year-old professor who specialized in water purification, was murdered with a chisel in his office. The police discovered that a lot of money, government bonds, and other valuables had been stolen from a storage box in the office.

Naturally, Captain Matveyev investigated the murder thoroughly. He recruited more informers and helped the police interrogate anybody who might know something about the murder. After six months, though, he still hadn't found the murderer.

Suddenly, however, the crime was solved. A man was arrested in Baku for selling government bonds on the black market. The serial numbers matched those on the bonds that had been stolen from Dr. Ignatov. A subsequent series of confessions revealed that Dr. Ignatov had been robbed and murdered by two students. They, in turn, revealed that the whole crime had been organized by . . . Captain Matveyev! He had learned about the miser's storage box from some of his informants and had then recruited a couple of students under his control to murder and rob the old man. The crime police arrested Matveyev at school and dragged him from his office through the narrow door, past the astonished students in the hall, and off to prison.

The quality of instruction at medical school suffered not only from political terror and enforced pseudo-science, but also because the Party Committee hired new teachers on the basis of Party loyalty instead of professional qualifications. Therefore, 50 to 75 percent of the teachers were members of the Communist Party, although only ten percent of Soviet doctors as a whole were members. Some Party members were talented teachers, of course, but the overwhelming majority of them were incompetents who owed their whole careers to political favoritism. This incompetence perpetuated itself and grew, because the worst teachers rose to the top and then hired and promoted other doctors with the same values. Excellence was a threat to the administration.

The quality of instruction also suffered from a lack of adequate facilities and equipment. All of the equipment at the school was twenty or thirty years old, so we didn't learn any of the precise new methods of analysis, diagnosis, treatment, or surgery. Our teachers could not even mention the revolutionary new medical equipment being developed abroad, because that information would have been considered "capitalist propaganda." We had to learn almost everything out of books and lectures because the school had so little equipment; theoretical knowledge was gradually emphasized at the expense of practical skills. We spent very little time learning to change bandages, make plaster casts, fix dislocations and fractures, lance abscesses, thump chests, listen through stethoscopes, read cardiograms, and interpret X rays. Only the 15 to 20 percent of the students who voluntarily worked at hospitals and clinics after school hours really learned any medical skills during their school years.

Despite all the bad things around us, though, we students were generally happy, optimistic, and romantic. And our girls and young ladies were beautiful!

6

I began writing poetry when I was five years old and kept at it throughout my high school years. I enjoyed the process of choosing the rhymes and the rhythm. My mother encouraged my hobby and composed a few little poems herself for me, making it a tradition to give me a verse on my birthday every year. I reciprocated and in my turn each year composed a poem on her birthday. My mother also read aloud to me from the works of Alexander Pushkin and Michael Lermontov, instilling in me great admiration for them: I learned many of their poems by heart.

My interest in poetry was further enchanced after I met several poets of distinction—Boris Pasternak, Alexander Tvardovsky, Michael Isakovsky, and Ilya Selvinsky. During 1941–43, my mother and I were evacuees and these poets were our neighbors. I was particularly impressed by Pasternak. These encounters whetted my desire to become a professional poet, although I still wanted to pursue my medical career. During my undergraduate and graduate years in medical school I continued writing poetry and was eager to see it published. I wrote poems late at night and early in the morning; they expressed my experiences of life and my budding love life. In class I often wrote spoofs in which I ridiculed our professors and my fellow students, and showed them to my friends, mostly girls. The girls giggled, boosting my writer's ego. However, for a long time I had problems with getting my verse into print.

In 1950, I wrote a poem about spring in Moscow and brought it to the medical newspaper office. The first four lines of the poem, roughly translated, were as follows: "The leaf was crowded by the bud/And the force of youth opened the bud/Everything is in bloom—/Spring has come to Moscow/And bestowed freedom on the leaves."

The editors liked my poem, but they suggested that I add some politics to it. "It's a good poem," they said, "but you should add something about a Soviet student, and at the end you should write something about Stalin. After all, you write about freedom, and there's really no freedom without Stalin."

I wanted very badly to see my poem published, so I wracked my brain to figure out how I would add the Soviet student and Stalin. Finally, I just gave up and wrote three separate poems: about spring, about the student, and about Stalin.

The poem about Stalin was the hardest to write. Thousands of poems had already been written about him by professional poets, so I didn't feel that I could say anything new or surpass the extravagant poetic praise he had already received. In addition, I was afraid of making a political mistake and getting into trouble. The subject scared me horribly instead of inspiring me. Finally, I wrote a poem about how satisfying it was that our school was named after him.

Why it was satisfying I didn't know, but I felt that nobody had written a poem on exactly that theme yet.

Two months passed as the censors continued to examine my poems. I waited with extreme impatience. Spring passed, and one poem was therefore out of date. I eventually discovered that my poems had to be approved at sixteen different administrative levels, including a special department of the Central Committee. This was standard procedure, even for a small paper like the school's *Soviet Medic*.

Eventually the poems were published. I continued to submit poems, but by now I had learned to try to add something ideological from the very beginning. I acquired the reputation of being the school's poet, and I especially enjoyed the praise that my female classmates gave me.

7

The tiny room into which our entire family was crammed was a source of increasing exasperation for all of us. Both my parents and I dreamed of a separate bedroom. I was growing up, my friends of both sexes came to visit, and we naturally wanted to be by ourselves. The situation was particularly unbearable whenever I wanted to be alone with a girl. I could not tell my parents that I planned to make love without overstepping the bounds of propriety, and so I had to suffer weeks at a time waiting for my parents to go to the theater or on a visit that would give me the precious opportunity to sneak my girl into our room. The room was chock-full of furniture, so for practical purposes our living space was nonexistent; besides, in addition to my father's medical library I had started buying books on history and art, novels, plays, and poems. I dreamed of becoming a writer as well as a physician and hence read voraciously: my daily quota was one hundred pages.

In the late 1940s, the government belatedly launched a small-scale housing program, and some of our acquaintances managed to procure apartments—tiny, but real apartments. My father, too, resolved to do anything at all to get an apartment, if only a one-bedroom, for his family. He wrote numerous letters to all manner of authorities and personally pleaded his case with bosses of various levels, claiming that as a surgeon and a professor he had to write research papers and prepare for the lectures and so he was entitled to extra floorspace. To be sure, under Soviet law he was indeed entitled to an additional twenty square meters above the regular nine square meters per capita. But in reality everybody ignored the law, and my father's petitions were invariably turned down, each time after a few months' delay. Every setback added perceptibly to the gloom in our room. After numerous refusals, my father suddenly hit upon the idea of writing a letter to Stalin himself. Rumor had it that some of the daredevils who risked a direct petition to Stalin got what they wanted.

As time dragged on, my father was increasingly enamored of the idea; besides, we saw no other realistic recourse. On the other hand, Father was carefully weighing all pros and cons. According to popular rumor's statistics, petitions to Stalin brought positive results in less than 10 percent of cases, whereas negative results could be very unpleasant. I for one would never have dared complain to Stalin that I needed to spend time with my girlfriend alone.

Lest our neighbors overhear us, our whole family conducted whispered discussions of the merits of such a letter. Our resolve was dampened by fear of the unforeseen consequences of such a daring undertaking. My mother and I insisted that we should cast the die, but father was vacillating. Finally he, too, made up his mind. One Sunday, when our neighbors went for a walk, all three of us gathered around our small table. Father spread good quality paper he had scrounged for the occasion. Since we did not have a typewriter (a luxury by Russian standards to this day), he wrote in ink. We watched his hand, discussing every word before he put it on paper. Our problem was too serious to take lightly; still, Mother and I were a little amused by Father's nervous agitation. He wrote: "Dear Joseph Vissarionovich! I am taking the liberty of appealing to you with a personal request. . . ." At this juncture, Father stopped and asked pensively: "Should I drop the word 'dear'? It sounds sort of unceremonious. . . ."

Mother and I tried to come up with acceptable alternatives.

"Why don't you write: "Dear and great Joseph Vissarionovich!' " Mother suggested brightly.

"No, it's a queer combination, 'dear and great.' What a ridiculous idea," I said.

"But what should I do?" Father asked in confusion. "Maybe I should just copy the official letters to Stalin from collective farmers as published in the papers? 'Dear Teacher and Friend of All Peoples.' This salutation is very popular."

"No, it's not the kind of salutation one uses in a personal letter," I said decisively.

"Some job I've taken upon myself," my father sighed.

"Listen," Mother said, "you should write this way: 'To Comrade Stalin, Chairman of the Council of Ministers.' "

But father failed to share her enthusiasm: "No, it's too cold. Besides, he's not only Prime Minister, but also Secretary General of the Central Committee of the Party, Generalissimo, and many other things."

"If you set about listing all his titles, you'll have no room left for your request." I laughed. "Besides, he's not going to read it himself—he has assistants to deal with this sort of thing."

Father flew into a rage at my words. "I fail to understand what's so funny," he said. He was obviously very nervous. Mother noticed.

"Why are we in such a hurry with the letter?" she asked. "Our request is clear, you've stated it many times in many letters. As for appealing to Comrade Stalin, why shouldn't each of us sleep on the idea and in a few days' time one of us is sure to come up with a suitable salutation."

The reprieve she suggested clearly pleased Father, and he brightened immediately.

"Surely, he's not going to read our letter himself, but still . . ." he said.

Hot-headed youth that I was, I was displeased with the deferral.

"What are you afraid of?" I asked. My mother stepped on my

foot under the table to let me know that I had to shut up. Father gave me a stern look and said, "You just don't understand."

The upshot was that the letter was never written, and we were the better for it. Mother's counsel was wise, because soon dangerous developments occurred in my father's life.

One evening in 1952, two ladies, one after the other, came to my father. Both served as minor clerks in our superintendent's office and both had the same story to tell. In the past, they had often come to seek my father's professional advice and he had helped them generously, treating them without charging fees and seeing that they and their children were admitted to hospitals for medical treatment. They, in their turn, esteemed his generosity and his professional competence. It was not medical consultation, however, that they came to seek this time. Each woman looked about her and spoke in a hushed voice.

"Secret police agents paid a visit to our office," they said. "They checked the roster of tenants and made inquiries about you. They asked about your *propiska* and about your comings and goings. They were also interested to know what kind of visitors you have and how often." Every Soviet citizen must have his or her *propiska,* an official permit issued by the police and authorizing him or her to live at this or that address. Without such a permit, no one can take residence in any area of the country. The secret policemen were not interested in the *propiska,* which was a binding regulation; they were interested in shadowing my father.

"They said they would come again," both women added, further lowering their voices and barely moving their lips, "and would ask questions about your visitors—who came to see you and when? They watch you and make me report on you. You may be sure I will never say one bad word about you, but you know their kind: if they are after something they just want it delivered to them. Please, be careful. . . ."

My father thanked them for their counsel and my mother asked them to stay for a cup of tea, but they refused and slipped out of the apartment.

Late that night, when I returned home, I found my parents very much upset. They were silently collecting different things, and around midnight they walked out into the night with several bundles in their hands. Surprised as I was, I was too preoccupied with my own affairs and problems to pay much attention. Only when I started making my bed did I notice that a small brown crocodile suitcase, my favorite, was gone. The makeshift bed on which I slept was made up of suitcases, and as I grew up I had to add a few more. The small brown one served as a headboard. In it I kept my souvenirs and mementos, including a genuine handgun with a broken firing pin that I had traded for when I was sixteen. I hid it from my parents, although I rarely remembered it was there. One other item was an old dagger of Damascus steel in a silver-encrusted sheath, manufactured by a Caucasian craftsman. A family relic, it had belonged to my grandfather on my mother's side.

My parents came back home shortly after 1:00 A.M. without the bundles and with the suitcases in their hands. Half-asleep, I grumbled at them, asking that they put the suitcase under my head, and then fell asleep. Early in the morning, I was awakened by the anxious whispers that came from my parents' bed behind the curtain. The strange events of the previous night sprang to my mind and I felt ashamed of my grumbling. All children, especially very young ones, are selfish, and I was no exception.

I hopped up onto the corner of their bed and Mother told me everything. Doctors everywhere were being arrested, she said. Late last night my parents had carried away those bundles to get rid of certain things that could be used as "material evidence" if the KGB came to arrest my father. My parents did not want me to get worried and so did not talk to me before they left. They hired a cab that took them to the other end of Moscow and there, in some dark street, they dumped the handgun, the dagger, and the letters and photographs of many friends who had been arrested or even executed into garbage cans in several backyards. Some of the letters were from the great Jewish actor Solomon Mikhoels and from the eminent Jewish doctor B. Shimeliovich, who have been killed by the KGB. They also dumped the beautiful samurai sword that my father had brought home after the end of the war with Japan.

While my mother was whispering her story to me my dad kept sighing and patting my hand with a helpless look in his eyes.

The story and my dad's looks sent cold shivers down my spine. I did not so much regret the loss of my handgun as the dagger and the sword. I also wondered if they had disposed of my hunting gun, a .20 Winchester that my father had given me when he had returned after the war. Yet I hesitated to ask. I sensed my parents' fear and felt helpless and unsure in the face of the future that now hinged on my father's fortune. If they arrested him they would not leave my mother and me alone, but would instead cart us off to some place in Siberia. I could then forget about my medical and writing careers, since we would become hounded and harassed "enemies of the people," like millions of other families some of whom we knew. The pattern was familiar. For this very reason my parents had not approached any of their friends for help. They did not want to put them in danger in case my father was arrested.

"We have to be ready for anything," my father said at last. "*Lapa* [an endearing nickname he used to call my mother], please, bring me two sets of underwear, a pair of socks, a shirt, a towel, and a muffler, so that I have them at hand if they come to take me away. They allow people they arrest only fifteen minutes to get ready, you know. . . ."

I fetched the crocodile suitcase off my bedstead and put it down near my parents' bed.

"Put the things that father wants in it," I told my mother. "In case they . . . I want you to have it," I finished, turning to my father.

He pulled my head to his lips and kissed me.

"Thank you," said he. "Your suitcase is too good for the camp and, sure enough, they'll take it. But who knows, maybe they won't. Now, about your hunting gun: we did not dump it. Try to figure out how you can stow it away for a while. Only do it today."

I felt both depressed and moved. On that morning, I warmed up toward my parents and my selfishness was gone.

The situation at home was near the breaking point. My father had all but lost his sleep. Nobody had come to arrest him, and he still continued as dean of the department of surgery and deputy director of the Institute of Surgery; but holding these positions was all the more excruciating since the administration more and more often rebuffed him for being a Jew and a non-Party member. In the meanwhile he had to go on supervising two institutes.

Late one night, around midnight, the telephone rang in our apartment. My father picked up the phone and almost immediately his voice sank and became thick with anguish. My mother and I anxiously listened to his monosyllables:

"Yes . . . I understand . . . I expected it. . . . Well, I will. . . . If that was the decision I cannot refuse. . . . Thank you for calling."

We watched him hang up the receiver in silence. He did not speak to us but first sat down on his chair, then stood up, then sat down again while we waited.

"My director called," he said at last, "to tell me that the Party Committee and deputy minister, Dr. A. Belousov, ruled to appoint another deputy and another dean to replace me. They want Party members in these positions. They've already selected their candidates for these jobs. I have to submit my resignation tomorrow. . . . If I balk they'll fire me. If I comply they'll give me the job of an assistant professor. This is two ranks below what I've had but it's not the worst that could have been expected. I shall receive lesser salary but we shall manage—for some time."

My mother reacted with absolute calm.

"Whatever God does he does it for the best, you know," she said. "You've put so much of yourself in these jobs, it would be a good thing for you to have a bit of rest. So don't get excited and let's plan how we'll spend your free time. I think we can afford to go to the theaters more often. As for the money, what we have will be enough; we'll trim our shopping list a little."

"Well, maybe you're right." Father smiled at her soothing words. "I really feel I cannot carry on as I did, under the circumstances."

8

The threat of arrest persisted. Now my father would come home earlier and I in my turn tried to leave early after classes. We would sit next to each other and discuss new rumors about new arrests. My father had known most of the newly arrested doctors for years as colleagues and friends. He was convinced that their arrests were unwarranted because his friends could not have committed any serious offense. Nobody would say that openly, however, and everybody waited for some sort of an official announcement. In Moscow and other major cities so many prominent doctors had been arrested that the government had to make some explanation. They did so on one cool winter day in 1953.

Since the West uses the reformed Gregorian calendar, and Russia before the Revolution used the somewhat inaccurate Julian calendar, Russian dates fell thirteen days behind Western dates. Russia celebrated Christmas on January 7 (according to the Gregorian calendar) and New Year's Day on January 13. After the Revolution, Russia adopted the Gregorian calendar, but many Russian still celebrate New Year's in traditional style on January 13. They begin to eat and drink on the evening of the twelfth and continue this feast for the whole next day.

On this unique, unofficial, but traditionally Russian holiday, the Soviet government often tries to provoke the drunk population with some type of reactionary news on the radio or television. On January 13, 1953, the newspapers and radio reported the discovery of a giant conspiracy to murder top Party and military leaders by means of medical maltreatment. This conspiracy was supposedly directed by an "international Jewish bourgeois nationalist organization" that communicated its orders "via the Moscow doctor, Shimeliovich, and the well-known Jewish bourgeois nationalist Mikhoels." Russians held meetings throughout the country to discuss the charges and to attack Jewish doctors.

Most people, even at the medical school, believed the accusations. The people who repeated the charges at the meetings often did so out of fear. "It probably did happen," my classmates told me, "there must be something to it." I will never forget the atmosphere. Every Russian doctor actively participated in the persecution. A doctor at the Kremlin made the original accusation of medical murder, and additional information was systematically and willingly supplied.

The Communist Party newspaper *Pravda* ran a story signed by its woman reporter Tatyana Tess. The story described a certain doctor, Lydia Timashuk, a Party member, who one day became suspicious of the prescription Professor Dr. M. Vovsi, her superior, had issued to a high-ranking patient. Since Dr. Timashuk was Professor Vovsi's disciple and much younger and less experienced than he, she first had her doubts, the *Pravda* story went on. However, the harder she tried to find out what had happened, the more she became convinced that Dr. Vovsi had committed an error that could have killed his patient. Stealthily, she checked up on his other prescriptions and found they were all harmful. Dr. Timashuk then felt it was her duty as a communist to report the case to the Party Committee of the Kremlin Hospital. The investigation confirmed, the newspaper alleged, that she was right and that doctors M. Vovsi, A. Feldman, E. Gelshtein, B. Kogan, M. Kogan, A. Grinshtein, and several other Jewish physicians had all tried to poison their top-ranking patients at the Kremlin Hospital. The newspaper cited the names of Russian doctors V. Vinogradov, V. Vasilenko, and P. Yegorov as their accomplices.

Dr. L. Timashuk was awarded the highest Soviet decoration, the Order of Lenin, for her outstanding "professional competence" and her "valor of a loyal citizen." She was made into a national idol, a savior of Russia, someone like Jeanne d'Arc.

This was the only information that came from the official source. It also added that the "doctors-poisoners" had plotted to kill all the government leaders, perhaps including Joseph Stalin himself.

After this story appeared in the press our classes at the medical school began every morning with the denunciation of the "doctors-poisoners." Dr. I. Murashov and Dr. E. Dubeykovskaya read out to us fresh articles on the subject from the Soviet newspapers and lashed out at their former colleagues, not stopping short of hysterical anti-Semitic outbursts. The Jewish students lowered their heads, their faces turning white. We felt miserable and terrified.

Every Jewish doctor had to condemn the "plotters," no matter whether he or she knew them or not. My father took it badly. He was convinced the allegations were false, yet he did not dare to say so aloud in his office; moreover he had to join the others in their condemnation and to demand at the meetings "to mete out the most severe punishment" to the people whose innocence he did not place in doubt for a single second.

"I'll never believe they're capable of poisoning their patients," he would confide to me in a low voice back home. "I've known them for over twenty years. They're the best doctors we have, the top men in the profession. Dr. Vovsi is a genius. I've never met another physician as skillful as he. All this is hogwash, believe me. Yet there's something behind it. I think they want to get all the Jews out of Moscow and then they'll kill us all."

Many different rumors circulated at the time. According to one of them several trains composed of wooden carriages used for the transportation of cattle and prisoners stood ready on the railways in one of the Moscow suburbs. The grapevine had it that they were assembled for the deportation of all the Jews out of Moscow.

The anti-Semitic campaign continued unabated throughout the nation, with particular repercussions in the medical circles. Every night we would listen intently to the steps in the doorway of our old wooden house: are they coming to take father into custody this time? My brown crocodile suitcase was now permanently placed by my parents' bedside. My mother put underwear, woolen socks, medication, and even our snapshots into it, just in case. My father had developed a habit of taking the suitcase up and holding it in his hand. "You ought to practice beforehand," he said.

Then the turn for the worst came: Stalin fell sick. In three days the death of Stalin was reported on the news bulletin at 2:00 A.M., March 5, 1953, and my father and I were horrified. We both surmised that his death meant the end for us. Father would be arrested and exiled because the secret police in their frenzy were now likely to vent their spite over the loss of the *vozhd,* the leader, on all the potential suspects. As for myself, I could then say good-bye to my M.D. degree and the hopes of normal life. So, when announcer Yuriy Levitan read out in his deep sonorous voice "Comrade Stalin is dead," my father wept like a child. I looked at him with tears in my eyes, well aware that he was grieving not over Stalin's death but over himself and all of us.

Only my mother remained calm, as was her habit. She found the right words to lift our spirits: "Perhaps it's not so bad after all that he died," she mused. "Perhaps this goddamned period in our life will now be over. Things must change for the better."

My father looked up at her and pulled himself together. "You think so, *lapa?*" he said.

"I'm almost sure of it," she answered.

"Well, maybe you're right," my father said with relief. We all quietly went to bed. It seemed highly unlikely that they would come to pick up my father on a night like this.

Dr. E. Dybeykovskaya, our professor of surgery, announced to us the next morning that the arrested Jewish doctors had murdered Stalin even after all the precautions that had been taken. She cried for several days and canceled all her classes.

The tears hadn't dried yet when, on March 20, the radio announced that the doctors weren't poisoners and that the accusations had been thought up by several KGB agents who had used "unallowable methods during the investigation"—i.e., torture. Later we learned that the whole conspiracy had been fabricated by one of Beria's deputies named Ryumin.

"Public opinion" didn't crawl back. Most Russians and most Russian doctors and medical students scratched their heads in puzzlement, shrugged their shoulders, and said, "Well, mistakes happen." But many of them said that with a tone of disappointment.

My mother was proved right this time, like so many other times before and after. The doctors had been exonerated, the anti-Semitic campaign subsided; we would no longer fear for my father. I brought back home my hunting gun from the hideaway and my parents said nothing. My father smiled and patted me on the shoulder.

I was happy because it meant living without the sword of Damocles above our heads. There was no more fear of being sent to Siberia in exile and I felt a sort of relaxation. However, the years of anxiety left a scar in my heart. I was only twenty-three but I had already acquired a lack of confidence and uncertainty to accompany me through my life. I did not trust the society I lived in anymore.

Stalin's sudden death brought universal relief. The new government, under Georgy Malenkov, took a liberal stance. General Ryumin was executed, to be followed by Beria. As for Dr. Lydia Timashuk, the instrument for the first accusation, she retained her job at the Kremlin Hospital. She only had to return her Order of Lenin. All the arrested doctors were released and dispatched to privileged government spas and sanatoriums; they were reinstated in their academic and administrative positions. The doctors had been beaten up during interrogations; Dr. M. Vovsi returned home in bruises, and Dr. B. Kogan died under torture.

Their detractors, who had denounced them in public and demanded that the "plotters" should face the firing squad, now had to back down and lie low. However, they could hardly stomach this unexpected setback. Although the public mood had changed, or so it appeared, the virulent anti-Semitic sentiments of many people, including many Russian doctors, remained intact.

The story of Stalin's fatal illness is still little known, and the fragmentary official information about it often deviates from known facts.

Stalin died at the height of an anti-Semitic purge of "medical poisoners," but he had been persecuting the Soviet Union's major doctors who had treated high government officials for thirty years. He had occasionally forced them to sign false death certificates to disguise the causes of death of people he had murdered or driven to suicide. A doctor who signed such a certificate knew too much and soon disappeared himself. In this manner, Stalin destroyed the elite of Soviet medicine. During his reign, the number of doctors and hospitals grew, but the quality of medical talent in the country fell. Soviet medicine has not recovered from these policies to this day.

Ironically, Stalin fell victim to his own policy of arresting all the best medical professionals. When he fell ill, there was nobody competent left to treat him.

The initial announcement of his ill-health had said that he had lost consciousness, that his right side was paralyzed, and that he could not speak. The announcements that followed were all vague: "The treatment of Comrade Stalin is being conducted under the constant observations of the Central Committee and of the Council of Ministers." The majority of common citizens accepted this assurance, but many doctors understood that constant observation by the Central Committee and the Council of Ministers is not a guarantee of good medical attention. Even as a student, I knew from the announcements that Stalin was not receiving any radical or sophisticated medical treatment. My father, a doctor with twenty-seven years' experience, assumed that the treatment was *very* poor. My father and I discussed these thoughts in only the quietest whispers.

Stalin's only personal physician, the skillful Dr. Vladimir Vinogradov, was at the time of Stalin's illness sitting in the basement of Lyubyanka prison with Dr. Alexander Grinshtein, a Jew, the best neurologist in Moscow. In fact, the families of these doctors had already been sent to Siberia.

Stalin was being treated from a stroke by a commission of eight doctors, who were all Party members but were nevertheless second-rate doctors. These doctors did not even have the chance to treat Stalin to the best of their abilities, for his illness had become a political event, not a medical one. Every action of the commission was closely controlled by two medical administrators, who had even fewer medical qualifications. These administrators were the recently appointed Minister of Public Health, Dr. Tretyakov, and the recently appointed head of the Kremlin Medical Directorate, Dr. Kuperin. They were so afraid of any complications that they refused to approve any type of radical medical treatment. They, in turn, were closely supervised by the members of the Politburo, but especially by Beria. All the doctors felt that they were in a dilemma: should they risk the life of their patient or should they risk their own lives?

At that time, the United States and other developed Western countries had a sophisticated method of examining and treating patients with cerebrovascular disease: X-raying the blood vessels in the brain to determine the location and size of the hemorrhage. The Soviet Union did not have such equipment and had not imported any, so not much could be done, since Stalin had had a severe stroke. Even had the commission been able to diagnose the hemorrhage, no neurosurgeons had been appointed to the commission, and in general Soviet neurosurgery lagged far behind the West's. The Kremlin did not even have any medicines for treating such hemorrhages, although such medicines were widely available in the West.

In addition, no foreign doctors were invited to consult on the diagnosis, not even from other Communist countries.

When he fell sick, Stalin was at his *dacha,* or summer house, in Kuntsevo, about fifteen miles out of Moscow on the Minsk Highway. There was absolutely no medical equipment there, not even any oxygen tanks. Stalin should have been taken immediately to the Burdenko Neurosurgery Institute in Moscow, but this institute was apparently considered too common to treat the great dictator.

The final government announcement, which appeared on March 7 (two days after his death), said that "the energetic means of treatment that had been undertaken could not give any positive results or prevent the fateful death." In fact, though, no "energetic means of treatment" were used at all. He only received treatment for his symptoms. He received injections to relax his heart and blood vessels. Suction cups and mustard plaster were applied to his chest. Leeches were even applied to his temples to suck his blood. It was the most ordinary Soviet medical treatment.

At the very end of his life, Stalin achieved the equal treatment that his communist teachings had promised. He was treated just like an ordinary old man in some remote area of the country. And he died.

Later I learned some details about his treatment from an observer, Stalin's maid and mistress, Valentina Vasilyevna Istomina, "Valechka." She was a typically warm-hearted Russian woman with high cheekbones, merry eyes, and beautiful blond hair. During the war, she had been my uncle's neighbor in an apartment on 51 Arbat Street in downtown Moscow that was occupied mostly by agents of the KGB. Valentina was almost never home. Officially, she was considered to be a kindergarten teacher, but unofficially everybody knew that she was a KGB agent with the rank of captain. She told people that she worked as a maid to "the great general." She boasted that: "My general said that nobody sews the white collars on his military jacket better than I do." She accompanied Stalin to the Teheran and Yalta conferences during the war. Valentina even received several medals for whatever role she played in these conferences.

At the time of Stalin's death, she was about forty, had served him thirteen years, and had given this evil old man her youth. She had served him in his kitchen and in his bed completely out of idealism. He never gave her anything in return. The furniture in her apartment was very modest.

Apparently, Stalin became impotent in his last years. Valentina married one of his guards, a young KGB major. She introduced her husband to my uncle and to my parents, and after Stalin's death, she told them of her personal relationship to the dictator.

On one occasion several years after Stalin's death, Valentina asked my father to examine her husband. He agreed and they came to our apartment in an official KGB car. That evening, Valentina told us how doctors Myasnikov and Lukomskiy had treated Stalin with suction cups, mustard plasters, and leeches. They performed these tasks very clumsily, because nurses usually did these things for the doctors. At the same time, the Minister of Health and the head of the Kremlin Medical Directorate had taken turns squeezing oxygen from a large rubber balloon into Stalin's face mask. Beria stood behind them looking around suspiciously as they did this.

Valentina said that ever since then she had lost faith in the Kremlin's doctors. That was why she had brought her sick husband to my father, an ordinary doctor and a Jew.

9

In spring 1953, memories of the "doctors' plot" were still fresh in our minds when I came to another critical juncture that directly affected all the students in the medical school: assignment after graduation. Our education had been free, but we were now obligated to take jobs assigned to us for at least three years, in any part of the country, by the specially appointed state commission.

I had just turned twenty-three and was happy to get my medical diploma at last. Now my immediate future hinged on the decision of the State Assignments Commission. On the eve of graduation everyone was jittery. I wanted to stay in Moscow but did not worry too much, having inherited calmness from my mother. Yet, this time she did worry. She did not want to let me go, and was afraid that I would be sent out to the provinces where I would starve because of poor food supply and would be uncared for. She also believed that I might marry, bashfully, a primitive provincial girl. She had surrounded me with so much care and attention that no girl, in her eyes, was good enough for me.

"I can see you in the provinces, sitting in front of the dinner table with stale food, a book, and a shoe brush," my mother sighed.

I was not uninitiated as my mother thought. I had had two affairs, one with a coed and the other with a divorcée with a child. I had fallen in love with one and then with the other and was thinking of marriage after graduation—if I could only procure a private room in the communal apartment. I was furious when both my paramours cooled off—fast—and began dating other men. After my two affairs had landed on the rocks, I became very wary and gave up the idea of marriage, shifting to short-time affairs instead. I realized that sexual loving was not enough and what I needed was spiritual partnership and intellectual rapport. So far I lacked both. Nevertheless, I was much more concerned with my future assignment than with my would-be love affairs.

When I was summoned to the dean's office before the Commission, I was told: "Motherland sends you to the town of Petrozavodsk. If you want to become a surgeon this is the only place where there is an internship vacancy." I knew next to nothing about the place. All the officials were silent. I reflected for one minute, and in the meanwhile I recalled my first day in grammar school and the silence when I had said I was Jewish. The situation was identical. I could read condescension and embarrassment on the faces of the officials. "You're a half-Jew and can expect nothing better, don't you understand?" they seemed to say.

I did understand. Silences can be many different things—exploratory, ominous, interrogatory. Silence in the dean's office was standoffish. I was in a vacuum. Had my father not lost his position he could have helped me stay in Moscow. But he had lost that because he, too, was Jewish. I dipped an old gray pen into the inkstand. A regular pen, nothing special. At that moment, however, it seemed to me a tool designed for me to sign the declaration of submission to being downtrodden and depressed. I signed the assignment to a job in Petrozavodsk.

Anya Alman, a Jewish girl with tender looks and a soul even tenderer who had stayed innocent and maladjusted through all the years at school, was given a job in Magadan. It is the farthest point on the map from Moscow, a city on the Pacific coast, the official capital of the camps forming the eastern portion of the Gulag Archipelago. Magadan crept with criminals just out of detention, most of them murderers, robbers, and muggers. They settled in the city because they worked in gold mines in the vicinity of Magadan; besides, they were not allowed to live anywhere else.

Anya was horrified, not so much for herself as for her ailing old mother. She could not think of leaving her mother for whom she was the only source of support and joy. But neither could she imagine taking her mother to Magadan. Anya wept and implored the placement commission to let her stay in Moscow or give her a job some place close. She tried to explain her circumstances, but the commission was adamant: "Our Soviet men and women live everywhere in our country, and you and your mother can live in Magadan as well as you do in Moscow," she was told.

Good assignments came to the students who had actively worked in political educational work in the Komsomol committee. Almost all of the active Komsomols were assigned to graduate programs in various departments of the Moscow school. Over the course of all six years of study, these students had spent most of their time not in intellectual halls, but at Komsomol meetings. Many of them became members of the Communist Party. Their careers began from the wooden chairs at the Komsomol meetings and ended in the soft armchairs of the medical elite.

The deputy minister of health, Dr. A. Belousov, came to our graduation ceremony. He gave a speech about how Soviet medicine was the most advanced, the most humane, the most free, the most etc. We took it all cynically, because for six years we had been systematically frightened and denied our rights. We had learned medicine badly, but we had learned well who was who.

And so at the graduation benefit at the Metropol restaurant, many of the students got drunk and started to get even with each other and with the teachers. Fights broke out, and the gala night ended with the beating up of our professor of political economy, N. Podgallo, in the early Moscow morning on Karl Marx Square. That was the last act of our student life.

10

The only way to reach Petrozavodsk from Moscow was on the Number 16 train to Murmansk. When I entered my sleeping compartment in August 1953, it was full of drunken sailors playing harmonicas and saying good-bye to their girlfriends. At that time, the Soviet navy was building a huge submarine base in Murmansk. There were only a few civilian passengers on the train, and it was in fact difficult for passengers to buy tickets.

While the drunken sailors caroused through the train, I lay on my bunk and thought about my past and future. A month ago, I had been vacationing at a special Black Sea resort, "Gagra," for Soviet writers. One morning, very early, I had walked on the still deserted beach and had seen a girl swimming in the distance. I dove into the water and swam over to her.

We were entirely alone. I asked her: "Miss, why are you swimming so far out alone?"

She only smiled in response. I remembered that smile, sweet and shy. I started circling her in the water, trying to show off what a good swimmer I was (in fact, I wasn't). Later we came out on the still empty beach and I continued to circle around her. Her name was Irina and she was a senior at the Moscow University, almost three years my junior. I introduced myself, and said I was a surgeon, although I hadn't yet worked a single day.

My maturity impressed her. She continued to smile sweetly, but not as shyly as before. I wanted to take care of her in every way. At first I invited her to take a place at my table for dinner; later I began inviting her to restaurants and cafés. She was very cheerful, athletic, and uncommonly smart. It was a pleasure talking to her, but even more pleasant kissing her. We fell in love with each other. And it all occurred in the very same place where, twenty-five years previously, my parents had met and fallen in love. I could not make my plans for the future, because I was soon to leave for my first place of work, and she had to return to Moscow for her studies. But the time with her was lovely, and I missed her dearly when I left.

My train arrived in Petrozavodsk two nights later at 2:00 A.M. The station was a small wooden building three kilometers from the city. A single light lit the cold scene. There was no public transportation or taxis. Fortunately, though, a woman I had met on the train offered me a ride with her husband, who had come to pick her up in a truck. They told me that they would drive me to the "Northern Hotel" Severnaya, which was the only hotel in the city.

I climbed into the back of the truck and rode off down the bumpy road into my future.

Although Petrozavodsk was the capital of the Karelian-Finnish Republic, it turned out to be only a small town. The dark, wooden, one-story buildings along the street made a gloomy and pitiful impression on me.

The hotel did not have any free rooms, so I settled down on the couch in the lobby to spend the rest of the night. The woman on duty felt sorry for me, though, and gave me an empty room that had been reserved for a deputy of the Supreme Council who had not shown up.

Early in the morning, as I drew aside the curtain to have a look at Petrozavodsk in the light of day, I was surprised to see Anya Alman walking down the street. I had never expected to see her there because I remembered how bitterly she had wept upon being assigned a job in Magadan, in the Far East. At first I even refused to believe my own eyes, but there was no mistaking her. However, something had imperceptibly changed in her: she was a beautiful woman conscious of her charms. "My, my," I thought, "so our ugly duckling has blossomed into a stately swan." But I decided against calling out to her. I was certain that I could find out from Anya herself how she had landed in Petrozavodsk instead of Magadan.

I eagerly went to the office building of the republic's Ministry of Health. Dr. Tatyana Belyakova, the head of the personnel department, met me with total lack of interest.

"Who told you," she said sarcastically, "that you would be working as a surgeon here?"

"The State Assignments Commission headed by the deputy minister of health."

"I don't understand how they could have said such a thing. We're sending you to work as a pediatrician in a rural area farther north."

I was shocked by this decision and by her whole attitude. I had majored in surgery; my goal in life was to become a surgeon. I then remembered a letter of recommendation I had from the wife of Politburo member Otto Kuusinen to Dr. Mikhail Isserson, the oldest and most respected doctor in Petrozavodsk. Otto Kuusinen was an old Finn, the vice-president of the Soviet Supreme Council and the president of the Karelian-Finnish Republic. His young Russian wife was a doctor and she worked together with my father.

"Where can I meet Dr. Isserson?" I asked.

"What for? He's already retired and can't help you," she sneered.

"I have a letter for him."

"Who from?"

"From Comrade Kuusinen."

"Show it to me," she said skeptically.

I took the envelope out of my pocket and showed her the Politburo return address, but did not give her the letter, because it was personal. Her whole attitude changed.

"Sit here, and I'll come right back," she said politely and left. She returned five minutes later. "The Minister of Public Health Dr. Mikhail Danilovich Zhuravlev is waiting for you," she said.

The first question that Dr. Zhuravlev asked me was, "Are you acquainted with Comrade Kuusinen?"

"No, but my father is."

Dr. Zhuravlev picked up the phone, called the hospital, and ordered that I immediately receive a position as a surgeon there.

The hospital was a two-story building erected fifty years before for 80 sick beds. The wards were spacious with large windows and high ceilings. There were 250 beds, occasionally 300, including cots. Many laboratories and ancillaries were missing; recovery rooms should have been differently shaped and fewer in number. As it was, the hospital was overcrowded, patients were placed in the corridors, there were not enough rest rooms, plumbing often collapsed. A building that was excellent in its early days was now totally unfit for dispensing medical care. The chronically overcrowded wards smelled of iodoform, pus, and feces, and the air was heavy and nauseating.

Still worse was the paucity of drugs and lack of medical equipment. There were no elevators, so to make an X ray we had to carry the patients upstairs on stretchers. The few available stretchers were all broken and there were no wheelchairs. We constantly ran short of X-ray film, there were no drugs in the pharmacy, and the list of prescribed medication was cut down to the bare minimum. Cotton, bandages, syringes, and needles were scarce. All the equipment in the operating room, brought from Europe at the turn of the century by the hospital founder, Dr. M. Isserson, was primitive and outdated.

Twice a month I was assigned to stay on call in the emergency room and another two times in the operating room. I also worked on night shifts five or six times a month. Thus I was on duty every third night.

My salary was 60 rubles a month, which I doubled by working overtime. I spent 20 of these rubles a month for a tiny room in an old woman's house without indoor plumbing or central heating. I brought my water in with buckets from an outdoor faucet, and I chopped my firewood in the courtyard. My immediate neighbors were ten chickens who lived in a coop in the kitchen on the other side of my wall.

I was luckier than other doctors, though, because I didn't have a family to support. Before I left home, my uncle had given me two bits of useful advice: don't join the Communist Party and don't get married. I liked this advice.

Despite the poor physical condition of my apartment, I did enjoy the privacy and independence of a separate room for the first time in my life. My only real confidant was my landlady's pretty daughter, a divorced nurse.

I had brought a large German Telefunken radio with me from Moscow to Petrozavodsk, and it served as the most important furnishing in my small room. I enjoyed listening to European and American music and was delighted that the reception in Petrozavodsk was excellent.

When I had lived in Moscow, I had only listened to the Voice of America a couple of times because it was heavily jammed and I did not like to try to listen through the static. In Petrozavodsk, I now found myself arranging my schedule so that I would not miss the night programs of the Voice of America and the British Broadcasting Corporation. I became very familiar with the voices of Sergey Markin from Washington and Anatoliy Maksimovich Goldberg from London.

They showed me a new world. The information that they broadcast differed completely from the information in the Soviet media, which I soon stopped paying any attention to.

I listened to my radio as quietly as possible so that my landlady on the other side of the thin, wooden wall would not overhear. To my surprise and relief, however, she said to me one day, "Those are interesting radio programs. The information in them is true. But don't worry; I won't tell anybody. My sons also listen to that 'American Voice.' "

One evening in 1955, I heard a BBC program on the life, arrest, exile, and death of Dr. Sergey Yudin, the Number One Russian surgeon. As the announcer said (I still remember his exact words), "Dr. Yudin was a surgeon of the same class as the famous Russian doctors Pirogov and Hertsen." I agreed with the BBC's description and I quickly realized my own way of thinking was much closer to these foreign broadcasts than to any Soviet sources of information.

The only time I turned off the broadcasts in Petrozavodsk was when my landlady's daughter came into my room. Then I tuned in a local music station so that the landlady wouldn't be able to hear anything that was going on in my room.

11

An ax blow had nearly severed four fingers of a worker's hand. The fingers hung to their base only by a mesh of soft tissue and crushed, exposed bone. I applied a tourniquet to stop the bleeding, but I didn't know what to do next. The simplest treatment would have been to amputate the fingers, but there was also a remote possibility that the fingers would somehow heal if I sewed them back on.

I looked with despair at my patient. After all these years, I remember the shudder that ran through my body and the quiver in my lips as I spoke with him. I have felt this sensation many times since in my work, and I can only compare it to what an actor feels when he steps out on stage. The patient was also upset, of course, but he nevertheless looked at me with a smile, in apparent condescension to my inexperience.

"You look a lot like my youngest son," he said.

"How many sons do you have?" I asked, trying to calm myself.

"Three, all engineers except the youngest, who's trying to become one. I also have a daughter who's a doctor in Minsk. They all have the education I never got. I worked forty years at a lathe."

"Still, you helped your children become engineers and doctors."

"I did, I suppose, but with the labor of my hands and now.
. . ." He looked at his fingers. "Are you going to amputate them?"

No, I thought. I would sew those fingers back on, no matter what. I had to save this hand, which had put four young people through college. And then the confidence flowed through me that I could do it, and that was the first time I really felt like a surgeon—perhaps it was divine inspiration.

"I'll try to sew them back on," I said, somewhat uncertainly.

"Do you really think it's possible?"

"I'll try."

"Well, you know best, Doctor."

I washed my hands in an old wash basin on a wooden stool in the corner of the room. A nurse sterilized instruments in another corner. The room was very small—only about a dozen square meters. It was actually a bandaging room, but over the years it had honestly earned the title "operating room."

I operated for more than two hours; if I were to watch such a clumsy operation today, I would surely throw the surgeon out of the hospital. At the time, though, I had never seen this type of operation, so I had to make up the technique as I went along. In addition, I had forgotten a lot about the anatomy of the hand and therefore had difficulty determining where exactly the tendons, arteries, veins, and nerves were supposed to run. The hardest job was to pull the severed tendons back out of the detached fingers, into which the contracted muscles had drawn them. I had no instruments for this. Finally, I stitched everything back together haphazardly with my thick needles and thread. During the whole operation, I frequently had to adjust the tourniquet and inject novocaine, since the patient was in such pain (fortunately, I had learned to use novocaine from my surgeon father, not from medical school). When I finally finished, I figured I would eventually have to amputate the fingers after all.

Exhausted, I moved the patient into a ward and then spent an hour writing the history into the log.

The next day, the hospital's main surgeon, Dr. Vasily Baranov, listened to my report with disbelief. He obviously considered me unqualified to perform such an operation successfully. My other supervisor, Dr. Mikhail Raudsep, told me plainly: "What the heck did you get involved in an operation like that for? It's clear to everybody that you didn't know what you were doing. You should have called in somebody more experienced. Now you've put yourself into a position where people will examine everything you do, because they'll be afraid you'll risk something even more dangerous in the future. What did you expect to gain from such a stunt?"

I expected no personal gain, of course. My state salary would remain 60 rubles ($90) a month whether I cut fingers off or sewed them back on. I had simply tried to make the best decision for the patient.

Unfortunately, the hand and fingers quickly swelled up and lost feeling, and the pulse almost disappeared. I was afraid that gangrene would develop, but I was even more afraid that the chief doctor would order me to amputate. I kept hoping that if we waited two or three more days the fingers might still heal.

In those days, I experienced for the first time the mixture of objectivity, anxiety, doubt, and hope that a surgeon feels throughout his career. I have recognized since then that hope is absolutely essential for a surgeon. Lack of hope paralyzes his will.

I never gave up. I kept repositioning the hand, changing the bandages, and injecting novocaine. Perhaps I did more than I should have, but the constant treatment reassured both the patient and me. After ten days, the hand finally began to improve, and after ten more days, I released the patient from the hospital. Although the fingers had lost much of their movement forever, they did heal. I had become a surgeon and had also gained a close friend.

My first success won me the respect of my colleagues, and they began to trust me again to man the emergency room by myself.

The hospital employed about five hundred people, and all of them were paid in cash on the fifth and twentieth of every month. The Soviet Union does not pay its employees with checks, so very little work gets done on these two days of *poluchka,* or "the take." Many of the employees of our hospital were alcoholics. Immediately after getting the *poluchka* they began to drink.

One of the doctors in the emergency room was a forty-year-old Russian named Dr. Khrenov who had become such an alcoholic that his hands chronically shook too much to operate. Since he was a member of the Party, it was decided not to fire him, but instead to put him on duty in the emergency room three or four days a week. He was strictly warned not to drink on those days. Like all alcoholics, he was powerless against the urge to drink. He was also a pleasant and witty man who had recently married for the second time and was always late to work.

"Why were you a whole hour late today?" I asked him one day.

"I had a technical problem," he answered.

"What kind?"

"Well," he said with an embarrassed smile, "our bed stands by the wall, and I sleep on the side next to the wall."

"What does that have to do with it?"

"Well, as I was crawling over my wife to get out of bed, I was . . . delayed."

Despite the orders, he still drank on the job. He would steal alcohol from the operating room or beg it from one of the nurses.

One day, one of the nurses asked me to change the bandages on a patient on whom Dr. Khrenov had performed a lengthy operation the day before. I read in Dr. Khrenov's shaky handwriting in the patient's records that he had sewn fifteen stitches to close up two wounds on the inside of the patient's hip. The patient complained to me of continuing severe pains, so I opened up the bandages and saw a large, wide cut—about ten by eight centimeters—with inflamed edges. The wound was not sewn up, but there were about fifteen stitches in seemingly random spots all around the wound.

I removed these stitches and then sewed up the wound correctly with fifteen new stitches. I did not need fifteen stitches, but I made them all in order to match what he had written in the patient's records.

12

In spite of being very much involved in my surgical duties, I was bored in the little town. I tried to read a lot and listen to classical records, but what I really missed was the company of a woman.

At about this time, I began to notice a young woman who cut hair in a barber shop. Whenever I was waiting in line there, I would secretly admire her tall, slender figure, her beautiful dark brown hair, and especially her shapely legs, which she covered with seamed silk stockings with the then fashionable black heels. I would also occasionally see her strolling with officers from the local base. All I knew about her, though, was that her name was Zhenya.

One night in the late fall of 1954, Zhenya was brought to the emergency room while I was on duty. I didn't recognize her at first; her face was pale and dirty. She had thrown herself in front of a train, and the wheels had cut off her legs at the knees. She was in third-degree shock, and she had lost almost all pulse and blood pressure. I treated her through the night until her blood pressure finally stabilized, and then as the sun was coming up, I amputated her legs to the middle of the thighs. I sewed up her stumps, wheeled her to a room, and then lay down on a couch in the interns' room, where unexpectedly I started to shake with emotional shock. When I calmed down I began to dream that she was running with her beautiful, shapely legs, and I woke with a start. I thought of her as a close relative.

As a matter of fact, I became her blood brother the next day, because I transfused five hundred cc of my blood into her body. At first, she thrashed around in her bed to resist the transfusion and protested that she wanted to die.

"You need more blood," I insisted.

"I'm Polish, and I only want Polish blood," she answered.

Fortunately, my ancestors were Polish, so when I showed her that the donor's name was the Polish-sounding Golyakhovsky—she still didn't know that was my name—she finally agreed.

Zhenya's stumps healed poorly and oozed. She always smelled like pus, sweat, and urine. Her temperature, anemia, and apathy remained critical. She shared a room with seven other patients, but she never talked with them or with anyone else. Her bed was by the window, so she stared out constantly at winter's passage. When I came with new bandages and my tray of instruments, she turned toward the window with stubborn determination.

I don't know what she was thinking about, but her tragedy caused me to think about the meaning of my own career. I wondered whether I could spend my whole life swimming in an ocean of intense human suffering. Moans, groans, grinding of teeth, and screams would become ordinary sounds. All my conversations at work would involve descriptions of illness and pain. To study, to perform, and to comfort every day and night for my whole life would take colossal strength. In our communist society, people did not open their souls to priests or to God; people could legally tell their troubles only to their doctors. For many patients—Zhenya was only one of the first —I myself would have to delve into spiritual and psychological problems that led to traumas or suicidal acts and then interfere in my patients' attitudes and private lives.

I treated Zhenya with special sympathy. I even brought fruits and chocolates, which were difficult to obtain in our remote, northern area, and secretly put them on her dinner tray. Gradually, she began to talk to me and tell me her life story in bits and pieces.

Zhenya had been five years old when Germany and the Soviet Union invaded Poland in 1939. The Soviets captured her father, a Polish officer, and executed him along with 12,000 other Polish officers in Khatinsky Forest in March 1940. In the meantime, a group of Soviet soldiers came and arrested his wife and young daughter at their home. An officer in the group advised Zhenya's mother to pack as many things as she could, but since Zhenya's mother couldn't understand Russian, the officer opened the shelves himself and began to throw Zhenya's father's uniforms and other things into their suitcases. Then the woman and girl were exiled to the Soviet Union, to the small town of Vorkuta, above the Arctic Circle.

Mother and daughter lived in poverty, hunger, and tyranny as "enemies of the people." Zhenya's mother was beaten and raped dozens of times by Soviet soldiers and lived in constant terror that they would also begin to abuse Zhenya. To buy enough food and wood, Zhenya's mother gradually sold the family possessions she had brought along. She was always thankful to the Soviet officer who had helped her pack, but she hated all other Soviets, and Zhenya grew up hating them too.

In the fall of 1953, after Stalin died, many exiles were pardoned. Polish exiles asked permission to return home, but the Soviet government turned their requests down. Zhenya and her mother decided to at least leave Vorkuta, but they only had enough money for one ticket to Petrozavodsk, so they decided that Zhenya would get a job there and then send her mother the money to join her. As a farewell gift, Zhenya's mother gave Zhenya her father's last parade uniform's dress coat, which was beautifully decorated with braids and silver epaulettes. They had earlier promised each other that they would sell this last memento only if they reached the edge of starvation.

Zhenya at first had trouble finding a job in Petrozavodsk because she could not even pretend to be pleasant with Russians, whom she hated fiercely. People thought she was insane. She finally enrolled in a hairdressing school, which paid a stipend of 15 rubles a month. For a third of this, she rented a corner in a hut next to the railroad tracks.

Almost every night as she walked home along these tracks, she felt the urge to lay her head down across the rail in front of a passing train, but the young life in her nineteen-year-old body beckoned more strongly. Petrozavodsk was much larger and more comfortable than Vorkuta, and for the first time in her life she felt free and independent. She wanted to dress up and have fun.

She had no boyfriends (or girlfriends) yet, but she was beginning to experience temptations. The officers from the local base would invite her out to restaurants. She accepted, because she saw that they were ordinary people, not like the guards who had kept her mother and her in Vorkuta. She had decided, though, that she would give her virginity only to a Pole.

Her coworkers at the hairdressers' shop were jealous of her when her admirers came there to pick her up for a date. The women called her a Polish slut, and the boss, an alcoholic war invalid, felt that she should share her body with him too. Zhenya sensed her coworker's hostility and refused to say a single word more than necessary to any of them.

After three months, she was due to take the test to become a master hairdresser. She was confident she would pass, because she had good taste and a talent for cutting and setting hair. With her increased salary of 45 rubles, she would finally be able to spare enough money to buy a train ticket for her mother.

The day before the test, her boss, drunk as usual, called her into his office at the back of the shop. After he had closed the door behind her, he grabbed her and began to pull up her dress. She struggled to break his hold.

"Don't resist, you dumb bitch," he hissed. "Think about it. Don't make trouble for yourself."

Zhenya immediately realized that this man was attacking her the same way the drunken guards had attacked her mother in earlier years. In horror, she shoved him away and ran out the door. She recovered her breath in the small passageway and then walked back out into the salon.

She didn't know what to do. She picked up a little pink comb. Tears welled up in her eyes, so she walked over to the window and pretended to look out so the others wouldn't see her cry. She nervously bent the comb back and forth until, crack, she accidentally broke it.

"What did you do that for?" one of the women yelled. "That was my comb! What did you break it for?"

The other women joined in: "She did it on purpose!" "What gall!" "She thinks she's better than everybody else!" "She's crazy!" "Polish slut!" They would probably have attacked her physically if customers hadn't been present.

The boss staggered out to investigate the commotion and, taking advantage of the sudden opportunity to avenge his recent sexual rejection, yelled: "You're fired! I'm not even going to give you the test. Get the hell out of here right now!"

"Stick it up your ass, all of you!" Zhenya screamed, furiously hurling the broken pink comb across the room. She tore off her white coat, threw it on the ground, and ran out the door. An impotent rage strangled her. On her way home, in despair, she decided to kill herself by throwing herself under a passing train. She hesitated twice, but then jumped. Perhaps her will to live still held her back just enough that she only lost her legs. . . . Legs only!

Zhenya's injuries finally began to heal in the spring. On March 8, International Women's Day, she greeted me for the first time with a smile, and I immediately noticed that she had curled her hair, manicured her nails, and sprayed herself with perfume. Her trade union had bought her the cosmetics as a Women's Day gift, although she still refused to talk with any of the union representatives.

"Big brother"—that's what Zhenya called me—"what will you do with me after I recover?" Dr. Dora Stepanova, a wonderful woman who had worked as a surgeon for twenty years in Petrozavodsk, had already told me that Zhenya would have to either enter an invalid home or return to her mother's care. Dr. Stepanova had also warned me that the invalid home was a cesspool of violence, drunkenness, thievery, perversion, veneral disease, degradation, and death, so I diplomatically tried to persuade Zhenya to return to her mother.

"Well, big brother," she answered, "I recently did call my mother on the phone. It took me a week to make the connection to Vorkuta, but I finally got in touch with her. I told her I had married an officer and was transferring with him to Sakhalin on the east coast. I told her not to follow me, but to go back to Poland and that I would eventually get back to visit her. I told her all kinds of lies, even that we went to a lot of dances. I told her I intended to send my father's uniform back to her, but she insisted that I give it to my new husband. I'm thankful that we were talking in Polish, so the other patients didn't understand what I was saying."

When the weather grew warm, I wheeled Zhenya out to sun herself in the courtyard. The male patients in their casts and bandages and with their crutches hobbled around to pay her homage. She sat in her wheelchair in their midst like a beautiful, proud Polish princess. She began to smile and laugh again. In the meantime, I filled out the paperwork to send her to the invalid home, which was located in a remote part of the forests outside the city. We hadn't told her about its horrors, but I think she realized she would perish there.

The day before Zhenya's departure, I was working alone in the interns' room when the door creaked open and she began to wheel herself through. I got up and helped her into the room, so we could have what would probably be our last talk in private. She had made herself up nicely and had even put on a pretty necklace.

"Kiss me, big brother," she said. Her face was inquisitive, watchful, and sorrowful. Her expression told me she wanted to make love with me, to have one romantic experience in her life. I glanced at her stumps, which I had sawed off myself. I kissed her politely. She embraced me and, leaning forward, pressed her body against mine.

"I want to give you a present," she whispered.

"I know," I whispered back, "but you're too much like a little sister to me."

"Please don't think of me that way."

"It's better that I do."

"But I've always liked you. I first noticed you when you came to the barbershop for haircuts."

"Really? I never realized." I was flattered, but remained cool to her offer.

"So"—she let go of me in disappointment—"now you know." She handed me a package. "Here. At least I'd like to give you my father's uniform."

"Thank you, really, but I can't accept that. It's your only remembrance of your father."

"I don't need any remembrances. The Soviets shot my father like a dog, treated my mother like dirt, and cornered me like a rat. Now, big brother, it's my fate to suffer for the rest of my life, so I'm mad at the whole world. But the most bitter insult of all, big brother, has been your rejection of me just now. You gave me your blood, but you wouldn't accept my body. If you had lost *your* legs instead, I certainly wouldn't have refused your last plea for love. I've accepted my fate, though, and I forgive you. I just ask that you never visit me. I've said good-bye to my mother, and now I say good-bye to you. I've already heard about the invalid's home, and I don't want either of you to ever see me there. I know I won't live there long."

She survived there two years. For the male invalids, she was a welcome present—young, attractive, and best of all, legless. . . . When her rations were cut because she refused to do her chores, these blinded, shattered, chopped-up men brought her bread, vodka, and their love. She became an alcoholic, and eventually died of a septic abortion.

The fate of this girl stayed in my imagination. I thought about her life and what it could have been if not for the clash of the conflicting social powers and the fatal sequence of events.

From time to time I told this story to my friends and gradually it shaped into the above story, which I even wanted to publish in Russia. My friends advised me not to do it and I gave up the idea. However, from this time on I started to write down real stories, which were in abundance in my medical practice.

13

I continued to write, even though I was very busy with my surgery. I would sometimes sit until two or three o'clock in the morning at my little desk by the window, which looked out onto a cliff over Onezhskoye Lake. During the white nights in the summer, I could read and write without a lamp, even at those late hours. I liked to look out at the cold gray waves of the lake. I remembered the girl Irina, whom I had met in the waves of the Black Sea, and I would write her poems in the style of Shakespeare's sonnets. In return, she would write me letters, "as I listen to a lecture on invertebrates in zoology class." She never said anything about my poems, though, and like any poet, I was crazy to find out if my beloved liked them.

I also began to write for children. I had no contact with children, but I liked to write clear and simple poems that they would be able to understand. I soon discovered that it was more difficult to write these "simple" children's poems than it was to write adult poetry. Adults have a basis for understanding poetic perception, especially in Russia, where poetry is so popular. Children aged three to five lack both this perception and a well-developed vocabulary. In my children's poems, I tried to create a poetic impression with the help of very simple words set into a playful rhythmic sound, as in the traditional English children's poetry.

As a surgeon, I was limited in my creative possibilities by the anatomy and physiology of tissues and organs. As a poet, though, I could create without limitations, choosing combinations from thousands of words. I think that both activities contributed to each other. Surgery helped me to write exactly, and poetry helped me to operate with more flexibility. Once, in 1955, I sent a packet of my poems to the well-known children's writer Korney Chukovsky in Moscow. I did not expect to get an answer from him, because I did not think that he would really like my poems. I was overjoyed to get a letter from him a short time later. I opened the envelope and read the greeting: "Dear Poet!" I was as nervous reading this letter as I was when I performed my first operation. I read and read and read, but did not really understand how it had happened that Chukovsky liked my poems. He wrote to me that he had submitted some of them for publication in a children's magazine and for a children's radio program. He also asked me to send him more poems.

I also submitted some of my poems to the local magazines and newspapers in Petrozavodsk, and they were published. I began to receive royalties. Emboldened, I began to draw pictures to illustrate my poems and submitted them too, and they were also published. Within a year, I had become a rather popular poet and artist in Petrozavodsk. My poems were even translated into Finnish and published with my pictures for children in Finland.

The poet and romantic that I am perhaps explains why I have never been able to do anything without devotion and affection. But falling deeply in love with orthopedic surgery during the second year of my work at Petrozavodsk came as a surprise to me. I knew almost nothing of orthopedics. Only four days were devoted to it in the curriculum when I was a medical student in Moscow. Now I assisted for the first time at bone-and-joint operations, and somehow preferred these operations to those of abdominal and chest cavity tissues. It was as inexplicable as all love is.

To an outsider, orthopedic manipulations on the bone may appear crude, like carpentry. Take, for example, osteotomy, or lengthwise dissection of the bone with a special chisel. The orthopedist hits the chisel with a hammer, breaking the bone. However, this is an extremely delicate operation, one which requires of the orthopedist great care and meticulousness in positioning the chisel, hitting it properly with a hammer, and accurately calculating the blow.

The great Danish sculptor Thorwaldsen once remarked that the art of sculpting is very simple, that all the artist needs to know is how to chisel away everything extra from a chunk of marble, to leave only the sculpture. Using this principle, one may say that the art of orthopedics lies in not chiseling away anything extra.

An orthopedist must develop a very fine hand for such precision. Orthopedics is a "power surgery," since bone is an extremely hard material. To drill even the smallest opening in the bone extreme physical force must be applied.

I decided that upon my return to Moscow I would by any and all means become an orthopedic surgeon.

14

One day in the spring of 1954, I came home after my working hours, cut wood in the backyard, set a fire in the stove, and went to the hydrant on the corner of the next block to draw two buckets of water. On my way back with the two heavy buckets I noticed a ZIM limousine, a government car belonging to the Minister of Public Health, near the gates of my house. I was told I had to attend an important gathering immediately. It was very unusual that they had sent a car to pick me up, and I wondered why. Knowing that you can never expect anything good from VIPs and important gatherings, I decided that I must be in for some trouble.

I was brought in the limousine to the building of the Central Committee of the Communist Party of the Karelian-Finnish Republic where I, a non-Party member, was issued a special pass to the office of the chief of the administrative department. When I entered the office I saw Minister Dr. M. Zhuravlev, and five young doctors, all of them Jewish. I wondered what was in the offing. The chief of the administrative department and the Minister greeted us with long perorations whose gist was that we were to be assigned new jobs in the remote areas of the republic, with promotions. I was supposed to take the position of head doctor in the rural hospital in the village of Loukhy, five hundred miles to the north of Petrozavodsk. Of course it was an exile, a part of the government's plan to which we had to submit.

I remembered that my Jewish ancestors, who were persecuted by the czar's government, had to reside in the specially assigned Pale of Settlement. That was 150 years ago. I also remembered that my father had to change cities and occupations, hounded by the government officials, before his medical career was launched. That happened twenty-five years ago. It looked like I was also to bow and follow in the footsteps of my ancestors. I determined that I would not leave Petrozavodsk. I was upset, angry, and full of mettle. I decided that I would put up a fight and win, although I had no idea what course of action to take.

I refused to sign the paper assigning me to the new job. The officials' faces contorted with displeasure. Then the chief of the department said, "You need not sign it today. Go home now, think it over, discuss it with friends. When you feel you are ready then you can come and sign. We shall send the car to pick you up."

The other doctors also refused to sign the order and the same car took us back. I asked the driver to drop me at the house of a friend, a young Jewish lawyer named V. Rosen.

I told him my story and asked for his counsel: what was I to do?

"Well, you're already in trouble," he said, and advised me to go to the law office of the Republican Trade Union Council to see his friend, Vasily Bronevoy, a young lawyer. Bronevoy, it turned out, was very nice, with a flair for drinking vodka and telling political and nonpolitical jokes. We soon became friends. As for my case, Bronevoy explained to me that I was entitled to stay in my present job because, according to the law, I had automatically signed a contract with the hospital on the day I began working for them. I was amazed when I heard this since I had not signed any contract and knew nothing about it.

Next day I was summoned to the Minister's office. He asked me again if I was ready to take up my new job at Loukhy. I said that I was not and that I did not intend to go there. The Minister called the Central Committee.

"Yes, he is in my office and tells me he does not want to go. Yes, I understand. Okay, you will see him soon," he grumbled. He put down the receiver and said the Central Committee official wished to talk to me; the car was waiting downstairs.

I met the Big Boss face to face. He asked me whether I was married. I answered that I was not.

"That is good. You will go to Loukhy and pick up a bride. After the war they have only a few men there, so you can choose a wife with a house and a cow. Your mother-in-law will bring you milk and will bake pies with mushrooms for you. Do you like pies with mushrooms?"

"I don't eat pies with mushrooms, have no desire to marry and get a cow, and I will not sign the paper," I retorted.

It all ended with the Minister issuing an order that removed me from my job in the hospital. Then my new friend Vasily Bronevoy compiled an appeal fully conforming to the existing Soviet laws and induced me to go to the courts and sue the Minister over the breach of contract. The Minister was dumbfounded: it was the first time that a young doctor had not only disobeyed his order but also filed a suit against him in the courts. I was idle for about a month in anticipation of the trial, went hunting, drank vodka with Bronevoy, and enjoyed myself.

During my free time I resumed my childhood hobbies. This area was a veritable paradise for hunters and anglers, an uninterrupted sea of forest interspersed with lakes. I had resolved to go hunting or angling at the first opportunity.

The best part of a hunting expedition is communion with nature very early in the morning. While it was still dark, around 4:00 A.M., I would creep into the small blind I had built from twigs the previous day and wait for daybreak. Birds and beasts woke up before dawn. I sat still and watched wildlife. My interest as an observer would naturally be mixed with the excitement of a hunter stalking his prey. I do not subscribe to the opinion that hunting is criminal killing. It is the oldest known way of procuring food.

After early morning hunting I would go to the nearest lake, where I had installed a fishnet the previous night. The morning fog still lingered over the quiet water while I rowed to the net in a small boat that I had brought with me. While I pulled the net, the sun would rise over the horizon, and I could admire the sunrise from the surface of the smooth water expanse.

Once, on a hunting expedition, I was rowing in my boat, vainly trying to peer into the thick morning fog hanging over the water. Suddenly I heard a loud splash, then another and another. I did not understand what it was, but obviously the splash was produced by something struggling in the water, not by the oars of another boat. I had never seen a big fish in the lake. What else could have produced a splash that big? I turned my boat and rowed in the direction of the splashes. As I was getting near, the sounds became louder. No fish would react this way to an approaching boat. But if not a fish, what was it? Suddenly, over the splashes, I heard loud guttural noises that sounded like rough grinding. I was sure I had heard such sounds before, but before I could identify the sounds my boat approached a large white swan. The bird was beating its wings, screeching. It wanted to fly or swim away but couldn't; something held it fast. And it was spinning, fighting, trying to break free and turning its head to me, awaiting the impending doom. I realized that the bird's feet were caught in my net, and recalled the myths of girls turned into swans by an evil spell. The most popular of such girl-swans is Odette-Odile, the heroine of *Swan Lake*. The prince's love broke the spell. So too I found myself in a situation where I had to set a swan free: never in my life would I kill a fettered prey. For some reason I was sure the swan was a she, maybe because it was very beautiful. Possibly, too, because I wanted to be a prince, bold and in love.

"Don't you worry," I told the swan, "you'll be free in a jiffy. Wait a second, I'll untangle your feet and you'll be free again. . . ."

The swan was jerking and bending its neck, but then, as if the bird understood me, it quieted down. I bent overboard and reached the net. The wet threads would not yield, and the cold water numbed my fingers.

At that instant something happened, I could not understand what: a tremendous blow hit me from the blind side. I was momentarily stunned, the light dimmed. Trying not to fall out of the precariously listing boat, I turned my head and saw another swan, wings spread, neck outstretched, attacking me.

So, I thought, you already have your prince and he, too, is enchanted. And he is protecting you like a hero, a real hero. The he-swan was out for my blood and was totally fearless. Meanwhile, the sun was rising and, bathed in its first pink rays, my birds also looked pink. My God, only Tchaikovsky's divine music was missing! And I did free her.

She swam some distance away and stopped, looking back at me. Bending her wonderful long neck, she was thanking me. Her champion approached her, they touched necks, and swam away side by side, the white-pink prince and princess.

To my surprise, I won hands down: the Minister revoked his order of my termination on the eve of the trial since all the laws ruled in my favor. I returned to my hospital and was even given money for the period when I had been away from the job.

As for the other Jewish doctors who had been scheduled to be exiled, some did sign the papers and had to relocate. Those who had refused to sign following my example all stayed in Petrozavodsk. For a brief period I became a kind of clandestine leader of the opposition to the authorities. Some people congratulated me, others were furious, still others expressed surprise. Bronevoy was so happy that he drank himself unconscious.

This episode had fortified my confidence in myself. I decided never to give up without putting a fight to the officials, no matter how highly placed. The decision was rather a bold one; everyone else I knew always got scared and surrendered when pressed by the authorities.

The Minister became my worst enemy and I had to make sure I did not provide him with an opportunity for revenge. Three months later he issued a new order assigning me temporarily to a job in the nearby town of Pudozh. That temporary assignment I couldn't refuse.

15

I reached Pudozh just before the autumn rains turned the ground to mud and made all travel impossible. Since we had no helicopters then, the town was completely isolated by mud every spring and fall. Even in summer and winter, Pudozh was culturally isolated by its remote location and primitive attitudes. The region had originally been settled by fanatic Old Believers who had fled all contact with the established Russian Orthodox Church and with the czarist government. Many times, whole communities would lock themselves into barns and burn themselves alive rather than compromise their religion. Even when I was there, most people had never seen a railroad or used electricity. There was no industry and almost no agriculture. The people lived by hunting animals and cutting lumber. The only intellectuals in the region were a few young college graduates like myself assigned there for an obligatory three years.

I checked into the town hotel, which was a two-story wooden dormitory with ten or twelve beds in each room. Fortunately, though, the hotelkeeper put me into a special room—it had only two beds—reserved for important officials. I was exhausted from my trip and fell fast asleep.

In the middle of the night, a nurse's aide knocked on the door and woke me up. Some lumberjacks had just brought in a man whose stomach had been slit open in a knife fight the day before. The woman led me to the hospital, lighting the way with an oil lantern.

The tiny wooden hospital had been built one hundred years earlier for ten beds, but we generally had about seventy patients. We had to sleep a lot of them in the corridors. The smell of pus permeated everything, including the old wood walls.

In the hospital courtyard, the lumberjacks were milling around a cart. They yelled curses and held up their lanterns to show me the groaning victim. He was a horrible sight. During the forty-kilometer ride to the hospital, his intestines had gradually slithered out and now lay piled on his stomach and strewn across the bed of straw. I was at first too shaken to act. I didn't even know how to carry him into the hospital without dragging his intestines across the ground.

The elderly nurse, Mariya Petrovna, sixty-five, began to organize us and give me advice. She even woke up two patients to help the cart driver and me carry the body while she and her assistants walked alongside holding up the intestines.

After we had laid him on the operating table, I examined him under the dim electric light. The intestines were cold and covered with straw and dirt, and some sections had turned black from necrosis. I pumped glucose into his bloodstream to treat his shock, enlarged the opening in his belly, and washed the intestines with a warm saline solution. I then began to cut out the dead sections and sew the walls together.

Mariya Petrovna was my only assistant. Since she was so short, she stood on a wooden stool on the other side of the table as she handed me my instruments and held the clamps in the wound. She constantly whispered: "Now let's cut this vessel. . . . First, we'll clamp it shut . . . then, let's put the thread around it. . . . Now tie it."

I followed her quiet advice, although we both pretended I was deciding everything myself. After we had finished the operation and filled out the patient's records, I thanked her for her help.

"Why thank me?" she asked in surprise. "Thank *you* for coming to help us. How could we manage without a surgeon?"

Mariya Petrovna was one of those typical Russian old women who radiate goodness and concern. These women have nurtured the souls and inspired the work of artists, social workers, builders, and scientists throughout Russian history. Mariya Petrovna had spent her whole, long life in the Pudozh wilderness and had taught a multitude of young surgeons serving their obligatory three years how to operate with almost no thread, bandages, medicines, clamps, or scalpels.

Not a single night during the three months that I spent in Pudozh did I sleep peacefully. Two or three times a night the aide, a powerfully built Karelian woman, clad in a padded woolen jacket and wearing a *babushka* shawl on her head and knee-high felt boots with gum soles, would knock on my window in the dark. She had an oil lantern with her when she came—the only light in the total darkness. On hearing her knock, I would wake up, come to the window, and wave to her, signaling that I would be ready in a minute. The *izba*, a wooden hut, was fashioned in the northern Russian style and stood high, so she called out from below, "Doc, please come, Mariya Petrovna says they brought a patient in."

That meant that Mariya Petrovna had made the initial diagnosis, as always the right one, and completed the necessary preparations for the operation.

I would throw on my clothes and walk out into the night, shivering in the cold. I wore a warm sheepskin coat and fur-padded high boots. The nurse's aide led the way with the lantern in one hand and a stick in the other which she used to keep away the dogs. You could hear the dogs bark on all sides and sometimes they would close in on us. We had to tread carefully, to circumvent snow drifts or pools of mud, depending on the season, and to shun the dogs. I had a stick in my hand too. It was a ten-minute walk to the hospital, and on some occasions I could watch an amazing sight in the skies, polar lights. An intertwined rope of blue, gold, rose, and silver light ribbons would illuminate the dark skies above my head. The ribbons wound and unwound, soared high up, assembled in circles, and then stretched into a straight line. I would watch this spectacle of lights only to step into a pool of water and then start at the harsh voice of my nurse's aide, who tried to shoo away a barking dog.

My patient with the exposed intestines died a week after the operation. His death didn't surprise me, of course, but I was worried that the autopsy would show I had failed to sew one of the excised sections up. The pathologist, Dr. Yefim Zakher, was the only Jew in town, and he sympathized with me.

"Don't worry," he said. "I'll write the report so that no health ministers or judges will ever find fault with the operation. If only you knew how much I hate all those stupid communist officials. I'm in the Party myself, and I have to attend all those idiotic meetings and vote for all those obviously ridiculous resolutions. Afterward, I go home and look at myself in the mirror with shame and disgust. Sometimes I've even struck myself in the face. Don't you ever join the Party for anything.

"I joined the Party during the war," he continued. "While we were advancing through Hungary, I happened to put two Jewish soldiers in the hospital for pneumonia, and the next day their whole company was wiped out. The company commander accused me of helping my fellow Jews malinger, and a military tribunal sentenced me to a suicide squadron. The commissar was a Jew, though, and he told me that if I joined the Party, he'd arrange to annul my sentence. At first I refused, but the commissar convinced me. He argued that I hadn't lived through the Leningrad blockade—my whole family except me starved to death there—only to be framed by an anti-Semitic Russian and shot by a fascist German. I finally agreed and so saved my life, but lost my conscience."

Listening to his story, sympathizing with him, I decided that I too would only join the Party if it was a question of life or death.

16

I was glad to come home to Petrozavodsk. The experience of being on my own in Pudozh had been very useful to me, yet I had to learn more from my more experienced colleagues. As all beginners I made many mistakes and was grateful to those who taught me.

I continued to live in my small room in Petrozavodsk, frequently visited by my friends, who came to chat, play records, and drink wine. Once one of them, Mark B., brought a guest, who turned out to be my former classmate Anya Alman. She was fancily dressed and her foreign-made makeup made her look glamorous and different from the casually dressed women in our town. I could hardly recognize her, she had changed, looked more mature and a bit nervous. We chatted about our years in the medical school.

"How did it happen that you came here instead of going to Magadan?" I asked.

She smiled mysteriously and remained silent. Later she said, "Sometime I will tell you; now let us drink wine."

At that time, the republic was renamed the Karelian Autonomous Republic and absorbed into the larger Russian Federal Republic. As a result of this decline in status, the republic officials in Petrozavodsk lost much of their salaries and prestige. It also became much more difficult for them to send their children to universities in Moscow and Leningrad, so they decided to invest in the University of Petrozavodsk and add a medical school to it. Since the university did not have the equipment or teachers for the medical school, though, the Karelian government invited Dr. Nikolay Vinogradov, the Minister of Public Health of the Russian Federal Republic, to Petrozavodsk in the summer of 1956 to discuss the possibilities of providing these resources. Dr. Vinogradov had previously served as the Ministry's personnel director and had gained a wide reputation as a corrupt, anti-Semitic despot. He was very handsome—tall, elegant, and intelligent-looking. His former mistresses were assigned to the best hospitals.

When Vinogradov arrived in Petrozavodsk, he got a grand reception. He was housed in a special two-storied country house, a governmental dacha surrounded by a fence and guarded by a police-man. He was also assigned three beautiful nurses from the elite Party hospital to look after his needs. Vinogradov eventually submitted to the local officials' hospitality and persuasion and agreed to approve the establishment of the new medical school.

My former classmate Anya Alman was very preoccupied with Vinogradov's visit. When she found out where Vinogradov was staying, she asked me to drive her in my new Pobeda automobile to the dacha. I had bought the car with a loan from my parents because the waiting time for a car was only a year in Petrozavodsk compared to three years in Moscow. Most of the Pobeda cars in Petrozavodsk were government cars, so the policeman let us through the gate without question.

Dr. Vinogradov was sitting in the dining room at a large table covered with bottles of champagne and cognac and drinking with the three nurses, all of whom were drunk. Anya had told me to come along but to do nothing and to be surprised by nothing I saw, so I stood and quietly watched as she entered the room and walked up to Vinogradov.

"Hello, Nikolay Arkadyevich," she said, "do you recognize me? Don't you remember that you arranged for me to be assigned to Petrozavodsk instead of to Magadan? I will always be thankful to you for that favor. This is my husband," she said, pointing to me. "We heard that you were here, so we drove out in our car to visit you."

"I don't remember you at all."

"Oh, but you must remember me. Don't you remember that you invited me into your office to drink tea and talk about my assignment?"

"I never drank tea with you. You're imagining things."

"So you think that I'm imagining it. I thought that we would always remain friends. Well, if that's the way it is, I guess my husband and I will be going. Good-bye."

Anya quietly chain-smoked on the drive back. As we were driving by a field, she asked me to stop the car, and we got out and sat on the grass under some tall pine trees. Then she broke into tears.

"That bastard raped me in the back room behind his office. Oh, I was so young. . . . My mother was sick and begged me to get my assignment changed, because Magadan is way out in Siberia. So

I tried for a long time to get an appointment to talk to Vinogradov.

"His secretary would never give me an appointment, though. Finally, once at the end of the day, I was in the reception room, and he walked through, and I asked to see him, and he agreed, since he had finished his other appointments.

"It was the first time I had been in the office of such an important man, and I felt intimidated. I told him about my sick mother and asked him to change my assignment to some place closer. He listened and didn't answer anything, and then asked me if I would like to drink some tea and led me into a small room behind his office.

"He closed the door behind us and sat me down on a couch. I continued to explain my situation, and then all of a sudden he stuck his paw up my dress. I resisted, but I was afraid to scream. He was very experienced and very strong and quickly subdued me. I wanted to bite him when he was lying on top of me. He told me to get undressed and submit or I would go to Magadan and never come back. At the same time, he promised that if I gave him what he wanted, he would give me a good assignment. I had no time to think, but I understood that I was completely in his power. He saw, and smoked and watched me while I got undressed. I didn't want him to hurt me, so I got undressed by myself.

"Forgive me for telling you all of this. I've never told anyone before. Anyway, he did with me whatever he wanted. He toyed with me. I was shocked. When he was done, he told me to get dressed and wrote out an order to change my assignment to Petrozavodsk.

" 'Did you like it?' he asked me. 'If you did, come again. I can even arrange an assignment in Moscow for you.' I didn't want anything else from him, though.

"I wandered the streets for a long time and then went home. When I told my mother that my assignment had been changed, she said, 'Oh, what a nice man he is. I hope you thanked him.' I almost told her that I had already given him a lot of thanks.

"Forgive me for having involved you in this trip," she said. "I just wanted to see the expression on his face when he saw me. But either he didn't recognize me or he's a great actor. I wanted him to think that I was married and happy, but he spoiled it all. I don't understand what I wanted out of this experience myself."

She broke into tears again, and I dried her face with a handkerchief. "Oh, I've messed up your handkerchief," she said. Then she smiled. "Have you guessed why I really brought you along?"

"Because of my car?"

"No, silly. Because I want you. I want you right now."

I acquiesced. . . .

17

In May 1956, the elderly postwoman came to my door with a large bag over her shoulder filled with newspapers and letters. He handed me a registered postcard from Petrozavodsk's military commissariat. The thin piece of gray paper informed me in a few poorly typed lines that in accordance with the law of universal military service I had to report to the commissariat. Every Soviet young man knows that this postcard means he is being drafted.

When I received my draft notice, I was upset, because I didn't want to interrupt my intensive and interesting surgical work. It was unthinkable to evade the draft, though.

I was sent to a three-month camp in the town of Sortavala, which is not far from the Finnish border. Until 1945, when the war ended, this town and the surrounding countryside of beautiful lakes, cliffs, and forests had been a resort center in Finnish territory. Now, even ten years after the war, the town was so full of people in military uniforms and insignia that you would have thought the war was still going on. The strong military presence was conditioned by Stalin's atavistic plans to reunite all of Finland with Russia.

Sortavala did not look like a Russian town. It stood on the bank of Ladozhskoye Lake and of a small river. Everything in the town had been built very comfortably and correctly. The architecture of most of the houses was modern, which was unseen in Russia.

The beautiful cottages made of gray granite seemed especially unusual to me.

I went to the headquarters of the base, which was located a little way out of town. The road there led past a Finnish cemetery, which had been abandoned. The cemetery had many beautiful marble gravestones. The large, tall monuments differed from the usual Russian wooden crosses in the same way that the stone cottages of Sortavala differed from the wooden huts of Petrozavodsk.

The base headquarters was on the territory of a rifle regiment that I was to serve in. A sergeant with a red armband in a wooden hut sat at the entrance point, and a soldier with a machine gun stood at the gate. Behind them lay military life with all its peculiarities. I showed the sergeant my draft notice and then passed through the gate to become a soldier. I was still not a proper soldier, however, for I did not present my documents to headquarters in the correct manner. The officer on duty ignored me for a while, then looked at the notice in my hands and lazily strolled off to tell the regiment commander of my arrival.

The headquarters was a large two-story wooden building to which adjoined a one-story stone barracks that served as the clubhouse. A network of wide roads covered with sand led to the headquarters from all over the base. The base in general was dreary. It had only a few sickly trees except in front of the headquarters, where stood tall and beautiful pines. The street where these trees grew was called the Alley of Combat Glory; there is such a street in every military base. Along the street were posted plywood signs with quotations from Lenin, the speeches of the Premier of the moment (at that time, Khrushchev), various Komsomol and military slogans, and large portraits of famous military leaders and war heroes. These posters are typical of all Soviet bases.

The duty officer told me to report to the medical point, under the command of the regiment's senior doctor, Major Bregvadze. I would hold the position of junior doctor.

Our regiment was soon supposed to deploy to its summer camp near another Finnish resort town called Lakhdenpokhya. Therefore I was temporarily housed in the clinic, which was a three-room wooden building. One room was the doctors' office; the second room was the examination and operating room; and the third room was a recovery ward with about twenty cots for patients with minor problems. In case of serious problems, the soldiers were sent to the district military hospital.

I ate together with the soldiers in the conscript refectory. The refectory was also a wooden building with long tables in two rows. Each table seated a platoon of forty people. The first thing I really noticed in the army was the poor food that the soldiers ate. The officers had a separate cafeteria and could buy decent meals, for example, butter, cookies, canned foods, sugar, eggs, and apples. The conscripts never saw anything like this, and were therefore chronically hungry. Their diet consisted mostly of various types of porridge made of barley, oats, or wheat. They were also served soup, a lot of black bread, old potatoes from the previous year's harvest, and a little bit of salted cabbage and salted fish. They got almost no meat. To drink they received hot tea with a half a tablespoon of sugar from a large pot. The soldiers who had money tried to buy some extra food, but the officers' cafeteria did not allow it. It is ironic, but elements of the discrimination that date back to czarist times are still present in the Red Army. The soldiers were also forbidden to leave the base. The only way they could buy any extra food, therefore, was to buy it from women who came to visit them at the entrance point on weekends or to buy it if they were ever sent into town on business. They even bought vodka in town, although this was strictly forbidden. The base patrol arrested any soldiers it found in the wine store, but the soldiers still managed to get drunk in town.

Each soldier earned only three rubles a month. They received a lot of packages from their relatives and friends, though. These packages were distributed only on Saturdays, and then the soldiers stuffed themselves with lard, honey, jelly, fruits, sugar, and candy. They could not bring food into the cafeterias, so they usually stuffed it all into their beds. The bunks turned into real banquet tables. The soldiers climbed onto their beds, spread out newspapers as tablecloths, and offered each other some of their food. These feasts reminded one of how prisoners in the labor camps ate the food they received in their packages. In many ways, army life was similar to prisoners' life.

I liked the beauties of nature where our regiment was located. I often took the clinic van and drove on an abandoned road into the depths of the forest. A lot of abandoned farmhouses that used to belong to rich peasants were located there. The owners had left the huts and fled the Russians. The houses were falling apart, the gardens were overgrown, and the fields had grown wild. The only things left around the houses were a lot of flowers, especially the pale pink Finnish roses. I used to pick bouquets of them.

There was one beautiful Finnish girl. Her name was Ayna. She was a typical Finn—large, erect, nicely built, strong. She had skin that was milky and rosy. Her nose was turned up. She had tender gray eyes, the same color as the Finnish lakes and cliffs.

I first saw her on the street, when I was riding my bicycle in my lieutenant's uniform. I was stunned by her slender figure and attractiveness. I turned my bicycle back and followed her. I had to start a conversation. She stopped by a public phone booth and began looking for a coin in her purse. Immediately I offered her one. She smiled. I stood aside and waited for her to finish her call, then I followed her. It did not escape me that she threw a glance at my epaulettes, and saw on them the medical symbol—the snake and chalice. Obviously, this appeared to her to be a sufficient recommendation. Then I began to speak. I told her I was a doctor, that I hadn't been here for very long, that I liked it here. By her accent I guessed that she was Finnish. I started telling her how much I admired the countryside. She listened graciously, majestically carrying her beautiful head. I finished by asking for a date. She played a little with her eyes indecisively, then finally agreed to meet me the following evening.

I cleaned my boots and brought her roses, which I cut especially for her, picking each one carefully. All night we walked about the edge of town, because I did not want my officer friends to see us and later ask me about her lovemaking. But I myself was curious. The first evening ended with a kiss. Her lips smelled sweetly of fresh milk. The following evening she let me enter her house when it grew dark. The decor was unusual, in every way different from the Russian: it was clean, tasteful, with a modern furniture style. On her finger she wore a wedding band, which she had not had on the day before. I was tempted to ask her if she was married, but didn't. My actions became more decisive. Ayna resisted sweetly, then at last she gave in to me.

As it turned out she was not married and only wore the ring to add boldness to my actions. This she confessed to me later, and we both laughed over it. She also confessed that she was having an affair with my main boss, commander of the northern army region, Colonel General Kalpakchiy, sixty years of age. He gave her expensive gifts and supported her financially. I was of course unable to do this. But my love was pleasant to her. To save us both, Ayna begged me to be careful, not to tell anyone about her and not to get caught by the general. I was not afraid of him, since I didn't consider myself part of the military. But for Ayna's sake I exercised great discretion in all I did. And we were happy.

The summer months passed, and I was scheduled to be demobilized, but whenever I talked to Dr. Bregvadze about this, he said that I would be released only after a replacement had been found. I waited until the beginning of the frosts, but there was still no replacement. I appealed to the commander of the regiment, Colonel Gavrilov, but he just sent me back to Major Bregvadze. I understood that Bregvadze just wanted to use me, although he had no legal right to hold me in the army. I couldn't leave without his permission, though, because that would be considered desertion, for which I could be tried and sentenced.

I became very angry and nervous. Dependence, dependence. . . . Everybody suffers from dependence. How could I escape it?

The first snow fell. We started to wear our overcoats. In that year, elections for local positions and for the Supreme Soviet were conducted. Before such elections, the population is always subjected to a long propaganda campaign. Since there's only one candidate, however, the whole campaign consists of a familiarization with his biography. And, of course, there is a lot of propaganda about the political and economic accomplishments of the Soviet Union under the leadership of the Communist Party. In the army, all this propaganda is conducted very strictly.

On the day before the elections, which always took place on Sunday, the whole base was carefully cleaned up and large posters were hung up that said, "Everybody participate in the elections for the Supreme Soviet!", "We will give our votes to the bloc of communists and Non-Party candidates!", "Forward to the Victory of Communism!", and so on. There was a snowstorm that night, however, and the whole road from the base to town was blocked with snow drifts. All the officers were supposed to arrive at the regiment at 5:30

A.M., before the voting began. The duty officers and the company commanders stayed in the barracks all night. The voting began exactly at 6:00 A.M. and was supposed to continue until midnight. The election committee opened the voting booths at 6:00 A.M. Exactly at that time, the soldiers were supposed to march in company formation to the voting booths and vote in alphabetical order. For this purpose, a row of tables had been set up in the clubhouse. The tables were covered with a red cotton cloth, and behind them sat the members of the voting committee, who had large books in front of them in which were written the names of all the soldiers, officers, and civilians older than eighteen who were supposed to vote in that location. Behind each committee member was a sign hung on the wall with the letters of the last names that he managed. Each member had five to six letters.

Along the tables on the floor was laid a special carpet that had been brought for this purpose from the Regional Party Committee. On the walls were hung portraits of the Soviet leaders: Khrushchev, Malenkov, Molotiv, Kaganovich, Voroshilov, Shepilov, Bulganin, Furtseva, and Zhukov. Bouquets of flowers, also brought from the Regional Party Committee, decorated the wooden sills on the other side of the room. At the far end of the club stood two large wooden urns under a large portrait of Lenin. At both sides of the urns stood two committee members, who monitored the actual balloting. To the side of these urns stood two small booths shaded with green curtains. Any voter who wanted to read his ballot and cross out the candidate's name or even write in another name could go into these booths. People understood that since only one person had been nominated for the position, it was practically impossible for anybody else to be elected. So there was no real choice except to agree. In addition, everybody was afraid of going into these booths, because it would appear that they were against the Party's candidate. Most of the soldiers were nineteen or twenty years old and were voting for the first time. Even so, they already knew that they shouldn't go into the booths.

At 5:30 A.M. I was walking along the snowy road from town to the base. I passed the Finnish cemetery and saw the marble gravestones covered halfway up with snow. I could still feel the warmth of Ayna's body, although a deadly cold was coming to me from those gravestones. Several other sleepy officers were walking with me to vote. Generally, they would have preferred to sleep a little more and then vote a little later, but the regiment was trying to finish its voting in order to be able to report to the Regional Party Committee and to the division that it voted 100 percent by eight or nine o'clock in the morning. The regiment's political deputy and commander considered that this would look good to their superiors. This is typical behavior in Soviet elections. The political leaders try to complete 100 percent of the voting as early as possible, even though officially the votes wouldn't be counted until midnight.

The voting in the regiment went smoothly. At six o'clock the first soldiers entered the voting area. Loudspeakers were turned on and began to broadcast from Moscow the national anthem, marches, popular songs, and selections from various operas and symphonies. Accompanied by the music, our soldiers and officers approached the tables.

The voters left the table with the ballots in their hands and walked along the carpet to the urn. They folded their ballots in half and then cast them into the slit of the urn. Nobody went into the voting booths. The whole procedure took each voter about two minutes. After the voter had fulfilled his duty, he exited the club, still to the accompaniment of the march music.

I returned to my Ayna. I wanted, however, to leave her and especially the regiment as soon as I could. As I walked by the cemetery, I thought about this. The sun was already shining on the snow-covered gravestones.

When I was back in Ayna's bed, Major Dr. Bregvadze came knocking on her door. The major asked me to come to the regiment headquarters immediately.

This was the first time that the commander of the regiment had ever called me in. On the road there, the major told me that an "unusual occurrence" (Ch. P. in Russian) had happened. (All soldiers knew that the term Ch. P. meant that somebody had died.) It turned out that two soldiers had been found frozen to death in the Finnish cemetery, and an autopsy had been performed by a civilian doctor named Eduard who was a friend of mine. The cause of death was basically clear; the soldiers had been drunk before they died. They probably passed out and froze to death. It was most important to determine the time that the soldiers froze, because the *zampolit* (political deputy) and the commander had already reported that 100 percent of the regiment had voted. The soldiers had been sent to town the day before and were supposed to have returned the same evening. By 10:00 A.M., though, they still hadn't shown up. The regiment commander wanted to report the completed voting so badly that the political deputy personally marked their names in the books and cast their ballots for them. When the report had been sent, the two soldiers were discovered at the foot of one of the gravestones.

The major did not go in with me to see the commander. I went in and reported: "Comrade Colonel, Lieutenant of Medical Services Golyakhovsky reports as ordered."

The colonel answered unusually politely. "Sit down, Doctor," he said as he moved a chair to me. He and the political deputy were in the room. They were obviously upset.

"Doctor, I know that you have a request to make of us. You want to leave . . ." the commander began. "The *zampolit* and I are very grateful to you for the help that you have given us here. I think that you will be able to leave soon, even though we haven't received another doctor yet. The only thing is . . ." he lowered his voice, ". . . we now have a request to make of you."

"An unusual occurrence has taken place in our regiment," the *zampolit* told me. "It has to be properly investigated, and conclusions have to be drawn. Two soldiers have frozen to death today. And this has happened on the day of the election of the Supreme Soviet!"

"I had nothing to do with that," I said.

"That's correct, you had nothing to do with that, but the commander and I are asking you to help us in this matter."

"But how can I help?" I asked in surprise.

"The autopsy has to show that the soldiers died later," the commander explained. "Major Bregvadze said that you are on friendly terms with the doctor who performed the autopsy. Therefore we are asking you to go to him right now—I will lend you my car—and then bring us a document that says that the soldiers froze to death today. Do you understand? If you do, we will discharge you immediately. I give you my word. The *zampolit* is our witness."

I understood the deal and wondered whether to agree or refuse. My refusal would not serve any purpose. My agreement would give me the opportunity to avoid a delay of my military discharge. I did not care about the colonels' problems, but I did care about my own fate. On the other hand, I did not want to take part in any improprieties. Nothing tied me to them, and I didn't want to have anything in common with them. It was difficult for me to make a decision right away—should I ask my friend to lie or shouldn't I? In any case, though, I could discuss the matter. I really did need somebody's advice, so I decided to at least talk with Eduard.

When I arrived at the pathology department of the city hospital, I told him everything that I knew about the case and how it affected me. Eduard thought for a while and then agreed to write that the soldiers had died between 4:00 A.M. and 8:00 A.M. It made no difference to him. Even if his conclusion was a bit mistaken, it would certainly never come to light, because by the time the bodies were exhumed it would be virtually impossible to say when they had died.

I brought the colonels a copy of the protocol, which I myself had written out by hand (there were no copying machines or even typewriters at the hospital). They were so happy that they almost kissed me.

It's possible that the whole matter might have taken a different turn for them if the relatives of the dead soldiers had tried to find out all the details of the deaths. But in the Soviet army, if "unusual occurrences" happen, the relatives always get one and the same standard announcement from the military unit: "Your son (or husband) has died the death of the brave during the fulfillment of his duty to the Fatherland."

The bodies of the deceased are never sent home for burial, and the relatives are not even informed where the burial took place. These particular two soldiers were buried in the Finnish cemetery where they died. And I was released from the service.

18

After three years of independent hard work in north Russia, I returned to Moscow to my parents in the winter of 1956. Our whole family—father, mother, ninety-year-old grandmother, I, and a large dog—still lived in the twenty-one-square-meter room.

I began to work in Moscow's largest hospital, Botkin Hospital, which had 2,500 beds. I expected that the conditions in the large hospital would be proportionately better than in the small hospital from which I had come.

This hospital had been built in 1910 with money donated by a wealthy businessman named Soldatenkov. For those times, it was a very good hospital. It was located in a park area away from the city itself. Its twenty wards held about four hundred beds. The rooms were spacious, the ceilings were high. Next to the hospital was a large church.

After fifty years, the city had grown around the hospital. Many of the trees had been cut down, and long, gloomy, wooden barracks were built in their place. The rooms of the hospital were filled up with four or five times more beds than the rooms were built for. Soon the progress of medical technology required more space for X-ray rooms, laboratories, and new operating rooms. So the patients' rooms became even more crowded, with ten or twelve persons in a room. The nearby church was turned into a dissecting room—the bodies were dissected on a marble table where the altar had been. Yet despite all these changes, the quality of the medical staff remained the best in Moscow.

When I began to work, I quickly learned that I had significantly less theoretical knowledge than the Moscow doctors, but much more practical skill.

I was lucky in that I had the opportunity to work with the most outstanding Moscow professors. Many of them were old veterans of the hospital and lectured on their experience to younger doctors who were trying to improve their skills. I met Dr. Miron Vovsi, Dr. Samuil Reynberg, Dr. Boris Votchal, Dr. Boris Rozanov, Dr. Anatoly Frumkin, and Dr. Nikolay Shereshevsky. These men were giants. I tried not to miss a single scientific conference in the department of roentgenology, because I wanted to hear everything that its head, Dr. Reynberg, had to say. His book, *Roentgen Diagnostics of Bone and Joint Illnesses,* was my favorite medical text.

I listened to the lectures of Dr. Miron Vovsi, the legendary doctor who had led the list of those who had been arrested in the doctors' plot in 1952. He returned to his clinic a half-year after Stalin's death, when he had recovered from the tortures, beatings, and degradations he had received in the Lubyanka.

I attended operations conducted by the famous urological surgeon, Dr. Anatoly Frumkin, the director of the best urological clinic in the country. He was a very emotional person. Everything that he touched sparkled in his hands, even urine. He knew how to demonstrate how the kidneys' product, urine, could become a magical substance.

Whenever Dr. Frumkin prepared to receive a foreign delegation of doctors at the hospital, he would throw a tantrum about the hospital's filthy toilets. The workers would lay out the red carpet used for distinguished visitors and begin to shove hospital beds from the walls into the already crowded rooms, when Dr. Frumkin would stomp up and down the corridors and yell: "Why do I need this red rug on the floor? I need clean toilets! Get rid of this stench and filth! This is a urology clinic, but I'm ashamed to let my foreign colleagues see my toilets! Culture starts with clean toilets!"

I enjoyed myself working with these men and tried to absorb everything I could see and hear from them. By far the most important school for me was their catalogue of professional mistakes—something no textbook contains.

Once during a night shift, we were awakened by the arrival of Dr. Alexandra Kutsidi, head of the diagnostic radiology department of our hospital and an experienced specialist and a very kindly woman. She was beside herself with anxiety: accompanying her was her husband, an old man, who had fallen victim to an unusual accident.

"My husband swallowed his large denture," she explained. "Look at this X ray. The denture can be clearly seen lodged in the abdomen!" She held out a fresh radiogram of the abdominal cavity, where a large metal denture was indeed visible. Its shadow was much larger than those of the trouser buttons also visible in the radiogram. There was no question that the denture could not possibly pass through the length of the intestinal tract and be safely evacuated from the body.

There was only one thing to do: operate. Dr. Boris Rozanov, professor of surgery and chief surgeon of our hospital, came without delay, examined the X-ray picture, and heard the story recounted by the patient's frightened wife. He palpated the patient's massive belly, eliciting moans of pain.

The patient was hurriedly prepared for anesthesia, and quickly the operation was underway. In general, an experienced surgeon, such as Dr. Rozanov, has no trouble removing any large foreign object from the abdomen or intestine. But Dr. Rozanov could find nothing either in the abdomen or in the intestines. The operation had been over an hour in progress, the surgeon's fingers were carefully moving about, trying to explore all cavities—and all in vain. Two hours thus passed until Dr. Rozanov tiredly told us, his assistants:

"That's it, guys, I'm sewing him up. There's nothing there."

Dr. Kutsidi was waiting in an adjoining room, confidently expecting the surgeon to complete the operation and show her the extracted denture. But he said: "I'm very sorry, but I couldn't find the denture in your husband's belly."

"What do you mean, you couldn't find it?" she asked in astonishment. "It's clearly seen in the radiogram."

"It sure is, but it's nowhere to be found in the body," the surgeon replied.

Dr. Kutsidi broke into tears: "My husband's going to sustain an intestinal perforation and die," she sobbed.

The patient spent several weeks in treatment. His condition grew worse, for he in fact developed peritonitis. Then he started to recover, and finally the patient was well enough to be discharged. That day X-ray technician Zhenya brought him his trousers and undershirt, which had been kept in her locker while the patient stayed at the hospital. He proceeded to pull the trousers over his considerably shrunken belly, when suddenly he shouted, "Here it is, here it is!"

"What?" his wife asked anxiously.

"My denture! It is in the small watch pocket. I must have shoved it there inadvertently. . . . Boy, what a prize fool I am!"

And he humbly extracted his denture from the small trouser

pocket. Then all the pieces of the puzzle fell into place: the patient had not taken off his trousers for the X ray and the denture in his pocket naturally showed in the film, seemingly inside the body. The patient was holding his head, endlessly repeating: "What an idiot I am! . . ."

Dr. Rozanov was summoned from his office. He came, had a look at the denture, heard the story of the watch pocket, and grasped his head with both hands. "What an idiot *I* am!" the surgeon said. "I made the worst of blunders by deciding on the treatment on the basis of a film instead of clinical indications."

And so they stood side by side, the surgeon and his patient, each excoriating himself: "What an idiot I am!"

19

I was sure Irina would not wait for me. I knew that by leaving Moscow for three years, I would lose her. So when I called, it was without much hope.

"Irina? It's me, Volodya. I've returned." My voice shook a little.

"I recognized your voice. Hello," she said. It seemed something had happened to her voice too.

"You recognized me?" From excitement, I started to say the wrong things.

"Yes." Her voice was definitely excited too.

"Well, how are you?"

"All right. I graduated from the university."

My heart leapt. Since she had started by talking about the university, she probably wasn't married yet.

"What are you spending your time on now?" I asked nervously.

"I'm trying to get a job."

Good, nothing about marriage.

"What else is new?" I asked, still asking questions like a fool.

"Lots of things are new." She seemed to be getting tired of the line of questioning, so I suddenly blurted: "Can I see you?"

"Is that what you want?" Now she was asking the idiotic questions. Oh, great Mr. Alexander Graham Bell, did you invent the telephone just for these simple-minded conversations?

"Of course, I'd like to."

"Then come on over."

"When?"

"Right now is all right."

I didn't just come over. I ran over. I galloped over. I flew over.

I can't remember a lot of what happened in that period of my life. I went to work, I listened to the radio, I talked to my friends, but I don't remember specifics. The only thing I recall is the whirlwind that flew around us both—the daily meetings, the laughter, the conversations, the theater, the concerts. It was our whirlwind only. All around us was emptiness.

For us nothing outside love existed, and we did not even consider having a formal wedding. We wanted above all to be together, only together; we could not even understand why we had to perform the ritual civil ceremony in the official cabinet of the ZAGS (the civil registry office), but marry we did, although we were living apart, she with her mother, I with mine. We told no one of our closeness. Each night after work I came to pick her up in my car and we went someplace outside the city, had picnics, and kissed and kissed. . . . Whenever Irina's mother went out or took trips, we were free to stay together in her two rooms.

My mother-in-law considered me unsuitable for her daughter. I was only setting out to be a doctor with a very distant prospect of material advancement. My mother-in-law had been widowed twice, by two writers, both of whom earned far more than the best doctors. She surrounded herself with people from the art world, the elite of the Soviet society. And all her friends married their daughters off to famous actors, artists, and writers. My mother-in-law was jealous of them, and disliked me. I felt uncomfortable under her disapproving glances. She did not like the flowers I brought Irina, large dahlias and tall gladiolus. The moment I handed them to Irina, she would grab them from her and immediately start breaking up the bunch, trying to place them in far-off corners of the room where they would not be seen. If it happened that we would all be sitting at the table together having traditional Russian tea, my mother-in-law would ask sarcastically, "You must be of noble descent?"

I answered, surprised: "I think so—fifty-fifty."

"Then why don't you take your spoon out of your cup when you drink?"

All in all living together with my mother-in-law was not easy. Irina and I did not speak on this subject; we bypassed it with silence. Indeed, we almost never discussed in depth details and plans for our future life. I feel that this was the best and most natural way of entering into marriage. Real love does not leave room for computations and calculations, it fills your entire being. To marry without calculation is the best calculation there is.

Irina was Jewish, on both her maternal and paternal sides. But she was entirely divorced from the mainstream of Jewish life because her parents, like my parents, were products of the post-Revolutionary break with tradition. Her father's name was Bermont and her mother's Eppelbaum. Irina's father, Yevgeny Bermont, who died of leukemia in 1948 at the age of forty-two, was a satirist, highly popular in the thirties and forties. I felt sorry for Irina because she had lost her father when she was sixteen. I was amazed to learn she was Jewish. She confided to me that she had been unaware of it before she was nine, till the day of the outbreak of the Russo-German war, on June 22, 1941, when malicious children her own age had told her: "This is it for all you Jews. The end is near, the Germans will kill you all."

Frightened, she ran home in tears and began asking her parents what Jews were and why the Germans were going to kill them. Only then did her parents tell her of her origins.

Irina's background was of no concern to me. I loved her and not her origins. But I was pleased to learn that even in childhood we had something in common: religious persecution.

On January 5, 1958, Irina gave me a son, Vladimir Golyakhovsky, Jr. I was sitting in the waiting room of the maternity ward when, at about one o'clock in the morning, I heard a little squeal among the other noises. The doctor on duty came up to me and asked: "Well, did you hear it?"

"What?"

"Your son's cry."

"Son? How is he?" I asked in confusion.

"Without any defect," the doctor answered professionally. And I decided for myself that this was the first characteristic of my son—"without any defect."

I walked the streets of Moscow, happy and excited, toward where my mother-in-law lived. I ran up the stairs to the fifth floor and rang the doorbell. My mother-in-law opened the door with an expectant look. She had wanted a granddaughter. I said to her, breathless from the run: "Congratulations on your new grandson!"

My mother-in-law replied dryly: "I never did expect any good from you."

Well, what was I to answer? I smiled and went to my parents, fifteen more blocks through empty streets of Moscow. They weren't sleeping, of course. Mama asked: "What is it?"

"A son, Vladimir Junior."

We kissed and drank a bottle of champagne.

Irina and I still had no apartment of our own; each lived at our parents'. Now, with the baby's arrival, we had to live together, no matter what. Otherwise, how would we bring up the baby? My mother-in-law stubbornly did not want to give up one of the two tiny bedrooms. Fortunately, my aunt offered to temporarily put us up in her communal apartment with seven other families and one kitchen for all. My parents, my grandmother, and my family, six people in one bedroom and a living room, moved there. Even so, the conditions were wonderful for us, because Irina, my son, and I could be together.

On a frosty January day, I came by limousine to pick my family up from the decrepit old two-story maternity home named for Krupskaya (Lenin's wife). My mother-in-law and her maid Nyusha were with me. These two women were bombarding me with advice on how I should hold my son, how I should give a tip to the nurse who would bring my son out, etcetera. I was nervous, awaiting my first encounter with my son, and said nothing. Before this very day I had not been permitted to visit my wife in the maternity home— this was forbidden for the fathers.

Irina jumped out the door, content, like a bird. Behind her a fat nurse was carrying a parcel: my son. I awkwardly handed her 10 rubles and more awkwardly took in my arms my son wrapped in a quilted blanket. My mother-in-law lifted a corner of the blanket covering his face and moaned with joy at seeing her grandson. Nyusha said, "Handsome!" I didn't find him to be so, in fact I thought he looked rather unappealing: red face, a small turned-up nose, and large lips. In the cab my mother-in-law asked: "How much did you give the nurse?"

"A ten."

She pursed her lips angrily and told me I had overtipped. But I didn't care because nothing was too good for my son.

A week after he was born, I proudly went to have him registered at the local Civil Status Records office. My main idea was to register him Russian because Irina and I did not want him to have the trouble we had as Jews. The office was empty; the young clerk, a girl of about eighteen, was clearly bored and inexperienced—indeed, it turned out this was her first day on the job. I handed her the maternity home certificate; she spent a lot of time searching for the requisite books and forms. I waited patiently, looking forward to the great moment when I would be issued the first document of my son. Finally, the girl was through. She sighed and told me: "It is better to register death than birth, because it is less complicated."

I was astonished at the idiotic simplicity of her pronouncement, though I said nothing. Any red tape is unpleasant. Anyway, my son is Russian, I thought.

From the onset our son possessed three qualities that have remained with him until today: good health, excessive appetite, and cranky character. He literally sucked Irina dry, and at any displeasure he would cause a ruckus, not giving us a moment's peace. My grandmother, his great-grandmother, who herself raised ten children, said: "A dignified child; he doesn't stand for anything."

I tried all I could to maintain Irina's strength, feeding her walnuts, black caviar, oranges, and pineapples, which were rather expensive and quite hard to come by. Irina took a leave from work to be with her son; thus we lost more than half our income. My mother fed us all, and tried to help Irina in every way. My mother-in-law came every day and in a businesslike manner commanded us all about. She had one obsession: cleanliness, and because of this she washed everything and poured boiling water over anything that was handed to the child, and made Irina and me do the same. There was nothing like "Pampers" in Russia, and still isn't; therefore, we had seemingly hundreds of diapers, which had to be washed and sterilized daily. My mother-in-law insisted that the diapers be ironed on both sides. Irina folded, I folded.

Once every two weeks a private pediatrician, Dr. Tselestin, came by my mother-in-law's invitation. Although there was no real need for him, she had no trust for the young woman pediatrician from the clinic. Dr. Tselestin was paid 10 rubles per visit.

Soon we began buying our son food supplements from our area's children's milk kitchen. I ran there every morning before work to buy bottles and jars. This was also not inexpensive. But once Irina discovered a large piece of glass in one of the jars, and after that we started buying everything from the private vendors in the market. It was double the price, but less risky.

Summer was approaching and we rented a dacha outside of Moscow so that the child could have fresh air. The dacha was a big problem. First, it cost 500 to 600 rubles a season and that exceeded my income by double. Secondly, goods would have to be brought almost daily to the dacha, because the stores in the outskirts of Moscow did not have a wide enough selection; you could still find bread and milk, but meat, vegetables, and other produce were not sold there. Thirdly, the move in itself was a nightmare, because we'd have to take the refrigerator, part of the furniture, and clothes for different weather.

This is when I felt the day-to-day drudgery of family life! But still we had it much better than most other young families, because my parents generously gave us money for everything.

Leo Tolstoy began *Anna Karenina* with the phrase, "All happy families are alike, and each unhappy family is unhappy in its own way." Somehow it is so, but one can also add: "To the extent that the so-called happy families are happy, they are to the same degree unhappy."

We rented two bedrooms in an old wooden house in a coniferous forest forty-two kilometers east of Moscow. My mother-in-law moved in with us, and helped Irina. I would bring goods from the city in a woven string bag, and Irina with our son in tow would meet me at the suburban train station.

On a rare Sunday, when I was not working, Irina and I would take our bicycles and ride to the neighboring town of Zhukovsky, where they had a large grocery store, to buy goods. The trip took two hours and it was pleasant, because we were alone together, sans mother-in-law. We then dreamed of having a daughter. It was difficult for us but we were young and full of energy. I said to Irina:

"You know, bringing up a son is a joy, but bringing up a daughter is an entirely different . . ."

Irina smiled quietly, possibly imagining herself the mother of many.

The fact that my parents helped me financially freed me from the necessity of slaving for a supplementary income, and gave me the possibility of doing scientific work and writing poetry. Without their support I would not have become what I am today; I would have been reduced to a clock-punching doctor, roaming hospitals in search of night shifts and consultations at the clinic. I would have been obliged to waste my brain and spend all my strength for a supplementary 100 rubles a month. I knew hundreds of such doctors, and thanked God that I was not one of them.

From my parents I acquired a simple truth, that there exists a reciprocity among generations within the family. Parents must help their children to stand on their own two feet, and not falter under the weight of life. My parents helped me to maintain my balance, and I will help my son to do the same. I hope that in the future my son will help either his son or daughter do the same.

But still, I felt uncomfortable accepting so much help from my parents. Where was my masculine responsibility? Why did I start a family if I was in no condition to support it? Our dreams of a daughter were not realized. It was too difficult bringing up one child, despite the material and physical help. Irina was pregnant several times, and each time it seemed inopportune. She had abortions, so as not to have more than one child due to the difficulties of daily life.

The years 1958–1959 were very good to me: my son was born, my first scientific articles on orthopedic surgery were published, my first book of children's poetry was published under the editorship of the master children's author Korney Chukovsky, I finished my residency as an orthopedic surgeon, enrolled in postgraduate studies, and began working on my Ph.D.

Seeing for the first time the fruits of thoughts and labors in print is a great moment for a creative person. The creative process is a long period of endless preparation, from the moment of a thought's conception to finally seeing it published as an article or poem. This process is not without its difficulties, disappointments, and joys. Interesting and original ideas may enter one's mind unexpectedly, but only a truly creative person knows how to convert such thoughts into a ready form.

My two first scientific articles were not very long; they were descriptions of clinical observations with discussions of what I had seen. But they were like two wings, which I felt behind me. I now have wings, and I can fly!

My book of poetry was also short, but it signified my officially becoming a poet. It required almost two years for the book to pass through the censors. Almost two centuries ago, Alexander Pushkin wrote that to pass through the tight Russian censorship was just as difficult as getting into the heavenly kingdom. Since his time it has become increasingly difficult, because after the Revolution all the publishing houses became government owned.

With the publishing of the book, I could count on my being accepted as a member of the Writers' Union. The privileged position of a writer held more promise for me than my position as a surgeon. But I wanted to become a writer and remain a doctor, like Anton Chekov, who liked to say that medicine was like his legal wife, and literature like his mistress. I can say the same: I love them both.

20

In the years 1957–1958, I often visited the small village of Peredelkino, about fifteen miles from Moscow along Minskoye Highway. More than one hundred of the most famous Soviet writers lived in government dachas there. One of them was Korney Chukovsky, my teacher, the editor of my first published poems and my first book "for the little ones." I brought him my new poems, which I continued to write after my surgical work, and we set off to stroll around the writers' village. As we were walking, Chukovsky would read my poems aloud and criticize or praise them, telling me what should be corrected and how. He also acquainted me with writers whom we met on our walks or who came to his two-story wooden house as to a literary salon. There I met the author of the novel *Doctor Zhivago*, the poet Boris Pasternak.

Chukovsky introduced me to him: "This young man," he said in a loud falsetto, "is already a very experienced surgeon and still a beginning poet."

Pasternak looked me over. "What hospital do you work in?" he asked.

"Botkin Hospital."

"Zhivago also worked at that hospital," he said, "and he was also a poet."

I was surprised that he spoke about the hero of his novel as about a real person.

"Could you treat me?" he asked. "My back hurts, my muscles ache, and also my arms, right here."

I had to examine him right there in the living room. He took off his shirt, stood bare-chested, and performed some movements for me—squatting, leaning over, shaking my hand—so that I could determine what his problem was. While I was examining him, I reminded him that we were already acquainted, but from long ago, when I was still a teenager. I had gone to school with his stepson, Stanislav Neygauz, who later became a famous pianist. At the mention of those past years, Pasternak smiled at me.

Boris Pasternak had come to our home once in 1942. It was in a small Russian town called Chistopol on the Kama River, in the depths of Russia, not far from the Ural Mountains. The war with Hitler's Germany was being fought, and the population of the major cities in the European part of the country had been evacuated to the east, away from the occupation and bombing. The Union of Soviet Writers as an organization had left Moscow for this town. The writers with their families fell into difficult and unaccustomed conditions there. After the metropolitan life in large apartments with nice furniture, they had to rent tiny rooms in wooden huts and limit themselves to poor iron beds, wooden cots, and old, crushed mattresses. Instead of armchairs made out of the beautiful wood of Karelian birch trees, they had one or two unpainted stools for the whole family. These common conditions of life for the Russian people were a burden for them.

Pasternak, his second wife Zina, and two sons aged fourteen and three squeezed into two semi-dark little rooms. The famous poet was very unhappy and bore the poor life of the simple people in torment. This life pressed on him physically and morally, and he suffered.

He visited us, because our house had practically the only piano in the town, and he wanted "to touch the keys." He was a wonderful pianist. My mother and I lived with the family of our old friend Samyil Samoylov, a popular, local, well-to-do Jewish doctor who had a two-story stone house decorated in the old merchant style. In the evenings, many writers and artists gathered in Doctor Samoylov's house, and they were treated there with a good dinner, which was also a rarity in those hungry years. Pasternak was fifty-two years old at that time, and had been famous for thirty years as one of the best poets of Russia.

That evening, Pasternak played Beethoven, Chopin, and Tchaikovsky for us, accompanying the famous bass of the Bolshoi Theater, Maksim Maikhaylov. Then Pasternak read several of his poems, and all of us listeners fell silent from their content and from the sound of the poet's voice. I was sitting in a far corner, awed by the unusualness of Pasternak. Of course, I didn't understand his poetry and could not appreciate its musical cadences, but I felt that this was a giant. And my mother and everybody else in the room treated him like a god.

Pasternak became interested in the life of Dr. Samoylov and visited us frequently. He looked into everything and asked a lot of strange questions. Writers' brains are always transforming overlooked facts of everyday life into future artistic images. This was probably what Pasternak was doing at that time. Many years later, when I read *Doctor Zhivago*, I recognized aspects from the life of Chistopol in many scenes and descriptions. Indeed, the description of the escape of Doctor Zhivago into the depths of Russia and his work as a doctor among the people of the nation had a lot in common with the fate of Dr. Samoylov.

In July 1943, we along with the Pasternak family returned to Moscow. The government made the steamship *Mikhail Sholokhov* available especially for the writers, and we sailed for a half-month during those hot summer days along the large Russian rivers, Kama, Volga, and Oka. It was pleasant to sail along slowly, although the danger of bombardment by German planes still remained.

The ship captain kept a memory book about the passengers. All the writers left their autographs in it, and some of them also wrote a short story or some poetry. The gloomy Pasternak wrote less than the others, only one line: "The weather is very nice. I dream of swimming—and of freedom of the press."

That line reflected his opposition to official policies. In the course of all the years of Soviet power, when many surrendered morally and many were physically destroyed, Pasternak never flirted with the government. He was the only Soviet poet who did not praise the Communists or Stalin. They did not break or destroy him in return, and in fact *they* had to flirt with *him*. Stalin himself called him on the telephone at home and talked with him, asking his opinion of this or that writer. He even promised him that he would save the life of another Russian poet, Mandelshtam, who had been arrested by the police. Stalin asked Pasternak to not "worry" about it, but did not keep his word. Mandelshtam died in a prison camp.

When the government stopped publishing Pasternak's books, he made a living by translating. He knew several languages—English, German, French, and Georgian. He translated Shakespeare, Goethe, Petefy, and the Georgian poets into Russian. And during this time he wrote *Doctor Zhivago,* in which he depicted the revolutionary epoch of Russia.

Pasternak made no secret of the fact that he was writing a novel about the Revolution in Russia, just as he never made any secrets of his creative work. Only a few of his writer friends and a small circle of the intelligentsia knew about it, however, due to the lack of printed information.

Pasternak tried without success to publish his novel in his homeland, but the ideological department of the Central Committee of the Party, headed at that time by Ilyichev, forbade its publication.

Pasternak was tormented with dreams of success as a writer, for he knew he was greater than any of the other Soviet writers. Despairing of his attempts to publish the novel in the Soviet Union, he sent the manuscript to the West. Pasternak also made no secret of this; I heard about it from the poet Ilya Selvinsky and others beginning in the 1950s. They waited with interest to see what kind of effect it would produce in the West and what kind of reaction it would call forth from the Soviet government. They did not condemn him, although the action had been unusual and officially condemned. The same writers who in friendly conversations expressed approval were required to slander Pasternak at meetings in the Union of Writers.

The novel was not published in the Soviet Union and still, twenty years after the death of the author, remains a forbidden book. Very few copies of the book came into Russia from Europe, and it was only possible to obtain it secretly, from close and trusted acquaintances. I know of cases in which people were arrested for reading *Doctor Zhivago* and sent to prison camps for five years. I myself received a copy in Russian, published in Italy in paperback, from my friend the poet Kostya Bogatyrev. He gave me the book to read for only two nights. The book was all wrinkled and soiled from many readings, but I was happy to receive it. Irina and I sat on the bed and read it together—one would read the left page, and the other would read the right page. We came to work without sleep in the morning, but inspired by the book. I believe that scarcely one-half of a percent of the readers of the Soviet Union have had the good fortune to read it. At the same time, I knew from one of the employees of the Party's Central Committee that several good copies of the book had been published "for official use only" on a special printing press in Russia. We wondered who read them.

Pasternak was never a dissident in the sense of the 1960s' development among the Soviet intelligentsia of a social movement against the Soviet regime. He never challenged anybody to anything, never agitated for anything, never criticized or condemned anything. He did not even speak at any official writers' conferences on the professional writer's topic of socialist realism. But he was the *only* one who did not submit to Communist propaganda, the *only* one who expressed his own credo in his works. This uniqueness made him the godfather of the free-thinking Soviet intelligentsia. Before Soviet people heard the names Aleksandr Solzhenitsyn, Andrey Sakharov, General Petr Grigorenko, and others, Boris Pasternak inspired with his firmness those willing to oppose the government. For progressive intellectuals in the Soviet Union in the 1950s, Pasternak was the Number One Person. People copied his poems and books by hand

and gave them to each other to read. It was impossible to obtain them in the libraries—one had to wait six months or longer on the waiting list.

In Russia, where there were never democratic freedoms and people could never express themselves, the carriers of these ideas and dreams were always the poets and writers. Therefore, they have a much larger significance there than in Western countries. In Russia they became the godfathers of the intelligentsia. And Pasternak during his life was such a godfather.

It was during this period that I met Pasternak at Chukovsky's home. During the fifteen years I had not seen him, he had improved physically, looked younger, and became almost handsome. His congenital myopathy almost disappeared with age, which is often the case with genetic defects. He led a simple and healthy life. In the mornings, he gathered firewood in the forest for his stove. On cold mornings he swam in the brisk, chilly water of a small stream, the Setun. During the summer, he planted vegetables in his garden, which he kept at his dacha, a wooden home next to the forest. He grew potatoes, carrots, beets, radishes. He watered and weeded them himself, and then fed himself with these vegetables. He could still run from the dacha to the railroad station easily in order to catch the train for Moscow (he didn't have a car).

However, on the basis of his congenitally ill muscles, he did develop myopathy of the back and shoulders. Therefore, I advised him to undergo some physiotherapeutic procedures.

"Where can I undergo these procedures?" he asked.

"Next to your dacha is the Writers' House of Creativity, where doctors and necessary equipment are available."

"No," he waved his hand. "The bosses won't allow me to be treated there."

"What kind of bosses do you have?" I asked in surprise.

"Those who sit behind desks—big desks, like the ones at the Union of Writers."

"But the House of Creativity is for writers."

"Only for Soviet writers. And Pasternak is not considered to be Soviet anymore. Since *Zhivago* was published abroad, I am not considered to be one of theirs. I am such a foreigner to them that they don't even want to see me in Moscow. Recently a group of writers from Europe came to Moscow, and they wanted to see me. So the head of the Union of Writers, Surkov, the First Secretary, wrote immediate instructions for me to take a trip to Tbilici and literally pushed me off, although I had no business at all to conduct there. I hung around for a whole month on the streets of that city, and I was furious the whole time. The Georgian writers kept asking me what I was doing there. I wasn't doing anything there. I was in exile, in disgrace."

In the fall of 1958, he won the Nobel Prize for Literature. He became the second Russian writer to receive this major prize—thirty years after Ivan Bunin won it. But Bunin wasn't a Soviet citizen. He had emigrated to Paris at the beginning of the Revolution.

Immediately after the announcement of the award on the Western radio station, dozens of foreign correspondents drove up to Pasternak's dacha. It turned into an unprecedented assembly of foreigners. However, other cars carrying KGB agents had arrived earlier, and these agents observed everybody who came. Many writers arrived to congratulate Pasternak. They thought that since he had won such an important prize he would be forgiven by the government. My teacher Korney Chukovsky came, and he gave an interview to one of the Western correspondents in which he praised the novel. The next day, though, all of the newspapers throughout the Soviet Union began a strong campaign slandering Pasternak. The Soviet people could not actually understand any of it, because none of them had read the book. Nevertheless, they were forced to criticize the book and its author at official Party meetings called together at factories, universities, and ministries. There had never been such a massive and brutal campaign against one person in the Soviet Union before. Khrushchev and all the members of the Politburo cursed him in their speeches. It seemed that the whole huge propaganda machine of the Party had crashed down on Pasternak's head. The massiveness of the persecution turned out to be counterproductive. People who had never been interested in literature began to ask their intellectual friends who Pasternak was, what kind of book it was, and if he was really so dangerous for the Soviet people. Once I took a taxi and asked the driver to drive me to the Literary House on Herzen Street, where a literary meeting was being held. When the young driver heard the address, he asked me, "What are you—a writer? Have you read Doctor Zhivago? Why are they criticizing Pasternak for it so much?"

In careful terms I answered that it was not so bad as they described it at all of those meetings. The driver was very pleased. "That's what I thought," he said. "I haven't read it, of course, but I think that if they criticize it so much, then it must at least be very interesting."

Pasternak was ordered expelled from the Union of Writers, and everybody who had congratulated him for winning the prize was called in to the Party Committee of the Union of Writers and sternly warned that they might also be expelled. This happened to my teacher Chukovsky. After that, the writers were afraid to visit Pasternak at his dacha, and he became totally isolated. But the rulers wanted not only to isolate him, but also to break his will. They forced him to turn down the prize and to write a repentant letter disavowing his book. They openly told him that if he didn't, he would be exiled from the Soviet Union, though they would not let his mistress, Olga Ivenskaya, leave with him. Previously, though, they had never exiled anyone, preferring to suffocate them in the Gulag camps. But they were afraid to do this to Pasternak. For the first time, their hands hesitated.

Pasternak hesitated for the first time too. He was old and tired, and could not handle his social or personal problems, which were drowning him. He was afraid of exile and preferred to stay in Russia, so he wrote the repentant letter addressed to the readers of the East and the West in 1958. In contrast to what he had shown in the novel, in this letter he wrote that the Revolution had "filled the present century with sense and content" and that "any military challenge will turn us all into heroes." He admitted his "mistakes and errors," and his "personal guilt," which had been inserted into the novel. He wrote about his "pride in the time in which I live" and about "the bright belief in the common future."

He had never known how to pronounce such words, had never occupied himself with politics, had never predicted military victory. It was clear that the words were forced, and many people understood that he had signed somebody else's words. In the Soviet Union, where the KGB destroyed 20 million citizens, everybody confessed their mistakes, and therefore nobody was surprised or criticized Pasternak. When they broke him, they arrested the woman he loved, Olga Ivenskaya, and sent her into internal exile. Pasternak unhappily lived out his days in Peredelkino. Sometimes he visited

Chukovsky, who did not break off his friendship with the fallen poet. In April 1960, I saw him there for the last time. He complained about his cough, which included blood, about pains in his chest, and about loss of weight. He looked older and apathetic. I examined him in the same living room. His condition was much worse. He already had a pleuritis, a very bad sign. I suggested he go to a hospital for an examination.

"I want to die," he answered calmly.

He had a cancer of the lung, and because nobody treated him anywhere, he died on May 30, 1960.

Across from his dacha was a large field, called "Unclear Field," as opposed to "Clear Field," where Leo Tolstoy had lived. Behind the field, on a hillock, was an old Russian cemetery, which Pasternak saw from his house every day. That is where he was carried in his coffin. There had probably never been such a mass private funeral in all the history of Soviet Russia. A hundred thousand people stood in the muddy field with bared heads. Nobody had announced the date of the funeral; they had simply all gathered.

His grave became a place of memorial for the nation, as for a saint. Every day, people came to his grave.

One of my acquaintances, a brilliant woman over fifty years old, came to his grave from Petrozavodsk, almost a thousand miles away. She was very poor and ill. I met her and took her to the cemetery in my car. When we returned, I asked her if she had really come all this way just to bow down at his grave.

She answered: "He was a poet for us all."

21

In the summer of 1959, my boss Professor Dmitriy Yazykov was ordered to come immediately to the Kremlin Hospital on Granovskaya Street to treat Marshal Semen Mikhaylovich Budennyy, who had broken his right shoulder in an automobile accident. Marshal Budennyy was now eighty years old, but as a younger man, he had become a legendary war hero in the Soviet Union. During the October Revolution of 1917, he formed the First Red Cavalry, which defeated all of the anti-bolshevik forces in southern Russia. Lenin appreciated Budennyy's accomplishments highly, and over the years many legends, books, songs, paintings, and movies were created to glorify the marshal. He was eventually awarded more than forty combat medals.

Dr. Yazykov fixed Marshal Budennyy's shoulder with a very thin steel surgical pin, the only available procedure at that time, even in Kremlin Hospital, but since the pin was thin and weak, Dr. Yazykov also decided to immobilize the joint with a cast until the X rays would show that the bones had healed. Marshal Budennyy was allowed to return to his special government dacha in Bakovka, about twelve miles outside of Mocow, but Dr. Yazykov visited him almost every week to check his progress, to change the bandages, and to adjust the cast. Dr. Yazykov could not perform these tasks easily, because he was old and had grown obese, weighing more than three hundred pounds. So he decided to bring me along.

On the day of the appointment, Dr. Yazykov and I got into Marshal Budennyy's bulletproofed ZIS-110. The license plate began with the letters MShch, which indicated that it belonged to the military directorate that served the Soviet Union's highest Party and military officials. The heavy car sped along Mozhayskoye Highway without hesitation, because it traveled in a special center lane reserved for the Party bosses' cars and because the police stopped all cross traffic along our route.

After we had traveled twenty-two kilometers along Minskoye Highway, we turned off onto a side road on the left and then drove about three minutes until we reached the heavy gates in front of the marshal's dacha. Our chauffeur, who was an officer, announced us to the officer on guard, and he saluted and motioned to drive on in. He did not check our identification, because he had been expecting us. The dacha was a two-story wooden palace set in several acres of trees and gardens, the whole park surrounded by a fence three meters high and painted government green.

The old but still muscular Marshal sat on the veranda of his dacha. I immediately recognized his famous bushy mustache and narrow, slanted eyes. A cape decorated with his marshal's insignia was thrown over his shoulders and cast.

His house was full of pictures and photographs. In particular, there were a lot of them showing Budennyy mounted on horseback. Some of the pictures dated back to the turn of the century. The newest picture was a large painting-in-progress of him seated on a horse. There were a lot of autographed photographs from past and present Soviet leaders such as Kirov, Kuybyshev, Khrushchev, Frunze, Ordzenikidze, Voroshilov, Kalinin, and Mikoyan. One special picture stood on the edge of the table in the study. It showed Stalin holding his pipe in his fist to the side of his face—a pose very different from the poses in his official pictures. I studied the picture and its autograph and message as if they were a rare museum exhibit. I had seen Stalin's genuine signature only once before—in the home of his secretary's widow, Mrs. Tovstukha. Stalin had died four years before and had already been denounced, but the power of his past influence was still magnetic. The message that Stalin had written on the picture obviously had a hidden meaning, but Dr. Yazykov and I couldn't guess it. Marshal Budennyy told us the story and even acted out the dialogue between him and Stalin.

In 1937 Stalin's terror was at its highest; the Minister of Internal Affairs Nikolay Yezhov arrested anybody whose glance Stalin decided was suspicious. Stalin would say: "Why do you have such a nervous expression?" or "Why don't you look me in the eye?" A little while later, that person would disappear. Usually they would be tortured and then shot. Marshal Blyukher, Marshal Tukhachevsky, and many other generals and government ministers around Stalin perished in this way.

One day in 1937, it happened to Budennyy. "It looks like you don't like me any more, Semen Mikhaylovich," Stalin told him with his threatening, slow Georgian accent.

"What are you talking about?" Budennyy answered. "I would follow you into fire or water. Just give the order."

"Why haven't you ever given me one of your pictures?"

"Oh, but I've wanted to for a long time, Iosif (Joseph) Vissarionovich! I was just thinking about it," said the cavalry hero nervously. He ran into his office and brought out one of his pictures.

"Could you please sign it for me?" asked Stalin. Budennyy sat down, dipped his pen into the inkwell, and then froze in indecision. It was easier for him to cut off a row of heads with a saber than it was to write a few words. He was afraid to write "Dear Stalin," because that might be too familiar, and he was afraid to write "To the most respected Stalin," because that might seem too cold. Budennyy could feel the whiskers of his mustache droop. In the meantime, Stalin paced around behind the chair puffing on his pipe, relishing Budennyy's indecision.

"Well, can't you think of anything to write?"

"It seems I can't, Iosif Vissarionovich."

"Then let me dictate. Write: 'To the great genius . . .' have you written that much? . . . then continue: 'who created the First Cavalry' . . . have you written that? . . . then continue: 'To Iosif Vissarionovich Stalin from Semen Mikhaylovich Budennyy.'" Well, now that you've written that, I see that you do love me. Therefore, I want to give you my picture."

He smiled mockingly, put Budennyy's picture on his desk, and took out his own. He took his pen and wrote on it: "To the *real* creator of the First Cavalry, S. M. Budennyy, from I. V. Stalin. 1937."

This story made an oppressive impression on me. Soviet citizens did not know anything about Stalin's personality. We only knew him as the public figure. It was deathly dangerous to tell or even hear any private anecdotes about him; people were sent to labor camps for as much. Almost anybody who had heard a story about Stalin reported it to the KGB for fear that the person who told it had been a provocateur. Even after Stalin died, we heard almost no stories about him that showed his personality. All we heard about were the results of the terror. I had always been interested in how much Stalin himself believed all the propaganda about his supposed greatness and genius. It seemed from Budennyy's story that all this praise was a game for Stalin and that he could even make a joke about it.

In January 1959, a well-known poster artist, Kokorekin, age sixty, was admitted in critical condition to the infectious disease unit of our hospital, a single-story wooden barracks presided over by Dr. Roodnev, a professor and academician. Although regarded as a leading authority in his field, Professor Roodnev failed to diagnose the patient. At first he was treated for severe influenza. To be sure, the artist had chills, high fever, and great weakness; he also suffered from headaches, muscular pains and backaches, and his skin exhibited numerous hemorrhagic lesions. His blood and urine samples were sent away for regular analysis. As usual, the laboratory took three or four days to come up with its results, but the patient had died before the analysis came back.

Since the case was unusual and the deceased was widely known, Kokorekin's death caused a stir among the hospital's physicians. Dr. Roodnev and his closest associates called a conference and debated the problem at length, but failed to arrive at any conclusion. A young woman junior resident shyly rose and, obviously uncomfortable in the presence of so many luminaries of science, asked doubtfully, "Maybe the patient had a case of smallpox?"

Her suggestion elicited an unceremonious and derisive response: "Are you crazy? You should think before speaking! There hasn't been a single case of smallpox in Russia for a century. And besides, the patient had been vaccinated against smallpox."

But no one attached any significance to the sinister rumors until it transpired that two of the hospital attendants at the carrier disease barracks, who had taken care of the patient, had died. Then many started to suspect an infectious epidemic, but which one, nobody knew.

The young woman was proven right: the patient had a fulminant, or "sledgehammer," form of smallpox contracted in India where he had spent a month, drawing indigenous life scenes in many towns and villages.

According to the rules, any person about to go to India or any other Oriental country known to contain endemic foci of dangerous infections was supposed to be freshly innoculated irrespective of the date of the previous vaccination. Customs officials demanded a vaccination certificate before allowing the person to go abroad. The artist Kokorekin did present such a certificate, but it was a forgery; Kokorekin had bribed a physician 100 rubles to avoid the shot. He was allergic to all kinds of shots, and besides he had recently married a young woman and did not want to feel sick and old with her. In India, he bought numerous presents for his wife, mostly clothes and beautiful fabrics. He returned home on board an Aeroflot TU-104 jet together with a hundred other passengers. No sooner had he embraced his young wife and given her the presents than he collapsed and was brought to the hospital.

When it was finally established beyond doubt that Kokorekin had brought smallpox to Moscow, a quarantine was imposed. That morning I came to the hospital at my usual hour, but left it only a month later, after the quarantine was lifted. The hospital gate was locked; its fence was patrolled by militiamen and special sanitary groups. No one was allowed to enter or leave. Our relatives and friends were allowed to bring food, but it had to be given to us through special intermediaries.

The police raided the apartment of the dead artist's young widow to place her under quarantine and confiscate all Indian presents. But the shrewd woman had foreseen just such a possibility and, unwilling to part with her late husband's presents, distributed them among her numerous friends all over Moscow for temporary safe-keeping. So the police had to hunt for the presents literally piece by piece, confiscating them at the apartments of the widow's friends and placing them under quarantine as well.

All the fellow passengers of Kokorekin and the crew of the airliner also had to be found and quarantined. Some of them by that time had left Moscow, and a nationwide search had to be instituted. The threat of a smallpox epidemic in Moscow or even in the whole country loomed large. Of course, nothing was reported in the media, but there wasn't a person unaware of what was afoot. Wild rumors, one more sinister than another, swept Moscow. A genuine panic set in. A vaccination program was hurriedly put underway in the capital.

The staff of the Botkin Hospital were the first to undergo vaccination, but the quantity of the vaccine was so large that the serum was prepared in great haste and consequently many batches were not clean enough, causing inflammations and serum sickness in many subjects. The first victim among us was my mentor, Dr. Yazy-kov: he developed high fever and pains in the joints, particularly in the wrists and feet. None of us could guess that the serum had not been properly prepared, and we were at a loss to explain the cause of large-scale severe reactions to the vaccine. We thought that the vaccine was ineffective and the smallpox epidemic was spreading.

I learned on the telephone that my one-year-old son had also developed a reaction to the vaccine and I was very worried. But he recovered soon.

We had a hard time bearing the quarantine; there was no place to sleep because all the patients were kept undischarged, filling the rooms and corridors to capacity. Together with a group of male physicians I slept in the X-ray room on the hard X-ray table. Fortunately, I had done without a bed for much of my life, so I didn't mind. Food was bad and we constantly harried our relatives with requests for parcels. We pooled the parcels and arranged communal breakfasts, lunches, and dinners. At night, we would drink wine, hiding from the patients who were prohibited to drink.

Worst hit by the quarantine was a young woman physician, Valya. The twenty-four-year-old girl missed her wedding because of the restrictions. Her fiancé, an engineer, was at home, while she suffered and called him at all times, now laughing, now crying. She was rapidly getting into a hysterical pattern. In order to distract her, we decided to organize a mock wedding. I was chosen to represent the bridegroom. Our ladies, doctors and nurses, set about cooking a sumptuous meal; we put on our Sunday best. Accompanied by the singing and applause of our colleagues, my "bride" and I entered the room and sat at the head of the table.

Russian custom dictates that the bride and groom kiss every time any of the guests shout that the food or drink is "bitter." The kiss will make it "sweet." So when we heard the first shouts of "bitter, bitter," Valya and I had to kiss, though we were both shy and embarrassed. Undeterred, the guests went right on provoking us into kissing with their "complaints of bitterness." Before long, we developed a liking for the admirable custom and started to kiss with relish. While we were thus engaged, the telephone rang. The real bridegroom was calling; he was shivering in the cold beyond the hospital fence, dreaming of his beloved. Valya took the receiver and gushed a stream of plaintive words, saying how she missed him, how acutely she was suffering and longing. Having given him an earful of complaints, she put the receiver down, took her seat next to me, and we resumed our feasting and kissing, amusing the guests and ourselves alike.

My wife Irina and I had no formal wedding; that mock ceremony was all the ceremony I ever experienced. As for Valya, in due course she married her fiancé. She had another, real wedding, but I was not invited for she wanted no reminiscences to spoil the happy occasion.

When the quarantine was lifted, I took my sick boss home. He was in poor condition, with persistent edema and wrist joint pains. His serum reaction gave rise to a complication: psoriatic arthritis, a disease of the skin and nails of the fingers combined with the deterioration of interphalangeal joints. It is a critical affliction for a surgeon because it robs him of the ability to operate. He was hospitalized at the Kremlin Hospital, where I enlisted the services of the leading specialists: Drs. Nesterov, Kartamyshev, and Tareyev. The consultants prescribed large doses of a steroid drug, Dexamethasone. The treatment had a positive effect on Dr. Yazykov's hands, but he developed deep hormonal disturbances. He was not to recover from that smallpox vaccination campaign. I know for a fact that the vaccination program resulted in numerous cases of severe reactions with a lethal outcome, but never has the smallpox epidemic been discussed or reported either in newspapers or in scientific journals, all of which are subject to special scientific censorship.

What did our doctors talk about most of all, aside from professional topics? Money. At the hospitals and outpatient clinics almost a million Soviet physicians talked exclusively of a sweet dream shared by all—an opportunity to earn a little more. No doctor could live on his or her salary alone: the starting pay of a doctor is 59 kopecks (90¢) per hour, and to buy a chicken at the peasant market, where it costs 10 rubles, the doctor must work for sixteen hours. Moreover, chicken prices go up very fast while salaries are increased very rarely and at a miserly pace. It takes three weeks' salary, for example, for a doctor to buy a pair of women's boots.

Most of the physicians at Botkin Hospital were poor and consequently given to a passionate debating of a coveted but, alas, unreal prospect of a raise. From time to time someone would bring a fresh rumor that we would be paid more. The news would spread with lightning speed through all staff rooms in all buildings, giving rise to a new outburst of discussions. Some of the polemicists tended to skepticism, others took the rumor on faith, still others were passionate believers, but no one was indifferent; everyone needed money.

And yet, compared to their counterparts in, say, Petrozavodsk, Moscow doctors enjoyed a high standard of living, reflecting the difference between the provinces and the capital. Moscow was better supplied with foodstuffs and consumer goods, and they were less difficult to buy at listed prices. In Petrozavodsk, just as in all provincial towns, food and consumer goods were always at a premium, and so salesmen sold them on the sly, naturally charging extra.

In Moscow, there existed additional options to earn a little more through doubling at other hospitals and outpatient clinics. None of the Botkin physicians held just one job; all of them worked at half- or quarter-load somewhere else, incessantly looking for more work though barely able to stand the fatigue.

The foggy prospect of a government-mandated pay raise could not be counted on as a way to enhance income, but the principle of patronage could. It is very popular among all professional groups, but reaches its ultimate heights in the relationship of doctors with their patients. We all loved to treat "good" patients, say a food-store salesman, warehouse man, or manager of an enterprise dispensing premium goods. With the right connections, one could buy a chicken at a state-run store for three or four rubles instead of at the peasant market for three times as much.

Woman doctors were particularly adept at getting "good" patients. Their connections extended not only to food and consumer goods stores but also to barber shops (hairdos ahead of the line), theater booking offices (tickets to any play), book stores (any book from under the counter). In short, they displayed characteristic abilities to grasp the realities of life and strike up useful friendships. Of course, cultivation of useful connections took much time, but who cared?

Male doctors, while clearly coming second to women in the ability to establish connections, equally clearly surpassed their female colleagues in the ability to get monetary remuneration from their patients. Naturally, it was done sub rosa. Soviet law views doctor's fees as bribery punishable by jail. However, hardly a single man could be found in the medical profession who did not charge patients for treatment. Some patients were not rich enough to pay, some others wouldn't, but a certain group, above all well-to-do intellectuals or affluent tradesmen, willingly paid their doctors. Jews and Georgians in particular made it a point of honor to pay for the treatment, even a small sum—25, 50, or 100 rubles.

Up to a point, I had never received money from my patients, although I was given bottles of cognac, crystal vases, and boxes of chocolates. My father occasionally received money from his patients, usually from well-to-do Jews. He told me: "I don't ask the sick for money, but if they want to give it to me, I won't say no. Especially, if I have to make a house call after working hours. If the patient doesn't want to come to the clinic for a checkup, that means he has the means to pay for the labors of a private doctor."

I agreed with my father, but it seemed to me that by accepting money, every doctor places himself in a position of dependence on the money-giving patient. Also, the law did not approve of this under any circumstances. Anyway, I was afraid.

My mother-in-law irritatedly told me several times: "Why don't you accept money from your patients? All good doctors do."

I didn't discuss this matter with her. But once she remarked: "My friend [the wife of a prominent theatrical administrator] asked me to recommend a good orthopedic surgeon for a private house call."

"Whom did you recommend?" I asked.

"You," she said dryly.

And so I went to visit that patient in her luxurious apartment. She had flat feet and a deformation of the toes. I gave her some suggestions and told her that she'd be better off having an operation.

"Could you perform this operation for me?" she asked.

"Of course."

As I was leaving, her husband shook my hand in the hall, and quietly slipped me an envelope containing money. Unaccustomed to such payment, I became quite embarrassed, and was about to protest, but he just tightened his grip on my fist containing the envelope and said, "This is for your effort."

I did not refuse. I opened the envelope in the car and found it contained a ten. This was not very much, but still, I had earned it for a half-hour's work. In the hospital I received as much for a hard night's duty with three to four operations. I was pleased to realize that, thanks to my qualifications, I could make money rather easily.

In several days I operated on the woman. The operation went well. She signed out in two weeks and asked that I visit her. When I arrived at her home for the second time, I expected to receive money again, more this time. I wanted to know just how much more. But I did not let on; I looked her over. Again her husband handed me an envelope, this time a thicker one. I opened it later to find that it contained 50 rubles. This was half my monthly salary. And all for just one operation.

So, with the help of my mother-in-law, I lost my innocence. But this loss was not much mourned.

In the summer of 1960 I operated on an American patient for the first time. He was a Mr. Perelman, a fifty-five-year-old from Chicago who had come to Moscow as a tourist, where he had tripped on the street and injured himself. He had strong pains in the knee joint of his left leg, so a special clinic for foreigners sent him to Botkin Hospital. I became his doctor. When I examined him, I found a rather rare injury—a tear of the side ligament of his knee. His leg had noticeably turned under the load. I suggested that he undergo an operation, and he agreed. The operation was planned at the usual conference of doctors at the clinic. I proposed to make a plastik of the outside ligament out of his own ligaments in a procedure that had been developed by the American surgeon Dr. Campbell. Frankly, I didn't want to treat the patient with a kapron netting, even though it had worked well in my Russian patients. Some kind of inner fear of possible complications in the foreign patient stopped me from using this artificial material. There's a Russian saying: "What's healthy for a Russian is death for a foreigner."

So I operated on an American for the first time, and after three weeks, I took off the plaster cast. The patient moved his knee around and soon began to walk without problem. We became good friends, and he told me about his country. He was surprised that he didn't have to pay anything for his treatment.

While there were no bad aftereffects for him, there were for me. The secretary of the Party Committee, Dr. Vera Paller, raised a scandal. She demanded to know on what basis I had operated on a foreigner, especially one from the United States.

"Did you know that he was an American citizen?" she asked.

"Of course I knew. It was written in his records, and everybody knew."

"Well, maybe he was a spy."

"Maybe he was." I shrugged my shoulders.

"What do you mean by that?" she shrieked.

"You yourself said that 'maybe' he was a spy. I didn't ask him."

"Well, did he ask you about anything?" She was obviously displaying the typical vigilance without which it's impossible to live in the Soviet Union.

"He didn't ask me about anything except his health."

"Do you know that in the United States a Soviet citizen wouldn't receive free medical care?"

"No, I didn't know that."

"Well, I'm telling you now. We have to pay there for treatment, but here they get treatment free."

"That's not any of my business. If he was supposed to pay, the head doctor should have collected from him."

"Did he offer you any money?"

"He didn't offer anything, and if he had, I wouldn't have accepted."

"I want to warn you, because you're still young and not a member of the Party. You can make a mistake very easily. By the way, why aren't you applying to join the Party?"

"I just haven't matured enough for such a step yet. You yourself said that I made a mistake in this whole matter."

"Keep in mind that if you do apply, I can write a recommendation for you. I've been in the Party for twenty years."

I pretended to be flattered by her offer. Later, I told my boss, who was not a Party member, about this conversation and he said: "The hell with her."

In the fall of 1959, I became an assistant professor and attending orthopedic surgeon at the Central Institute for Advanced Medical Training based at Botkin Hospital. One day I was summoned without explanation to the personnel department of the institute. The summons failed to surprise me; what did was the time of the appointment—8:00 P.M., when everybody was supposed to have long wound up for the day. However, I reasoned that an urgent meeting might have been called.

The institute is housed in Vosstanija Square in downtown Moscow in an old palace built a century ago as a nursing home. A wide, beautiful stairway led to the second floor. I entered the personnel department and found that nobody was there. I was about to leave when a nondescript man, about forty and wearing a gray suit, entered the room from a side door. He gave me a sullen, attentive look, as if studying me, and asked: "Your name is Golyakhovsky?"

"Yes, that's me."

"Take a seat, I want to have a talk with you."

He did not introduce himself, nor smile nor offer a handshake. He even forgot to mention what it was he wished to talk to me about. He sat down at a desk across from me. The man in gray took a gray folder from his bag and put it on the desk. It was my "dossier," containing all documents pertaining to my person. The man slowly and pensively leafed through the folder, occasionally casting a sharp glance at me, but did not attempt to start a conversation. About ten minutes passed. I felt uncomfortable under his glance. By that time I had figured out the identity of the man with the bland face; it was not too difficult to place him even in the absence of prior personal contacts with KGB agents. I heard a lot about them; all anecdotes featured just such men as the one I now faced. Too, I knew that personnel departments were their favorite information-gathering spots. But I could not figure out his intentions with regard to me.

I tried my best to seem carefree under his sullen look, pretending that I was neither surprised nor interested, while frantically searching my memory for a clue to his visit: what had I said or done that had put me in bad grace?

He closed the folder without undue haste, fished for a cigarette, took his time tapping it on the desktop, slowly lit it, and all the while looked at me in a searching way. I was very nervous and tried my utmost to conceal a facial tic.

"Why haven't you joined the Party?" he asked me at length.

I was ready for this question, for it was not the first time it was asked, though the previous inquisitors did not represent the KGB. I gave my standard response: "I thought it would be a premature act; I must first mature politically, read some more political literature. Unfortunately I have been too immersed in my surgical duties and could not devote sufficient time to my political education."

It was impossible to read on his expressionless face whether or not he believed my explanation. But I was sure that was merely an introduction; surely he would not have summoned me to discuss my Party affiliation.

"Well, you should join the Party if you know what's good for you," he said after a pause.

"You're absolutely right; I've been giving it a lot of thought lately." Another standard line. I had no intention of arguing with him. And I felt a surge of relief as it dawned on me that he had nothing to charge me with. Otherwise he would not have raised the question of the need for me to join the Party. He said, "What are your plans for the immediate future?"

"I'm going to complete my doctoral thesis and then write a scientific book—along with my regular duties, of course."

"And what would you say if you were offered an opportunity to work abroad?"

I was thunderstruck. Some of my colleagues did get foreign assignments, but all of them boasted impeccably Russian ethnic pedigrees, all were Party members, and all were Party activists, devoting much time to what is known as "public functions." I did not fit any of these qualifications and consequently had never thought of the possibility of being sent abroad.

"What country would you offer me?" I asked, not so much because I really wanted to know as to gain some time.

"How about Cambodia?"

My mind was racing, weighing all pros and cons. I knew that Cambodia was in the throes of civil war, that some other Asian countries were involved, but that the Soviet Union had nothing to do with it officially. It was thus easy to see that the mission of a Soviet doctor sent to a country with a complicated political and military situation through the services of a KGB agent entailed a dual purpose, professional and political. Or maybe, the priorities were to be reversed: first political, and only then professional? But why had the KGB chosen me? The only explanation I was able to come up with was that they needed a proven professional absolutely unknown as a political figure. I tried to imagine the faraway country, with its jungles, its climate, its exotic life-style. I itched to have a look at Cambodia at first hand, to travel. But what would my wife say? We had a son who was only twelve months old. Would he be able to stand the Cambodian climate?

"Can I take my family with me?" I asked.

"Of course."

"For how long would we be gone?"

"Two or three years."

"When am I supposed to give you an answer?"

"Now," he said, and for the first time a ghost of a smile flitted across his face.

"What kind of work would I do?"

"I won't describe everything now," he said, "but in a nutshell: you'll be a surgeon at a Soviet hospital catering to the civilian population. And you'll draw a salary in foreign currency at three times your present pay."

I understood that he would not tell me all the functions I was expected to perform. But to find out if they really intended to use me for their purposes, I asked an indirect question: "Do you think I'll have to join the Party immediately?"

"You can take your time," he replied, "but you will eventually have to. And one more thing: we will have to certify you as an officer of the reserve."

"But I *am* an officer of the reserve."

"I know," he said (of course, he did), "but we'll transfer you to the reserve of another agency."

It meant that I was to become a captain of the KGB. All Soviet physicians working abroad were recertified as KGB officers.

I was offered a chance to radically change my life and become a KGB agent. If I said yes, I would get a chance to visit an exotic country, and later on maybe others. Yes, the career I was offered promised far better remuneration than I had or could dream of ever having. For this I would have to cut off my surgical career all but completely, give up my dream of a doctoral degree and the authorship of a book, and sooner or later join the Party. In short, I was to sell my soul to the KGB. An enticing but scary proposition. . . . I told the agent I had to think it over and talk to my wife. At home Irina and I had a lengthy discussion, weighing all relevant factors. Both of us yearned to travel and see the world, but we were leery of selling ourselves out. Besides, Soviet newspapers were reporting at the time that the Cambodian river Mekong was swollen with blood. I did not want to add our blood to those streams. And so I turned down the offer of the man in gray.

22

My boss, Dr. D. Yazykov, pulled a few strings and had me included in a delegation of orthopedic surgeons that was to attend an international conference on the treatment of scoliosis in Czechoslovakia in May 1960. I had to hurry to secure a recommendation, *Kharackteristika,* from the District Party Committee and fill out a very detailed questionnaire, and rushed from one office to another until finally I had all the requisite documents processed and approved. Each of the twenty members of the Soviet delegation was subjected to a thorough security check by the KGB starting two months in advance of the trip, and no one could say with certainty whether or not he or she would be allowed to go. At long last, the list of delegates was approved, and we were all summoned for briefing to the Party Central Committee External Relations Unit on Kuybyshev Street. Properly cowed by the long wait and the forthcoming briefing by a high Party functionary, we were not a little edgy. The atmosphere was coldly official, so much so in fact that we were even afraid to talk out loud and communicated in semi-whispers.

Finally, a Central Committee instructor appeared, a young man in a well-tailored, dark suit, whose looks and comportment unmistakably bespoke his high station in life. He took a roll call of those present and opened the briefing. Although facing a group of physicians, some of whom were venerable professors of considerable renown, he addressed us as a group of kids.

"You, comrades, are going abroad where you will represent our great Fatherland and our advanced medicine. You should all be aware of the tremendous responsibility devolving on you as representatives of our Fatherland. . . ."

While he was carrying on in a loud voice and crisp phrases, I recalled the political indoctrination sessions conducted by the political commissar *(zampolit)* of our regiment in the military camp—the same manner, the same curt turn of phrase. The briefing boiled down to a few points underscoring our duties in Czechoslovakia. We were required: (a) not to walk the streets singly, but always in threesomes or at the very least in twosomes; (b) on no account to enter into contact of any kind with foreigners, including Czechs, unless an embassy representative or some other Soviet official was on the scene —to avoid likely provocations; (c) to be constantly on our guard and watch one another carefully ("Maintain your vigilance, comrades," the instructor said); and (d) to report to the Party supervisor without delay any infraction or suspicious act on the part of any other member of the delegation.

The Party supervisor had already been appointed—a thirty-six-year-old orthopedic surgeon, Katya Abassova. She was a pretty, single woman with kindly gray eyes and light hair pulled tightly in a bun at the back of her head. I had only a nodding acquaintance with her though she had always greeted me courteously at scientific meetings. I distrusted her as I did all other Party women, but now I doubled my caution because I knew she would be watching all of us. As a matter of fact after the briefing we all feared one another, willy-nilly trying to guess who would be squealing on whom. The practice of ratting was quite widespread in intellectual circles, with official blessing and encouragement. And now so highly placed an official as a Central Committee instructor himself ordered us: squeal, comrades!

I emerged from the briefing, choking with impotent rage. My whole being revolted against the brazen control of my personality, with its recommendations, security checks, restrictions, and demands that I spy on my colleagues! One would think we were a platoon of saboteurs about to be parachuted into the enemy territory on a dangerous mission, rather than a group of physicians planning a tourist trip to a friendly satellite country. And to add insult to injury, they have assigned that female to watch us, I thought indignantly. However, I took pains not to let my anguish show; I smiled, exchanged small talk, traded jokes with the other physicians. Departing from the group, I smiled pleasantly at my new supervisor and the rest of them, those who were likely to spy on me. To hell with them! I decided.

Nevertheless, when the group went aboard the Moscow-Prague train, we were all in a festive mood; everybody wore their best clothes, the ladies arrived carefully coiffed. Katya seemed a nice, kind woman, not our Party boss. But it transpired immediately that the group included a new person whom we had not seen at the briefing, a queit and smiling man of about forty who kept to himself.

Each of us decided that he was a KGB agent assigned the task of spying on us. Our mood soured. Even Katya turned gloomy each time her gray eyes turned to the newcomer.

Almost none of us had previous experience with trips abroad and consequently we anticipated the forthcoming encounter with the customs officials at the border with anxiety. No one knew for sure what we were entitled to take out of the country and what was forbidden to import. Thus, I carried five bottles of Stolichnaya vodka and five small tins of caviar to entertain my Czech counterparts or present to them as gifts if need be. But I was not sure if it would all be confiscated.

We had paid for our trip in rubles and received only 100 rubles worth of Czech koruna. But every one of us had a long shopping list for Czechoslovakia, and we discussed the expected prices and availability of consumer goods even more hotly and at greater length than the forthcoming scientific conference.

We passed the border town of Czop at night without any customs inspection. Were we glad! Everybody cheered up noticeably. Soon unaccustomed scenes opened up to our eyes beyond the windows. It was spring, trees were in full bloom; everything was strikingly different—village houses, railway terminals, everything. We even felt different; everyone was in holiday spirits.

I stood at the window next to Katya, exchanging impressions with her: "What a beautiful house!"

"And look at that field; have you ever seen a field so neatly tilled?"

"Everything is so clean and bright. . . ."

"Everything looks so different! . . ."

While we were thus chirping away, the car swayed and our shoulders touched. A pleasant sensation shot through us and we both smiled, drawing apart. Then we stopped drawing apart and stood, tightly pressing shoulders. From time to time, Katya glanced up at me languorously. She was a smallish woman.

In Prague we went to a third-rate hotel, the Flora. But we liked it because it was considerably neater and more comfortable than Russian hotels. We were put up two to four persons to a room; only Katya was accommodated in a room all her own. We walked the streets, all twenty of us together, trying not to stray from the group. Our "stranger" accompanied us, but nobody talked to him.

Katya watched us with a distracted smile because she was in a dreamy mood; the night before we had been alone and had kissed each other, although it did not last long for she had to process our documents. She was in love and could only think of another opportunity to be alone with me instead of attending to Party business.

I liked Katya, but my sentiments were laced with residual resentment against having her *diktat* imposed on me. It was not so much desire that propelled me into the affair as an urge to prove that I was a man, a human being requiring no meddlesome supervision. I would rather she loved me than spied on me. Our romance evolved on classic lines: from an exchange of glances to smiles to touches to kisses. Still, I could not shed the obsessive thought that I was embracing my Party boss. Such were my feelings when we slept together the second night.

The spring air of Prague blowing through the open window was laden with desire. Katya was burning with impatience and pressed against me, waiting to be undressed. And, guilty toward Irina though I felt, I was impatient, too. But I could not help a little mischief. After undressing her completely, I suddenly stopped and asked her with a laugh, "Aren't you afraid that while we're making love, people will wander off in all directions?"

"To hell with them," Katya whispered sibilantly. "A-a-h, come on!"

Czechoslovakia dazzled us as a land of plenty after Russia, and Prague seemed a miracle city compared to drab Moscow. We gazed in amazement at the abundance of food and consumer goods in the stores, the lack of lines, the throngs dressed in what seemed to us incredible opulence. Even more amazing was the absence of drunks: no winos dotted the pavements or staggered through the crowds and accosted passersby, as is the custom throughout the whole of Russia. We kept our observations to ourselves, however, because any praise of Czechoslovakia could be interpreted as criticism of Russia. Prudence dictated reticence. But we freely shared our impressions with those we completely trusted, admiration flowing unrestrained. Katya was enraptured by Prague and frankly confided it to me. But each time she saw me to the door of her room after a love tryst she never failed to admonish me: "Be careful and keep your big mouth shut!"

At the Brno terminal, we were met by Dr. Miloš Janeček, a

distinguished-looking and handsome gentleman, wearing a wonderful dark suit and light-colored kid gloves. At that time I possessed just one light suit my mother-in-law had procured from a black-marketeer. Though made in France, the suit was rather shabby from long wear, and the presence of the dapper Dr. Janeček made me feel inferior in my capacity of "representative of our great Fatherland."

Once, during an intermission at the conference, I found myself next to the Czech physician and he engaged me in a conversation, talking to me in a fluent and animated Russian. I enjoyed his company, but I could not help casting occasional wary glances around to see if anyone of my Soviet colleagues was watching. Meanwhile Dr. Janeček told me a political joke: "What is a sputnik? It is the only satellite that succeeded in breaking away from the Soviet Union." It was surely a funny joke, particularly coming as it was from an inhabitant of a satellite country. And though the situation clearly warranted caution, I could not restrain myself and laughed. Then I reciprocated with my own joke, also of a political kind: "What is genuine communism? It is like being in a pitch-dark room with the aim of catching a coal-black cat by the tail. And though you are aware that the cat is not there, you shout out loud: 'I've caught it! I've caught it!' "

Dr. Janeček laughed so uproariously that I was sure somebody would definitely rat on me, though no one could hear my joke. He liked my frankness, a rare trait in a member of socialist society; he liked my courage, and so he said, "I'd like to invite you to my place for dinner. The invitation is for you alone, but perhaps you'll be less than willing to come all by yourself because you Russians are required to do everything collectively. So bring somebody else along if you must."

I was pleased by his invitation but it put me in somewhat of a quandary because to leave the hotel alone at night for several hours was a serious violation of the rules. Still, I was not eager to have somebody tagging along; my overriding concern was to demonstrate my independence to Dr. Janeček. He could think what he pleased about Russians in general, but I was bent on proving to him that I was not bound by the collective restraints. I accepted his invitation.

Late that afternoon, I told Katya, "Dr. Janeček invited me for dinner and I want to go. What will you say?"

Katya looked at me lovingly. She was willing to absolve me

of any sin. "If you promised to come, you must keep your word," she said. "Don't worry, I'll think of something to distract the others; for instance, I'll call a meeting of some sort. Everybody knows how you hate meetings, so it will give you a good chance to sneak out unobserved. And even if your roommate reports your absence, I'll be the one he'll be reporting to." She sighed. "You are playing with fire, baby. You're in trouble because you don't want to be submissive like everybody."

I ironed my only pair of trousers, put on a fresh shirt, took a bottle of vodka and a tin of caviar as gifts for Dr. Janeček, and slipped out of the hotel when Katya called her meeting and my colleagues, cursing under their breath, dragged themselves to the hall.

Dr. Janeček lived much better than Soviet doctors did. His apartment was much larger and furnished better than ours. In fact, I had never been in such a luxurious apartment before, and I was shocked to learn that Dr. Janeček owned the whole seven-story building, which stood on Mendelev Square. He had inherited it and now rented the apartments out. Even after paying for employees and materials to maintain it, he earned a significant income from it. This would have been impossible in the Soviet Union, especially since Dr. Janeček was a member of the Communist Party.

I asked him how he combined capitalism with communism. He smiled and answered: "We have a different idea of communism than the Russians do." This was a totally new idea to me. I had never been abroad before, so my understanding was limited to the Soviet model. I now saw for the first time that communism could be something besides an ascetic, fruitless ideal; it could be real, normal, and beneficial.

I spent a marvelous night at his home. Both of us possessed the Slavic gift for friendship and we became fast friends for life.

Before my departure, he told me, "This coming summer I'll attend a surgeons' conference in Moscow."

"I'll welcome an opportunity to reciprocate your hospitality."

"Thank you. I have a business proposition for you. In Moscow I'll need Russian currency. If you wish, I'll give you koruna now and you will pay me back in rubles when I come to your country."

He offered me 3,000 koruna ($450), far more than I expected.

I was literally dying to accept the deal, but my desire was mixed with fear. It was a direct infraction of currency regulations.

He watched my hesitation with a smile. "Come on, make up your mind. Take the money and pay me back in rubles later. Don't worry, I'll not report you; squealing's not one of our customs."

"Well, here goes!" I took the money.

Now I had a new worry: how to buy things in such a way as not to arouse suspicions among my colleagues that I was spending more money than I was supposed to have. I told Katya about my secret, and from then on she accompanied me on shopping expeditions, to create an impression that we chipped in for what I bought. Katya was watched less strenuously than the rest of us, but she was afraid just the same, particularly of that strange man. However, he turned out to be an orthopedic surgeon from Leningrad, Dr. L. Zakrevsky. His identity was revealed when he delivered his paper at the conference. The paper was solid, and he himself proved to be a nice guy. On the way back to Russia he shared my compartment and we became so close that I confided in him: "Do you know that we all thought you were a KGB spy assigned to the group? You weren't present at the Central Committee briefing, that's why we suspected you."

He smiled modestly. "I was late for the briefing and had to undergo it separately," he told me. "But I also tried to spot the spy among you. Once I saw you leaving the hotel in Brno late at night all by yourself. Then I decided that you were the spy, for who else had the authority to go out alone?"

23

If a woman slaps a man in the face, that is her right, and it remains a private matter between the two of them.

Dr. Lyudmila M. was put on trial for slapping one of her

patients in the face. She had been the surgeon on duty in the reception room one evening, and as she was examining a man who had been brought in as an emergency case, she slapped him. Several other patients who were waiting to be admitted saw this through the door. One of them, a seventy-year-old retired communist who had served as a military commissar, immediately raised a scandal about it.

"What's this?" he yelled. "She was beating a Soviet patient! This has got to stop. Let her bear the punishment."

The other doctors on duty tried to settle him down by telling him that he didn't know what had taken place between the doctor and the patient before she slapped him.

"No matter what happened, she had no right to strike him," he insisted.

"Look, the guy's drunk. He could have said anything."

"So what if he's a little drunk? Maybe he was celebrating something and had a perfect right to drink. He doesn't deserve to be beaten for that. No, I insist on filing my complaint."

The doctors then turned to Lyudmila, who had been sitting and listening to this conversation. "Why don't you explain what happened," they said.

"There's no explaining to him."

She was a large, blond woman about forty years old, a good specialist and a good person. She had worked at this hospital ten years as a surgeon, and all her colleagues understood that she would never strike a patient unless there was good reason. But she refused to explain.

The whole matter might have been dropped, but the retired communist began to take his complaint around to various government agencies. He emphasized that the doctor had slapped "a Soviet patient" and finally managed to bring the case to trial.

At the trial, Lyudmila admitted slapping the patient, but would not explain why and would not apologize. She was given a six-month suspended prison sentence and a written notice of the sentence was sent to all doctors in Moscow to warn them of the seriousness of mistreating any Soviet patients.

Lyudmila had been very somber and reticent before the trial, but after the trial she unexpectedly cheered up and became sociable and began to crack all kinds of jokes. In order to celebrate the return of her good nature, we doctors all chipped in to buy a bottle of vodka and went together to the apartment of Dr. Tatyana Velskaya to have a little party. When we had all drunk enough, Lyudmila stood up.

"Do you want to know why I slapped him?" she asked. "When I was examining him and feeling his abdomen, that drunken beast said to me: 'Suck my cock.' Wouldn't you all have slapped him too? Now I'll tell you why I didn't say this publicly. At first I thought that they wouldn't bring this to court, but as the court day approached, I started to wonder whether those bastards would convict a woman doctor if she refused to go into why she had slapped a man. Well, they did it, and now I know that all their talk about respect for the labor of women doctors isn't worth the paper it's written on. Nobody appreciates or defends us. . . . Let's all have another drink."

Almost two-thirds of the doctors in the Soviet Union are women. They did not oust men from Russian medicine; men themselves had to abandon the field because the authorities turned the occupation into one of the least attractive ones.

After the 1917 Revolution, the number of female physicians started growing in the Soviet Union in inverse proportion to the diminution of doctors' earnings and deterioration of living standards. In the late 1920s, increasing industrial and military potential became a top priority of Stalin's administration. Engineers and technicians were kings, and were remunerated at twice or thrice the level of physicians. Faced with the task of supporting their families, men opted for high-paying occupations. The Revolution and the Stalin purges, which cost the lives of over 20 million young men, also contributed toward the vacuum at medical schools.

The vacuum was rapidly filled by young women. Many of them dreamed of becoming doctors because the occupation conferred status, tuition was free, and medical education required meager background. The emancipation policies of the government filled women with pride at the opportunity to enter the medical profession, an almost exclusively male occupation before the Revolution.

In general, women had to shoulder almost the entire burden of labor-intense occupations. For close to a quarter of a century, from the early thirties to the mid-fifties, they constituted the mainstay of the country's work force. Thus, the prevalence of women among doctors was not strange. Medicine has long been a typically female occupation, and with good reason. Indeed, the female touch, womanly diligence and thoroughness, selflessness and warmth, made women, if anything, better fit for coping with the many hardships of the medical profession than men.

Women have learned to treat patients well. However, they lag far behind their male colleagues in the ability to draw benefits from their occupation. While men account for less than 30 percent of all Soviet physicians, they have appropriated for themselves practically all well-paying jobs, leaving drudgery to women. Thus, in the highly paid medical categories, the ratio of men to women is the reverse of the general. This also reflects the preoccupation of woman doctors with family matters, leaving them just enough time and energy to perform routine duties. Most Russian woman doctors are strikingly passive; they have no time for enterprise or initiative. However, they fit nicely into the system of socialized medicine.

24

One day in the fall of 1960, Dr. Yazykov invited me into his office and closed the door.

"Bring your internal passport to work tomorrow," he whispered with a smug smile. "We're going to go examine a leg of . . . whom do you guess? . . . Khrushchev! Don't breathe a word about this to anybody."

Dr. Yazykov had long been the Kremlin Medical Directorate's only consultant for orthopedics. The Directorate trusted his skill and discretion, but since he had psoriatic arthritis now, he needed an assistant. He had chosen me and secretly assigned me the work he couldn't do anymore himself. The most important requirement for my position was to keep quiet about what I saw and heard, so I've never told anyone about my high-ranking patients.

The next day we rode with Dr. M. Khutornenko, the head doctor of the Central Kremlin Clinic, to our appointment in a large limousine. We drove forty kilometers on Mozhayskoye highway, past the suburb of Barvikha, and turned off onto a forest road marked "No Trespassing." Security guards stopped our car twice along this road and checked our documents. We finally reached a gate, where guards checked our documents again and then transferred us to another car. A KGB officer rode with us some distance farther until we reached a large dacha. The officer transferred us to another KGB officer, who checked our documents again and then led us into a waiting room. Surprisingly, nobody searched our pockets during this whole procedure, but apparently the head of the Kremlin Clinic, who was a colonel in the KGB, had already vouched for us.

We arrived at about noon and waited without explanation until about 6:00 P.M. The furnishings in the room consisted of rugs, expensive polished furniture, landscape paintings, and frilly white curtains. I had earlier seen exactly the same type of furnishings in the Party sanitoriums at Sosna and Barvikha. We were tense the whole time, because Khrushchev could appear at any moment. Dr. Yazykov was suffering from his aching joints and difficult breathing, and we were both hungry. The room grew dark, and we turned on the lights.

Khrushchev flew into the room as if pushed. He was still talking with somebody behind him, but an officer closed the door, so he immediately turned to us.

"Well, dear professors, my leg hurts. I limp especially badly in the morning, but it eases up later in the day. My wife Nina nags me to see the doctor, but when do I have time? I've just spent all day with the other Presidium members preparing reports for the next plenum. [The Presidium is now called the Politburo. A plenum is a meeting of the Central Committee.] Forgive me for the long wait, but I just couldn't get away. In any case, can you help me?"

Khrushchev flashed his gap-toothed peasant grin and pulled up his pant leg. Dr. Yazykov kneeled down with difficulty because of his arthritis, so I got down immediately beside him and began to remove Khrushchev's shoe. Khrushchev protested that he could take off his shoe himself, but I nevertheless helped him. The shoe was a simple slip-on; I later wondered if it was the same famous shoe he banged on the podium at the United Nations.

Khrushchev stood barefoot on the rug with his cuffs rolled up as I helped Dr. Yazykov feel his ankle's pulse and points. Khrushchev answered the doctor's questions with the respect that uneducated people always accord physicians. Dr. Yazykov and I saw almost immediately that Khrushchev was suffering from arthritis at the base of his toes, made more painful by flat feet. We saw similar cases almost every day, but Dr. Yazykov slowly and thoughtfully felt the soles of both feet and pretended to take a long time to reach a firm diagnosis. The head of the Kremlin Clinic stood by and took notes on what he said.

After he finally allowed Khrushchev to put his shoes on, my boss fixed his gaze on his patient's gold cuff links. Khrushchev noticed his interest and asked, "Do you want to swap my cuff links, Professor?" He was obviously amused at his own proposal and curious how the old doctor would react. Dr. Yazykov played along. "Sure, Nikita Sergeyevich, let's swap," he answered as he began to undo his own cuff links.

Khrushchev burst out laughing. "You think these are real gold, Professor? Heck no, they're even cheaper than yours are!" We all laughed along, but I noticed that the guard only smiled politely. He was apparently used to this simple-minded humor and had perhaps already heard this same joke several times.

"Thank you, professors," Khrushchev said seriously. "Some of the comrades don't believe in medicine, but I do. Thanks to the hard work of you Soviet doctors, our citizens are healthier and live longer. I hope you can fix me up, because I still need my feet for my work. I move around a lot. I hurry all the time, because there's so much I still want to do. Now, you'll be paid some extra money for this trip [the head of the clinic nodded to us], but in the meantime, allow me to invite you to dinner, because you're probably hungry. We in the Presidium work hard and then eat well. Follow me."

He flew out of the room as forthrightly as he had entered it, and we hurried after him. Dr. Yazykov had so much trouble keeping up that it seemed he should have been the patient. He nevertheless nudged me happily and winked, obviously honored by the invitation. The communist dictators usually treated their doctors like servants, but Khrushchev treated us like equals.

When we entered the dining room, he announced to the indifferent members of the Presidium: "I've invited these professors to eat with us. They came to look at my legs." He turned to us:

"These are the members of the Presidium. You'll recognize them all from their pictures. Let's eat and drink. What will you drink?"

"Cognac," said Dr. Yazykov.

"So, professors like cognac just like us. Pour it for them." The servants, who despite their simple black pants and white jackets were at least majors in the KGB, offered us a tray of glasses of cognac. We chose the smallest glasses and sipped from them.

"No, no," said Khrushchev, "that's not how we drink cognac here. I'll show you how." A servant filled a water glass with cognac up to the very rim—at least 250 grams (about nine ounces). Khrushchev grabbed the stem earnestly, took a deep breath, carefully lifted the glass to his lips, and drank it all in one gulp. He wiped the glass out with his finger and licked it off and then stood up and shook the empty glass upside down over his head to prove he had drunk every drop. "That's how to drink cognac."

The other Presidium members also drank a lot, but not so boastfully. They didn't discuss politics that evening, perhaps because they had already done that all day, perhaps because Dr. Yazykov and I were present. Khrushchev relaxed and chatted with his tablemates, among them Yekaterina Furtseva and Leonid Brezhnev, and continuously illustrated his points with exuberant gestures of his short arms and stubby fingers. I watched everybody as attentively, yet discreetly, as I could. This was a rare opportunity.

There were ten men around the big table beside us, but half the seats were unoccupied. Apparently other occasions were graced by a greater number of guests. No one was accompanied by his wife; it was a typical business meal. The waiters were anchored behind each of us, never departing. Judging by the speed and dexterity with which they worked, it was clear they were exceptionally well-schooled in the tastes and manners of their charges. Also present in the room were several waiters' aides who passed the dishes around the table. Nothing was carted around; all food was passed from hand to hand.

As Russian custom dictated, the numerous appetizers were set on the table and one could either help himself or ask the waiter to serve a particular delicacy. Silver plates were filled with heaped caviar and salmon roe, lox, salmon, sturgeon, ham, small pickled cucumbers (called *nezhinskiye* after the Ukrainian town where they are grown), pickled mushrooms, and black olives; and there were a mixed red beet salad and fresh vegetables in large cut-glass bowls. Two deep china bowls contained Georgian ethnic specialties: chicken and mutton Chakhokhbili, cold stew in a special piquant sauce with tomatoes and nuts. Long china plates displayed several varieties of bologna and salami, exuding a pungent yet subtle aroma. All the delicacies on the table were cooked at a special Kremlin shop of the Mikoyan Food Plant in Moscow from the best and freshest provisions, ones never supplied to regular shops.

The waiters offered us menu-cards to mark the soup and main course each of us desired. All the menus were personalized, with the name of a Presidium member printed at the top. I got hold of the Pospelov menu (Pospelov, a Secretary of the Central Committee, was not present at the table). I do not know where he was at the time, but I had the meal of my life on his behalf. There were several soups to choose from. I chose *Troinaja Ukha,* a triple chowder, with a *kulebyaka* fish patty. I had never tasted triple chowder, although I heard that before the Revolution rich merchants and bishops had been particularly fond of this Russian specialty. To the best of my knowledge, triple chowder is prepared by successively boiling three different varieties of fish in the same water in a specific order: first, the small fish (ruff or perch); then the small fry is removed and a sterlet is put into the pot, followed in a like fashion by a pike perch or sturgeon. While the fish is boiling, spices are added liberally.

Only the soup proper, the triple fish broth, is served, while the fish is baked in dough into long patties together with ground sterlet chordal gristle. These long patties are known as *kulebyaka.*

It was impossible to buy all these varieties of fish in regular stores; pike perch, for example, would be sold only on extremely rare occasions, mostly in special restricted stores for the big wheels. As for sterlet, it had never been openly sold. This kind of fish can be found only in the Volga and its tributaries, but its population dwindled rapidly when the river was contaminated with petroleum products and when hydroelectric dams were built. Therefore, it was officially prohibited to fish for sterlet to protect the species from extinction, but it did grace Khrushchev's table. And the chowder was stupendous. For the main course I ordered shish kebab Kars style and received a large slab of the softest mutton imaginable with rounds of white onions and gravy.

The dinner lasted over two hours. Finally, though we had

thoroughly enjoyed the food, my boss whispered into my ear that he could stay no longer. We exchanged glances with the head doctor, he gave us the "let's-go" look, and we left the table without saying good-bye. In fact, nobody paid attention to us; everybody was preoccupied with eating and talking.

The dinner that evening was an ordinary meal for these communists, but it was the richest, most delicious food I'd ever seen. Normal Soviet citizens don't even know such foods exist. I stuffed myself as if it were a last supper. And I sensed that all Khrushchev's disciples at that Last Supper—every single one—were Judases.

When we were brought outside the dacha limits and climbed into the Kremlin Clinic limo, the chauffeur was finishing a sandwich, which he had brought with him. Nobody bothered to feed him the whole day. His sandwich emanated a salami aroma. It smelled a lot worse than the "government" brand.

25

After five years of work as an orthopedic surgeon, I began to feel that I was mastering the art of surgery. I accumulated experience and various technical skills and methods, and it became increasingly easy for me to perform operations.

At the onset of my surgical career, I made errors, as do all beginner surgeons. My incisions were not directly above the area of tissue that was to be operated on; my manipulations of bones, joints, and ligaments were crude and time-consuming.

I have always considered surgery to be an art. While the surgeon is examining the patient to determine the diagnosis, he is a scholar, applying his knowledge. But when he makes an incision and manipulates with his hands, he is an artist, a performer. And I attempted to polish each technical element of my operations, as an artist perfects each line or a performer polishes each phrase. The only difference is that artists and performers have an opportunity to rehearse as much as they need, while I had to operate on my patients without rehearsals.

May patients forgive young surgeons their inexperience!

Operations that were new to me I tried first to perform on corpses in the morgue. Rules allowed this to be done without the consent of the relatives of the deceased; but all incisions had to be made so that any trace of the operation would be covered by the clothing in which the deceased was then handed over to the relatives. Thus, for example, you could not operate on a woman's corpse below the knees, but it was possible with male corpses. Unfortunately, there was not always enough time to go to the morgue, which was housed in a beautiful former church at the end of the hospital's grounds.

Since I could not always rehearse the operations before performing them, I devised for myself a method of mental rehearsals. On the eve of each operation, I sketched a line of the projected incision on my skin and then, with the aid of an anatomical atlas, I imagined penetrating deep into the tissue. I tried to think out every possible variable of unexpected anatomical or surgical deviations beforehand. For this, I surrounded myself with textbooks of orthopedic surgery and read different authors, comparing what they had written. Alas, it is difficult to describe an operation in full detail.

Since we were very short of instruments I was sometimes obliged to improvise beforehand. In my mind I pictured the exact spot where I, my assistants, and an operating nurse would stand. I thought out each plaster cast to be applied after the operation, for they were almost always needed. As a result of these preparations I felt I was approaching mastery of the surgical art.

In essence, surgery is a craft. A surgeon operates on tissue, as does a carpenter on wood, a potter on clay, or a mason or sculptor on granite or marble. But the point is that the surgeon operates on live tissue. Each surgeon develops his own feel for it. This is the surgeon's sixth sense, the ability to feel tissue through steel instruments.

The basic Hippocratic rule of medicine—*Do Not Cause Harm* —most vividly manifests itself in surgery. The danger inherent in an operation is sometimes great, and only a genuine surgeon can perform the operation in a way that will not cause harm to the tissues. In the hands of such a surgeon, craft becomes true art.

There are surgeon-craftsmen and there are surgeon-artists. There are far more craftsmen; I saw hundreds of them. I strove to become a surgeon-artist.

I love orthopedic surgery, as I love poetry, for its beauty and precision. It seems to me that it would be easier for me to put up with a wife I do not love than with work I do not love. As soon as work ceases to interest an individual, his intellect immediately weakens.

I liked to dedicate my operations, as a poet dedicates his poems, to friends and beautiful women. Sometimes I told them of this, oftentimes I did it just for myself. It simply added romantic overtones to my identity as a surgeon and helped my art. Surgically, I was lucky, for not one of my patients died through a fault of mine.

No patient can appreciate the art of his or her surgeon. He can be pleased or displeased with an operation, but can not understand its art. That is unfortunate because people do understand the art of a painter or a performer. As all surgeons, I did not receive applause or other rewards for my art. However, on one of my rounds in the 1960s, a girl of about twenty was brought in a cab with a bouquet of flowers in her arms. She had a severe break in the ankle-bone, and I had to restore the fragments like a jigsaw puzzle and fasten them so she would not have a limp for the rest of her life. Satisfied but tired, I went into the surgeons' duty room after the operation to rest and eat my by now cold dinner. On the table I saw that beautiful bouquet she had brought in an enameled pail. "What a grateful soul that girl has!" I thought. But a little later when I thanked her for the flowers she was embarrassed.

"The bouquet was not mine. I was on my way to a funeral and was taking it to put on the coffin. I turned my ankle instead. Where was I to put them? I decided to give them to you."

So, you see, surgeons sometimes do receive flowers for their art.

Thanks to my hyperactive nature, I wrote a Ph.D. thesis and a textbook. But simultaneously I had been collecting enemies.

The official ceremony where I defended my thesis was held at the ancient palace on Solyanka Street that housed the Academy of Medical Sciences. The thesis was concerned with "The Surgical Treatment of Recurrent Shoulder Dislocation." I had proved, in experiments on dogs followed by clinical tests on fifty patients, that an artificial ligament I had invented made of capron fabric yielded good results. The thirteen professors making up the Scientific Council of the academy unanimously voted for awarding me a Ph.D. degree.

Once their decision was approved by the Supreme Certification Commission, I was to start drawing 300 rubles per month—good money, or at any rate not less than an average bus or truck driver's wages. But all my work was nearly wiped out by a letter of denunciation received by the academy. It was written on a small sheet of paper torn out of a school pad, in an awkward scrawl, and signed with a woman's name. The author purported to have been my patient, though I had never had a patient by that name. The letter said that my doctoral thesis was a pack of lies, because all I had done for her was a skin incision for which I charged 100 rubles, and later another 50 rubles. Then, the victim of my "professional perfidy" claimed she went to Dr. Dubrov, a well-known orthopedist, who operated on her a second time. It was in the course of that surgical intervention that Dr. Dubrov discovered I had done nothing save a skin incision, said the denunciation.

But that was not all. The author also insisted that neither I nor my father "deserved" the lofty title of Soviet doctor; she was at a loss for an explanation of why we were both tolerated at Soviet hospitals and institutions of learning. It was a purely political accusation, hinting at our Jewish identity and lack of Party membership.

When Dr. N. Krakovsky, Secretary of the Scientific Council, showed me the letter, I was dumbfounded at the unexpectedness and viciousness of the charges it contained. But since the letter was signed and had a return address, the procedure of my certification was suspended. Dr. Krakovsky, a very old friend of my father's, told me: "You must have cunning enemies. You were lucky that the letter had been lost for several days in the academy red tape and failed to arrive before your defense. Otherwise we would have had to cancel the proceedings. Their calculation was impeccable: to trip you at the last moment. Sure, I know that the letter is ridiculous, but I'm obliged to check the facts."

Even leaving aside the political accusations, the charge that I had extorted money and engaged in fraudulent activities was enough to put me on trial, strip me of the doctor's diploma, and send me to a Siberian concentration camp. Fortunately, however, the author of the denunciation committed several tactical errors. I went to the building indicated in the return address and easily found out that no one by the name shown on the letter lived there. Dr. Dubrov, who was my official interrogator at my doctoral defense, had never operated on a patient by that name, and such a patient had never been admitted at our hospital. I obtained certificates to support all my findings and brought them to the academy: once you are called a camel, no matter how nonsensical it is, you have to prove that you are indeed not a camel. And I did, and received my Ph.D.

I told the whole story to my boss, a man of the world. At that time he was in very poor health and I had to perform his duties with increasing frequency.

"Look around you for the one who tried to destroy you," he told me. "The culprit must be very close."

I was no Sherlock Holmes and for a long time could not unravel the mystery. But at long last the truth was out: my "well-wishers" were two women, Dr. Antonina Belova, forty-five, a Party member, and Dr. Natalya Gracheva, thirty-five, who did not belong to the Party. What had made them resort to squealing I never learned because neither of them would admit to the authorship of the letter. However, they began to quarrel, accusing each other in the process of being the mastermind behind the letter of denunciation. Most likely, they both tried to take revenge on me for my successful career, my boss's confidence in me, and my professional achievements.

"The women are full of shit!" My boss was beside himself with rage. "Don't you worry, we'll get them yet, though I wish I were as strong as I used to be. Listen, maybe you ought to join their idiotic Party. Otherwise you'll never be safe from bitches. They'll always stalk you, believe me!"

But I shook my head. "There's no way I'll join," I said. Not even this pressure could make me change my mind.

26

One night in late October 1960 I was on a regular call as chief surgeon-traumatologist at Botkin Hospital. Suddenly the telephone rang and I heard the anxious voice of an unknown man: "Comrade surgeon, here is military surgeon Colonel Ivanov. In a few minutes a severely burned patient will be brought to you. Stand by to administer emergency aid. I will be accompanying the patient."

Such a warning was out of the ordinary, so I guessed that there was a good reason for the doctor's anxiety. Several minutes later, a military ambulance entered the hospital gate followed by five or six Volga cars, painted official black. The cars disgorged a crowd of military officers, almost all of them colonels and many with medical insignia on the shoulder straps. The colonels rushed to the front car from which a stretcher with a patient was being unloaded. They carried the stretcher up a short flight of stairs and into the admission room, where I was waiting. The patient on the stretcher exuded an odor of singed tissue. Silently, I helped them carry the patient to the shock treatment room. A nurse and an intern helped me take off the blanket and sheet covering the patient and I couldn't help shuddering: the whole of him was burnt. The body was totally denuded of skin, the head of hair; there were no eyes in the face—everything had been burnt away. It was a total burn of the severest degree. But the patient was alive and even tried to say something through burnt lips. I bent down close to his awful face and managed to decipher what he was trying to say:

"Too much pain . . . do something, please . . . to kill the pain. . . ."

He desperately needed an immediate intravenous injection of liquids, but I could not find a single vein on his body. Only the skin on both of his feet remained intact. Finally I managed to insert needles into foot vessels and started injecting glucose and sodium chloride solution. I also gave the patient a shot of morphine and his labored breathing eased a little.

After that I had a chance to talk to Dr. Ivanov, the senior of the group of physicians. He told me that the patient had been brought straight from the Space Research Institute near the Dynamo subway station, about ten minutes' ride from our hospital. That was why he had been rushed to us: our hospital was the closest. The patient had sustained a burn an hour previously while undergoing a test in an altitude chamber. The chamber was maintained at elevated pressure and its atmosphere was heavily laden with oxygen. All of a sudden a fire broke out and the subject found himself in an atmosphere of burning air. He tried to put out the flames and actuated the alarm; but it took about half an hour to decompress the chamber, and all the while the patient was burning. Initially, his protective suit safeguarded him, but after a while the suit melted down. Only the special shoes withstood the fire, which accounted for the intact skin on his feet. Having finished his story, Dr. Ivanov added pleadingly, "Do something for him, save him. He is not an ordinary man. . . ."

"What about that altitude chamber he was in?"

"I'll tell you, but it's strictly confidential," Dr. Ivanov replied in a whisper. "It was a model of a manned spaceship. And the patient, Sergeyev by name, was undergoing tests because he was training for the first manned space flight."

Now I could see why the military doctors were so agitated. Until that time, nobody had flown into space, except the dogs Belka and Strelka. It was clear to me that a fire in the model of the first manned spacecraft was a serious blow to all who worked at that institute, and the lethal burn of the first cosmonaut was fraught with grave consequences for many of the institute brass. Unfortunately, Sergeyev was doomed. Dr. Ivanov and all the others in his group were aware of this. And yet, all of us were eager to do something, anything, to alleviate his terrible suffering. The military doctors were constantly on the phone, and the brass called back incessantly.

Dr. Ivanov summoned me to the telephone. Chief Surgeon of the Soviet Army, Professor and General Alexander Vishnevsky was calling: "The chiefs demand that we transfer the patient to our burn department," he said. "But how can we move such a patient? I'd rather send Doctor Shreiber with assistants and our special secret liquids to your hospital."

I was glad to have the benefit of an expert's advice, but I yearned even more for the special solutions that our hospital lacked. I had at my disposal only the simplest of solutions and several protein preparations, but that was pitifully inadequate for the burned twenty-four-year-old Air Force lieutenant. I urged Vishnevsky to send help, and in due course it arrived.

The burned flyer lived for another sixteen hours. Whether he was exceptionally strong or the Vishnevsky solutions were exceptionally potent, I don't know, but it was a miracle he lived so long.

Nothing has ever been officially said about the death of the first spaceman.

While several physicians and nurses were busy trying to alleviate the suffering of Sergeyev, the colonels who had brought him stationed a liaison officer at the sole telephone in the emergency room to answer the incoming calls. The young officer was sitting on a wooden stool in the corridor, a white gown over his military tunic, softly reporting the state of the patient:

"The condition is very serious. . . . The doctors are doing everything possible to save him. . . . yes, Comrade General . . . right, Comrade Marshal . . . check, I will, Comrade Chief Designer . . . The patient is still unconscious, Comrade Minister. . . ." He had a pleasant face, an open high forehead, a handsome, though sad, smile.

The next morning, when the patient died, I saw the young officer, a lieutenant, again. He was sitting all alone on the sofa. As I came up to him, he jumped up and stood at attention, looking at me expectantly. I said, "Please sit down." I sat next to him. "Were you friends?" I asked.

"Very close friends," he told me. "We served in the same unit."

"How did the fire happen?"

"A lapse, just a stupid mistake," he explained. "Sergeyev was undergoing three days of tests inside the ship to condition his body for the flight. The tests proceeded smoothly and were almost over. Shortly before the end of the testing program the cosmonaut was supposed to heat up his supper on a small electric stove. Sergeyev turned it on, but failed to see a small rag, actually a bunch of thread, at its side. When the stove grew hot, the rag burst into flame. The cosmonaut grabbed a fire extinguisher and proceeded to put out the flame, but it was too late. The air in the cabin caught fire. What a stupid mistake! Thank you, Comrade Doctor, for all you tried to do for him."

We silently shook hands. He was very small in stature and his wrist was thin as a child's, but he gave me a strong man's handshake.

His face stuck in my memory, and six months later I saw his photograph in the newspapers: his name was Yuri Gagarin; he was the first man in space.

I saw Yuri Gagarin several times afterward. In 1962, Dr. Vishnevsky performed an appendectomy on him. I came to visit him at the Institute of Surgery. We recalled our first meeting during the tragic death of his friend. Of course, I was eager to hear from Gagarin his personal impressions of his historic space flight.

"Were you scared, really scared?" I asked him.

"You bet I was," he replied. "While I was sitting on top of that giant rocket waiting for the takeoff, I was acutely aware of the thousands of kilos of fuel beneath me, and not just plain fuel. That mass of fuel was to be ignited, and once ignited who knew what would happen? Then the scariest moment occurred as the craft orbited the Earth and started a reentry maneuver. When the ship entered the dense layers of the atmosphere, her skin was ignited by friction. When I saw through the window a wall of fire all around me, I was scared out of my wits. That's when the memory of poor Sergeyev came back to me. How could I know if my craft would withstand the flame? But when the parachute opened and the ship jolted and started rocking over the ground, I calmed down. What I could not imagine was that I would be scared on the ground again. Try to see it: my ship touched down near a farm field, and the rescue team was on the way in its helicopter. I was beside myself with joy at the thought that I was alive and everything had come to a happy end, when all of a sudden I saw through the window a crowd of Virgin Lands peasants, approaching with pitchforks and wooden stakes. They intended to take me prisoner, just as the U.S. pilot Gary Powers had been taken prisoner the year before. The peasants had read about the American spy but knew nothing about my flight, because they were in the field and had not heard radio announcements. Naturally, they decided that I was another enemy of the Fatherland dropping from the sky onto their field. Add to this their feelings about my none too ordinary ship: an American spy definitely, if not a Martian. Luckily, no sooner had they surrounded the craft than the rescue helicopter landed nearby and the boys unpacked me and started embracing and congratulating me. The peasants had the shock of their lives at the sight of the 'spy' turning into the first cosmonaut."

In 1967, I chanced to examine Yuri Gagarin as a patient. Our mutual friend, chief test pilot of the MIG program Colonel Georgi Mosolov, brought him to me. Two years previously he had sustained a frontal bone fracture with an extensive wound. The newspapers did not report Gagarin's misfortune, but in 1965 his photographs disappeared from all publications. Only a year later, his photograph appeared, showing a cicatrized dent in his forehead and a scar across his brow. The photograph gave rise to wild rumors: an automobile accident, an air crash, a political assassination attempt, and even a scuffle with the cuckolded husband of a movie star (no name, of course). It was even said that Gagarin had been beaten by his cosmonaut colleagues to let some air out of his puffed-up persona. Such a rumor mill is only too natural for Russia: where information is at a premium, disinformation takes its place.

In truth, Gagarin had indeed become the victim of a romantic escapade: while staying at a select governmental sanatorium, he came to a young nurse's room to spend the night, but the lovers were interrupted by the husband appearing out of the blue, so the first cosmonaut had to climb out of the window and jump from the second floor. Yuri landed on his forehead and was lucky at that: had he hit the ground at a slightly different angle, he would have lost an eye.

The story was kept under tight wraps. Gagarin was taken to the exclusive Hospital #6 set up by the Third Department of the Ministry of Public Health for the cosmonauts, and there his wound was treated. The outer table of the frontal bone was found to be fractured and bent inward; the wound was contaminated. The surgeons feared that the infection had extended to the front sinus. However, the cosmonaut's young and strong body easily coped with the trauma. But it did leave its mark.

Gagarin complained to me that the surgeons had been unable to make his face scar invisible. I examined and felt the scar. To be sure, it was the epitome of crude surgery. The skin was mottled and the scar soft, but it crossed the eyebrow in an ugly line, extending downward in a stepwise fashion. The forehead dent was totally exposed.

"You ought to go to the West. Experts there in plastic surgery could correct the defect."

"I have no foreign currency to pay for such an operation," he said.

"I'm sure the government will give you as much money as you need."

"No way. The days when my former master Nikita Sergeyevich [he meant the fallen Khrushchev] indulged me are long past. I tried to talk about it to the honchos in the Politburo, but they told me to forget it. They even slapped me with a Party reprimand."

"Any surgeon will be glad to operate free of charge," I suggested. "For him it will be of inestimable promotional value. He'll be able to advertise himself as 'personal surgeon to Yuri Gagarin, Cosmonaut Number One.'"

"Hell, no," Gagarin said. "I was told to keep quiet about that incident so as to avoid unfavorable publicity in the West. So there's no way I could go for treatment there. But can I get treatment in any of our countries?" He meant one of the countries of the Eastern European bloc.

"Why don't you go to Czechoslovakia? The great plastic surgeon, Doctor Burian, is no longer alive, but his disciples and associates are still active. They'll be able to make your scar disappear."

But Gagarin was not allowed to get his surgery even in Prague. The famous "Prague Spring" was in full swing; Czechoslovakia was brimming with democracy and crawling with Western newsmen.

Yuri Gagarin died at thirty-one under mysterious circumstances. On a warm spring day, March 27, 1968, he set out on a test flight in the company of an experienced flight instructor whose name was Sergeyev—the same name as the very first cosmonaut who had burnt to death. Their specially designed two-seat sports plane was in excellent condition. Less than an hour after takeoff, the ground controllers lost track of the plane. A search helicopter found its debris in the forest 150 kilometers east of Moscow, halfway to the city of Gorky on the Volga. A memorial was erected on the site "where Yuri Gagarin died."

The circumstances of his death are shrouded in mystery and never discussed by the Soviet press. With information conspicuously lacking, its place again was taken by rumors: Gagarin was killed on Brezhnev's orders because he was a Khrushchev creature.

27

My boss Dr. Yazykov died in 1962; an infection from contaminated smallpox vaccine killed him. Before his death, he stayed at the special Kremlin Hospital on Granovsky Street, where I often visited him. Almost the entire time he was ill I had to substitute for him as head of the department and chair of orthopedics. I had no experience and had to rely heavily on his advice. Once, several months before his death, Dr. Yazykov told me that he wanted me to be his successor as director and professor.

I had a premonition that the Ministry of Public Health would not appoint me to the vacated position because I was too young and was not a Party member. That is exactly what happened. But the director of the Central Institute of Traumatology and Orthopedics (CITO), the largest orthopedics center in the country, offered me the positions of senior research associate and senior attending surgeon. It was the best possible job, enabling me to combine practical surgery with scientific endeavors under the best of all possible conditions. I dreamed of major scientific work; I had original ideas of new surgical procedures that would take at least ten years to be developed. And so I gladly accepted the offer.

My monthly earnings increased five- or sixfold, and reached about 400 rubles per month. This income gave us a higher living standard than a common Soviet family enjoyed. The conditions of all of us and of society were unmistakably improving.

Most significantly, the practice of indiscriminate terror stopped; people no longer disappeared as they had when Stalin was alive.

Khrushchev's administration instituted certain democratic changes in the hierarchical structure. The system of one-party dictatorship was still in place and free elections and demonstrations remained a dream, but some signs of relaxation were obvious. People were no longer mortally terrified of the government and one another. After Beria was executed in 1953, the secret police lost some of its hitherto absolute power. People loosened up visibly; conversations acquired an edge of frankness.

Even in print there appeared bold stories and poems criticizing the recent past. The most momentous event in literary and political life came with the publication, in the late fifties, of Alexander Solzhenitsyn's novella *One Day in the Life of Ivan Denisovich.* Within a week, there was hardly anyone left in the country who had not read it, and the jubilation was almost universal: at long last a writer emerged who was capable of writing truthfully and allowed to publish his works. The next critical and very poignant literary work was Alexander Tvardovsky's poem "Tyorkin in the Nether World," a scathing attack on many of the negative aspects of Soviet Party bureaucracy. It was an open secret, of course, that quite a few critical books and speeches were suppressed by the new administration. But the few works that did manage to find their way into print gave hope that the thaw, as the writer Ilya Erenburg aptly called that period, was really coming to fruition.

Western exhibitions came to Moscow and other major cities. The pathfinder was an American exhibition at the Sokolniki Park in 1958 inaugurated by the then Vice-President, Richard Nixon. Millions of Soviet people thronged the exhibition, and almost all of the visitors had a chance not only to see the products of U.S. industries but to talk to Russian-speaking American exhibitors. For many, it was their first chance to be exposed to real American life. I, of course, visited the exhibition and had my first taste of Coca-Cola.

I was to learn even more about America than the exhibition showed, because in May 1962, my father's elder sister, Luba Churchin, came from New York City to see us on a ten-day tourist visa. At that time she was seventy-two. My aunt had left Russia in 1913, and since then had known next to nothing of her six younger siblings—three brothers and three sisters. Only the youngest of the sisters, a housewife all her life, had written to America—and even then barely ten letters in all—while the others, including my father, had been afraid of corresponding with Luba. During the reign of Stalinist terror everybody knew only too well how dangerous it was to write or receive letters from relatives abroad; there were many documented cases of people being kicked out of their jobs or even thrown behind barbed wire on charges of espionage based on just such a flimsy pretext. I knew that I had relatives in America and Europe, but I never mentioned the fact when filling in official forms. Had I told the truth, I would certainly have lost my job, because my father's elder brother, Arkady

Zak, had been the Kerensky Provisional Government's ambassador to the United States in 1917, and when the Bolshevik Revolution broke out he stayed in New York.

My mother's cousin, Colonel Nikolai Limansky, had been the czar's military attaché in Washington prior to 1917, and he, too, chose not to return to Russia, but stayed in New York. None of our relatives mentioned these two names on official forms and all their lives they trembled at the prospect of being found out. For some reason, our secret had not been discovered, and now we were all able to come to meet Luba at the old, small Sheremetyevo Airport on the outskirts of Moscow.

Through the glass wall of Customs we watched her belongings being examined most thoroughly. Luba approached the glass wall and stared intently at her siblings, who had grown old over the long years of separation. She was pointing her finger at us, calling our names. Her voice was not audible, but reading her lips we could see that she had managed to recognize us all.

Luba was also met at the airport by an official representing Intourist, a young, gently smiling man who spoke fluent English. There could be no doubt that, like all Intourist employees, he was a KGB officer. I asked him to let Luba go to her hotel in my car, not the official car sent by Intourist. I explained to him that she had not seen her relatives for close to half a century and they wanted to ride with her. The officer agreed on condition that I follow his limousine. When we all climbed into my car, the tension generated by his presence dissipated and everybody heaved a sigh of relief. But we were too overwhelmed by the occasion to engage in smooth conversation, and the air in the car was filled with a mixture of laughter, tears, excited exclamations, shouts of surprise and joy. Bursting with emotion, I drove carefully on the tail of the limo, straining to hear snatches of conversation behind and beside me.

From the very first day, Luba and I developed a warm relationship. She liked the idea that her nephew was an up-and-coming doctor. "I remember that your name is Vladimir," she told me, "that you are Yuli's son and that you were born in 1929. You can address me with the familiar 'du' pronoun." We talked a lot. I listened to her stories of the American way of life, and particularly of American medicine. For me it was all new, a glimpse of a totally unknown world.

Luba was not rich, but she did bring cash gifts to all her relatives: $200 to each. She had no way of knowing that Soviet citizens had no right to own dollars. To convert the cash into commodity gifts, she took each one of us to the special Beryozka Shop, where goods were dispensed only to foreigners and only dollars were accepted in payment. The goods at the shop were far superior in quality and much cheaper than the wares offered by regular stores. It was my first trip to the Beryozka Shop and I was shocked at the difference. I felt ill at ease in the store because I was sure that we were being watched. Luba spent my gift to buy three suits, two pairs of shoes, a Japanese transistor radio, and American cigarettes. Never in my life had I possessed three suits and two pairs of good shoes; never had I smoked American cigarettes either.

Those new possessions were not only a nice gift but also symbolized the fact that I could meet my American relative. They represented a tangible process; an element of freedom.

My aunt Luba was booked into Intourist's National Hotel, across the square from the Kremlin, reserved exclusively for foreigners. I knew that each room in the hotel was bugged, and all visitors were secretly photographed, their contacts rigorously watched. Therefore, the very first day, while we were riding from the airport, I warned my aunt not to talk openly to us at her hotel room and not to be surprised at our incongruous answers should the conversation take an undesirable turn. Luba had guessed as much and fell in with our scheme. We engaged in frank discussions only at home, in my car, or during strolls when nobody was around. Luba proved to be much better informed about our life than we were about life in the United States. Still, from time to time, she would be astonished to learn from me some aspect of life in the Soviet Union she had not suspected before.

A day before she was to leave, we went for a walk in a beautiful park close to the Khimki river port near the northern border of Moscow. It was a warm summer night. We sat down on a bench under birch trees, and, somewhat abashed, Luba started talking: though I openly told her of my critical attitude toward Soviet rule, she tried not to wound my civic pride.

"I apologize in advance if I'm being offensive," she said. "I don't want to sound insulting. But tell me: if an opportunity to go to America presented itself, would you find the courage to take it?"

Her question was totally unexpected; I had never thought of it. At the time emigration from the Soviet Union was nonexistent; it was not to begin until the early seventies as a concession for the sale of American grain.

"I've never thought of leaving," I replied, "because it's simply not feasible. But even if I could, I don't think I'd want to leave Russia for good. I know that life in America is better than here: freer, richer, calmer. But for me the most important thing is not my surroundings, but my inner world, what's in my soul. I'm content with my life; I'm used to living here. I have great plans; I hope to become a really good doctor; I want to become a true scientist; I hope to become a popular poet. And I'm almost sure that I'll be able to achieve my goals."

"You're still young. You could gain what you want in a different country," Luba rejoined.

"I'm thirty-two. It's no age to start a new life. I prefer to carry on what I have already started."

"Many American doctors begin their careers at exactly your age," said Luba. "And in ten or fifteen years they become rich."

"I can't imagine what being rich is all about," I said. "But I do know the meaning of happiness: it is to set oneself a goal and to try to reach it. I hope to achieve much in my country."

Luba did not raise the subject after that, she was polite, like all the Americans. The next day she left for home. Once again we stood at the glass wall, watching Customs officials go through her personal effects. Luba was not allowed to take two cans of caviar I had given her; they were returned to me.

Walking into the interior of the airport, Luba turned around and waved to us. Her brothers and sisters were in tears. It was easy to appreciate their feelings: having met their sister for the first time in nearly fifty years, they had no hope of seeing her again. I was sad too, recalling my previous day's conversation. In some strange way our sudden talk had touched off unexpected emotions. Wouldn't it be interesting after all to enjoy the life I was not accustomed to— freedom, peace, affluence . . . ?

28

When my father turned sixty and was about to retire, he was finally given for the first time in his life a state-owned apartment: two tiny bedrooms and one smallish living room in Cheryomushky, a distant Moscow suburb. They had considered giving him an even smaller apartment, but I and my newborn son both had a residency permit to live with my parents, and so he got the larger space. Irina was registered at her mother's. So finally, after years of worrying and waiting, my parents were given their own place.

We were all quite pleased: this was already a real apartment, and not a room in a communal flat! Around New Year we moved into it and had a housewarming: our guests sat on unopened boxes of my books instead of chairs, because we hadn't any yet. The very first thing I did was to get my parents two good beds, which I managed through acquaintances of a patient friend. They had slept their entire life on one old 1 1/4 sleeper brass bed. They were extremely touched.

Irina and I couldn't have a double bed, because our bedroom was too tiny to even fit a single adult and one child's bed. I slept in the living room on a pull-out armchair.

Although my mother-in-law continued to dislike me, she told me of some cooperative apartments being built for a House of Writers. "It's expensive," she said, "and the apartments won't be completed for three or four years. But the building will be in a nice area of Moscow, near the airport subway station. The apartments there should be nice. For writers, they do their best."

"How much is it?" I asked.

"Two hundred rubles per one square meter. If they make you an apartment, it'll be approximately fifty meters."

This depressed me; I didn't have that kind of money, and would not have it for quite some time.

My mother-in-law eyed me skeptically. "You need only to put down a fifty-percent deposit."

That was also inconceivable. Nevertheless, I discussed it with Irina. The possibility of having our own apartment was our most cherished dream.

We whispered together until my mother finally asked: "What is it?" I told her. Without further questions my mother understood, in her own way.

"I'll ask Papa for money," she said. My father was thrown into confusion by the sum, but Mother insisted: "Yulya, but our children need . . ."

In three years we got that apartment. Although I had paid for it in advance, they still did not want to give it to us because the secretary of the Union of Writers wanted it for himself. History was repeating itself; the same thing had happened nearly thirty years ago with the apartment my parents had had in the city of Gorky, when the head of the local KGB took it from them. Our hopes had almost shattered. But after all these times were different, and I found a number of friends and patients who were able to get me into the office of the secretary of the Regional Committee of the Party, Yevgeny Pirogov, an impressive and powerful figure, who pleaded my cause. So I won a half-year battle, and in the spring of 1962 we moved into our apartment. Irina's and my joy was rapturous, even though my mother-in-law moved in with us. She took the largest room for herself, and left us the two smaller bedrooms. Irina and our son moved into one, and the second I converted into a library with a bed. We had been married for eight years, but still did not have a bedroom of our own.

Since our building was earmarked for writers under a special government decree, it was built to a much higher standard than regular housing: large rooms, ceilings twenty inches higher than normal, wide windows, spacious corridors and kitchens. The interior finishing was equally impressive: parquet floor without a crack, imported Polish and Czech plumbing, imported wallpaper. In terms of quality, our building could be said to occupy an intermediate position between the poor housing built for the general populace, and the luxury dwellings the government built for itself.

Next to the building there was an exclusive clinic for the writers and an exclusive kindergarten with a beautiful playground for their children and grandchildren, safeguarded from Peeping Toms by a tall fence. Also close to the house was an underground garage, an unheard-of luxury for Moscow. While car owners account for a mere 2.5 percent of the Soviet population, about 75 percent of the writers have them.

Thus in the sea of poorly built, standard five-story barracks without elevators, inhabited by ordinary folk—"the people"—there rose an island of ten-story luxury buildings for men and women of letters. It became known as "The Nest of Nobility," after Ivan Turgenev's classical novel.

No other professional group enjoys such a good life since none is so close to the rulers. The Union of Writers is part of the state propaganda machinery, one of the most important links of the huge ideological chain fettering the entire country. Aware of their importance, established writers can wangle material concessions from the authorities; of course, doctors cannot even begin to dream of attaining the writers' exalted status on the social scale.

Although I had three books of nursery rhymes published in a total of 400,000 copies, I had little access to the writers' milieu—my books were not propaganda. But Irina and I enjoyed our unusually comfortable living conditions. Our son went to the writers' kindergarten and I bought a place for my car in the writers' garage. Both feats took some wheeling and dealing. Fortunately, my mother-in-law was wise to all intrigues, and managed to make the necessary arrangements. All I had to do was shell out the money.

I disliked my new neighbors. Each of the writers held an inflated opinion of his own talent, and all of them showed excessive zeal in maintaining the rules of subordination within their union. Almost all were Communist Party members, in most cases activists.

A writer's popularity in the Soviet Union depends not so much on talent as on standing with the union brass, that is to say Party bosses. And mediocre writers are often more popular than their gifted colleagues and are published more extensively. Some of them are Jews writing under Slavic pseudonyms in order to protect themselves. I did my best to avoid them, in part because they rather unceremoniously tried to take advantage of my being a physician. Pampered by the powers that be, they took it for granted that everybody should fawn upon them.

"Listen," a neighbor would say, "my wife needs such-and-such medicine unavailable even in our writers' pharmacy. Can't you procure it for me?" Or: "I'm planning to go to a good hospital for examination. Tell me which one I should go to and help me be admitted there."

It was not easy to meet their demands, particularly since each request entailed new ones.

There was a small group of dissident writers among our neighbors. They were not Party members, preferring to listen to the dictates of their consciences. Accordingly, their books were rarely published, so they were poorer than their servile brethren and virtually unknown. They formed a closed circle inaccessible to outsiders.

Every evening, my neighbors promenaded in small groups, endlessly talking among themselves. "Will they ever tire of chatter?" I often wondered.

Their wives, too, spent much time either outdoors, attending to their children and grandchildren, or at their exclusive clinic, tormenting the doctors with vague complaints of strange aches and ill-defined disturbances. They loved medical attention, maybe for lack of anything better to do. Almost none of the writers' wives work —an oddity in the Soviet Union—the median income for writers is twice the national average.

Neither Irina nor I acquired any friends among our neighbors; with one exception: Konstantin (Kostya) Bogatyrev, forty-five, our fifth-floor neighbor, a poet and German translator. He was an interesting and pleasant conversationalist and never beseiged me with medical inquiries or requests. On those occasions when I had a few hours of leisure, I would invite him for a walk to listen to his stories. In 1948, he was sentenced to ten years for plotting to assassinate Stalin. Several dozen Moscow University students were charged with the same crime; one of them, a girl named Nina, lived in Arbat Street. She had a spacious apartment in an old, stately building, and her friends never missed an opportunity to party at Nina's. On the way from the Kremlin to his country house Stalin usually rode past Nina's building, so the entire area crawled with KGB agents and many of the girl's neighbors were police informers. One of them informed the authorities of the frequent gatherings in her apartment.

They were all arrested, along with a group of students from several other colleges. Three of them were executed, the rest had their death sentences commuted to ten years' imprisonment. But Kostya preferred to speak of other things. He was an active member of the dissident movement and a friend of its leader, the physicist Andrei Sakharov (Kostya had gone to school with Sakharov's wife, Yelena Bonner, and they had remained friends ever since). He liked to tell me what a wonderful man Sakharov was and related numerous episodes from Sakharov's life. Though not a dissident, I nevertheless felt profound respect and admiration for those who had embarked upon that path of sure martyrdom. Though he never took part in demonstrations and shunned other dissident activities, Kostya was often visited at his apartment by Western writers, notables of the world of art and active champions of democratic liberties, mostly West Germans. Since Kostya was officially known as their translator, the KGB reluctantly tolerated such visits but watched them with unrelenting vigilance. Among Kostya's guests was Nobel Laureate Heinrich Boll, with whom he was on friendly terms. During the sixties, when Boll was extensively published in the Soviet Union, he frequented Moscow.

Each time Western guests came to see Bogatyrev, a Volga car with KGB license plates and three or four plainclothesmen inside would park for hours at the entrance to our building, with the police captain whose beat included the writer's house hovering nearby. He always hung around our house and knew everything about everybody, but foreign guests added to his troubles.

Kostya feared nothing. And really, why should he be afraid of anything after surviving a death sentence?

On many occasions, I heard his name mentioned in the Russian-language Voice of America and BBC broadcasts, and so realized how prominent he was. I learned from those programs that an increasing number of dissidents' manuscripts were being smuggled to the West and published there, and could not help noticing that the publication of each new book almost invariably followed a visit of foreign guests to Kostya Bogatyrev's apartment. Was he involved? Aware of the tremendous risk he ran, I never asked him that question. But I was sure nonetheless that it was he who was passing on the manuscripts to the free world. Later those books in printed form would turn up in his hands and he would give me some of them to read—for one or two nights only, because a lot of people waited for their turn.

So, life was in full swing in our house: the writers promenaded, chattering about trifling matters; their wives were busy with real and imaginary ailments; foreign guests came and went, carrying away forbidden books. And the hawk-eyed police captain watched it all.

29

■ My mother brought me to the university for the first time when
I was just ten days old. Since then any university or other center
of learning or science has filled me with trepidation. That was exactly
my feeling one day in 1962, when I entered the Central Institute of
Traumatology and Orthopedics (CITO). At thirty-two, I was the
youngest member of the senior staff. But for all its advantages, my
situation had some disadvantages too, for the veteran doctors, who
had not achieved comparable status until their fifties, met me with
a good deal of antagonism.

The CITO was a large institution: four hundred orthopedic
beds and a lot of scientific laboratories. It was housed in an old
four-story brick building erected almost a century ago as a hostel for
women workers of a textile factory in Tyoply Pereoulok. After the
Revolution the factory was nationalized and renamed Red Rose. Our
quarters were indescribably cramped and inconvenient.

Jews accounted for a fairly large proportion of the staff—
about 15 percent, many of them filling important positions of heads
of departments or laboratories. It was an exceptional situation
wholly attributable to Dr. Nikolai Priorov, the former director of the
institute. A pure ethnic Russian of peasant stock, Dr. Priorov, far
from being anti-Semitic, even gave refuge and comfort to Jews fired
from other institutions. How he managed to get away with this
highly unusual practice is a mystery. An even greater mystery is the
fact that he was not an anti-Semite. At the CITO, I met a group of
Jewish professors who had been fired from my medical school long
ago, when I was still a student: A. Kaplan, V. Shlapobersky, M.
Mikhelman, R. Ginsburg, and A. Dvorkin. They set the scientific
tone for the Institute.

The laboratory equipment was scanty and obsolete; the research by and large boiled down to a recapitulation of what had been
done in the West fifteen or twenty years previously. Still, it was by
no means useless, for without it our backwardness would have been
much more pronounced. Thus Professor A. Kaplan wrote a book on
the treatment of fractures that was largely a rehash of the world-
renowned textbook by Sir Reginald Watson-Jones, the giant of Brit-

ish orthopedics. But were it not for Dr. Kaplan's book, Russian orthopedists would have learned the Briton's ideas much later. Similarly, Dr. V. Shlapobersky pioneered Russian research into skeletal tumors at a time when the West abounded in textbooks on the subject. But without him, we would have been further behind. Besides, none of them cared to mention that many of their "findings" had been borrowed from Western counterparts. Thus, through their plagiarisms, they fostered belated scientific progress in orthopedics. I am sure that given different circumstances and better conditions, those professors could have mounted a successful challenge to Western supremacy; it was their misfortune, not their fault, that they had to follow trails blazed by others.

Scared by their previous experience, they were extremely cautious and tried as best they could to avoid any semblance of conflict with the institute's management and Party Committee. On seeing me for the first time, Dr. Shlapobersky immediately pressed a finger to his lips and eloquently hissed: "Tsh-sh-sh-sh! . . ." implying that keeping mum was the name of the game for the Jews.

Over a decade had passed since the high point of Stalin's anti-Semitic tidal wave, marked by the jailing of the "Kremlin doctors" and the firing of thousands of Jewish physicians, but they were still deeply demoralized. It was a lifelong psychic wound. And they knew that the horrible past could very well recur. Their protector, the old CITO director, was dead, while the new director, Dr. M. Volkov, was not to be trusted: at the height of the anti-Semitic drive, when they were being kicked out of the medical school, he had been secretary of the Party Committee. And though now he treated them with utmost deference, the Jewish professors knew that they were not guaranteed against a fresh outburst of persecution.

The CITO's residency program included about twenty young physicians, of whom only two were Jews though many more applied for positions. The new director turned them down. On the other hand, young Party members were openly favored and everything was done to further their careers. One of the residents was twenty-seven-year-old Dr. Anatoly Pechenkin, a stocky blond fellow who had no surgical experience but did have a Party member's card. For this reason he was pampered as no other resident: an easy work schedule was worked out for him; he was relieved of many duties compulsory for the rest of the residents; and he was forever away attending an assortment of Party conferences, meetings, and gatherings. Later he was made a member of the Party Committee—a huge step forward. Since that momentous event he has all but stopped working as a physician. But nobody minded. On the contrary, the pampering, if anything, intensified.

Once I witnessed a ludicrous scene. Dr. Pechenkin entered Dr. Kaplan's office and asked him to lend him a hand in drawing up an outline for a research paper.

"But of course, dear Dr. Pechenkin, of course." The old professor jumped up from his chair. "Let's do it right away."

"But you're busy with Dr. Golyakhovsky."

"Never mind, it's a trifling matter," Dr. Kaplan said hurriedly, though in fact we had been discussing urgent business.

"I don't know how to start," said the inexperienced Pechenkin.

"That's exactly what we'll do; we'll discuss the beginning and go through with the whole thing."

"Much obliged, but I can't do it now. I have to attend a Party Committee meeting."

"Oh, I see. . . . You know what? Why don't you go to the meeting and leave your notes here; I'll take care of the rest."

Pechenkin put his notes on Dr. Kaplan's desk and left. Kaplan carefully shut the door behind him and said sarcastically:

"So?! You know what? I'll have to write a paper for this illiterate free-loader. How do you like it? I have to do it for this good-for-nothing ignoramus. And he will never know anything, because *he doesn't need knowledge.*"

Admittedly, Pechenkin was not generously endowed with brains. But the way he was pampered made even the most elementary working ability irrelevant. He was turning into a sloth and rapidly putting on weight; his face acquired the cast of total indifference characteristic of an up-and-coming Party hack.

Another young resident, Dr. Vladimir Mikhailenko, was my assistant, but as secretary of the Komsomol Committee he was rarely available for medical duty. Because of that we clashed frequently. He heard my reprimands in stony silence. Once I asked him, "What are your plans for the future?"

"My plan is simple: to join the Party and try to land an assignment abroad for a couple of years. I think it can be done; I've already put out the feelers. Then, when I come back, I'll buy a car and a cooperative apartment and start looking for a better job."

Unquestionably the plan was realistic and firmly rooted in his philosophy: to advance in life with the help of his Party affiliation. There was no medical factor in his plan; never once did he mention that he would "study," "acquire the know-how," or "learn." His aim was to take without giving anything in return. The Party was an excellent school for proponents of such an attitude.

At long last, our institute was given new accommodations: a large six-story building on Priorova Street in northwest Moscow. It took us six months to move into our new quarters. The builders who had worked on the site were recalled for some other crash project and left the building uncompleted. When we came there for the first time, we found that the rooms were full of litter, no doors were hung in doorways, closets were half-completed, and half of the building was unpainted. The physicians and researchers together with the nurses, laboratory technicians, and technologists had to take over where the construction workers had left off. For six months I worked as a carpenter, specializing in the completion of closets. Every morning as I arrived at the institute, I donned soiled overalls and took up the tools of my new trade: a saw, a plane, a hammer and nails.

The old professors, too, scraped off paint from windowsills and carried litter from the rooms. When there were only Jews around, Dr. Kaplan would say, "You know what? I see almost no difference between what I am doing here and what my coreligionists were forced to do in concentration camps under Stalin and the Nazis. No, it will never end. . . ."

And Dr. Shlapobersky would press a paint-smeared finger to his lips and hiss:

"Tsh-sh-sh-sh! . . ."

30

When our son grew up a little and went to kindergarten, Irina landed a job, the position of a lab technician paying 90 rubles per month at a laboratory set up for the study of allergies. It was the first and only laboratory of its kind in the whole country, founded some thirty years after similar institutions had mushroomed in the West. The laboratory director, Dr. A. Adoh, was regarded as Russia's pioneer in the subject, although his papers by and large rehashed old Western research. Still, he should be given credit for having pressured medical bureaucrats into permitting at least a semblance of such studies.

The laboratory boasted its own accommodations—an old stable at the century-old Municipal Hospital #1 on Lenin Prospect. It was a squat building that had subsided into the ground over its long life. The horse stalls were converted to lab rooms. The laboratory was appointed scantily, to put it mildly: all apparatus was Russian-made and almost nothing worked properly. Returning from work, Irina told me that her centrifuges jerked spasmodically instead of turning; the refrigeration chambers refused to maintain constant temperatures; and they were short of all materials including graduated glass pipettes. Yet the laboratory enjoyed a high rating at the Academy of Medical Sciences because it generated a steady stream of research papers and doctoral theses. The researchers conducted experiments, and if their results were at variance with what had long been common knowledge in the West, they simply scratched their results and entered the correct Western figures in their reports.

While escorting his foreign counterparts from Eastern Europe, where the study of allergies enjoyed a higher standing, Dr. Adoh liked to banter: "See, here they once kept horses. Yes, sir! And now you see my horses sitting at their microscopes. Yes, sir!"

The laboratory director was notorious for his nasty disposition, and almost all of his staff developed a "moral allergy" to him, that is to say they hated his guts. My Irina was sometimes so exasperated that she came home in tears. Dr. Adoh's temper was offset to a certain extent by a very knowledgeable and calm man, Dr.

Alexander Poner, who helped Irina a lot and did much to brighten up her life on the job.

At home, a sea-change occurred: at the age of fifty-seven, my mother-in-law married a sixty-seven-year-old musician, a violist. It was an incredibly lucky break for us: at long last—and not a moment too soon—we got rid of her. Irina was even happier than I.

My mother-in-law moved in with her beloved in a nearby building, and now the whole apartment was completely at our disposal. Thus, after twelve years of marriage, we finally had a true-blue separate bedroom that we could call our own. And an added benefit: Mother-in-law no longer scampered about the apartment, treading on our nerves with her presence and remarks.

We acquired new friends: a Russian couple from Holland, Lev and Natasha Sanitsky, both past fifty. They had been born in Russia, but soon after the Revolution their parents fled to Europe and they were both raised in Holland. They had spent many years outside Russia, but were addicted to all things Russian. In Holland, Lev was employed at a large construction company that had extensive business dealings with Moscow. Since he spoke Russian, the company frequently dispatched him to the Soviet Union to escort Dutch experts, negotiate trade deals, and conduct joint research with Soviet experts. Accordingly, he was the ward of the State Committee for Science and Technology, a cross between a scientific agency and an intelligence outfit, staffed almost exclusively by KGB operatives.

We were introduced by our neighbor, Kostya Bogatyrev. Lev and Natasha were nice people, and Irina and I enjoyed having them to our home. For their part, they often brought along other Dutchmen who came to Moscow on business. In this way almost all the employees of Lev's company marched through our apartment. Needless to say, it was dangerous because our neighbors could rat to the police, or our police supervisor, a captain, was likely to find out. In fact, he probably did find out about our "unauthorized contacts with foreigners."

The Sanitskys told us much about Europe in general and beautiful Holland in particular. We dreamed of visiting Holland one day, though we knew that our dream had no chance of coming true. The Sanitskys brought free-world magazines and we marveled at Western life, so unlike ours. They also brought wonderful toys for our son, the likes of which Russia has never seen. Lest our son tell his pals about the origin of his gifts, we deceived him by saying that the toys came from Nikopol, a small town in southern Ukraine. At his tender age he did not care where the toys came from as long as they were his to play with.

Lev photographed us in the country where we took him in our car, and later brought us the color prints of his snapshots. Color photography was all but unknown in Russia, and the pictures were so exotic that even we looked like foreigners in them.

Lev also kept me supplied with aromatic Dutch pipe tobacco unavailable in Russia, and for many years I puffed at my pipe filled with it. For ten years our friendship had grown steadily, to the point that we started addressing each other with a familiar Russian pronoun used only among very close friends.

"Have you gotten anywhere in your negotiations on scientific cooperation between your firm and Russian scientists and engineers?" I asked him.

"They're dragging their feet."

"Believe me," I'd say, "they don't care a hoot for any kind of cooperation; what they're after is contact with your people to secure one more foothold in Holland."

"Yeah, looks like it," he would agree. And we would both laugh. We were absolutely frank with each other.

In order to feed our Dutch friends well, I scrambled to buy special provisions and, above all, good meat. I procured it from one of my patients, a butcher named Slavka. He was a giant man, almost six foot seven, weighing over three hundred pounds. On each of my visits, I crept surreptitiously through the back door into the room where he cut meat. Hundreds of people stood in line in the store, while down below Slavka chopped and cut the choicest pieces for me. With his daily rations of close to half a gallon of vodka, he was forever drunk. Whenever he saw me he never failed to open a fresh bottle and insist that we have a drink together. I hated the prospect of either drinking or chatting with Slavka, but I needed meat and had to succumb.

The butcher's occupation is very profitable in Russia. Slavka sold at premium almost half the meat he handled and in consequence was far more affluent than I. From time to time, the police raided the store and beseiged the butcher with questions on how much meat

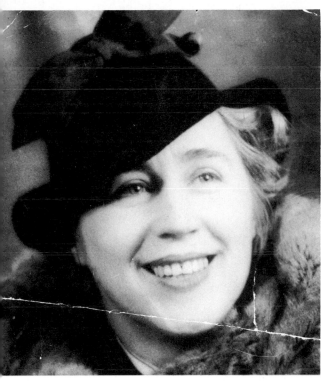

My mother, 1939.

My father,
a World War II veteran,
1975.

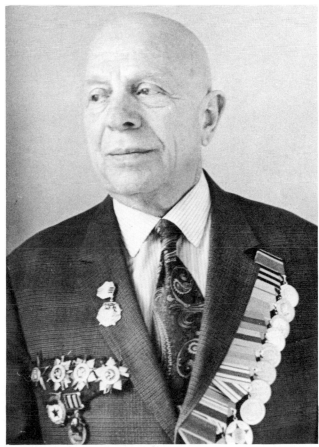

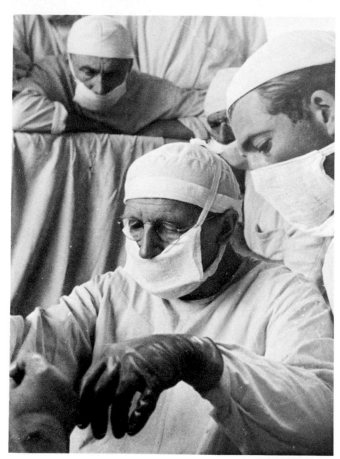

Doctor Sergi Yudin
performs an operation.

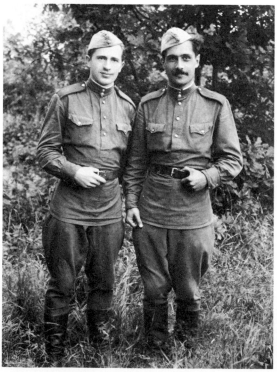

The author *(left)* with a
medical student as short-term
army privates, 1952.

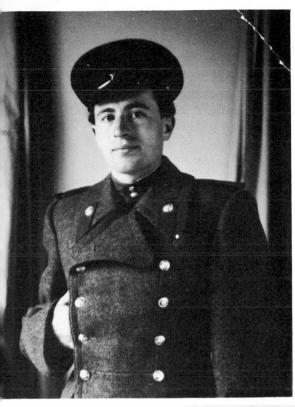

The author as junior doctor
of the regiment, 1954.

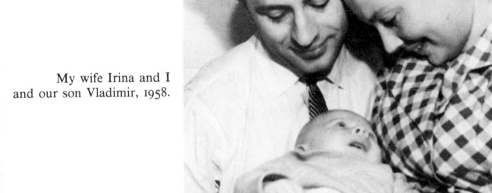

My wife Irina and I
and our son Vladimir, 1958.

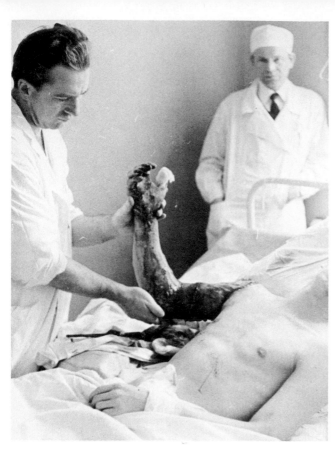

At the bedside of the
first patient whose arm
I reattached, 1969.

The funeral of Boris Pasternak at Peredelkino, 1960.

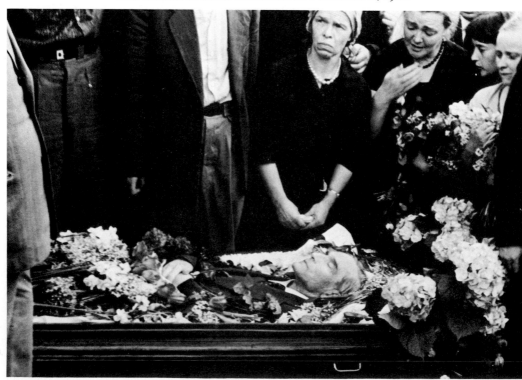

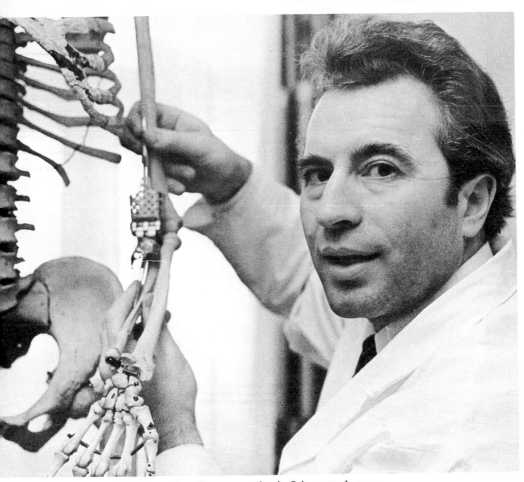

Holding the elbow prosthesis I invented, 1971.

Examining the patient after the replacement of the
elbow joint with the prosthesis, 1971.

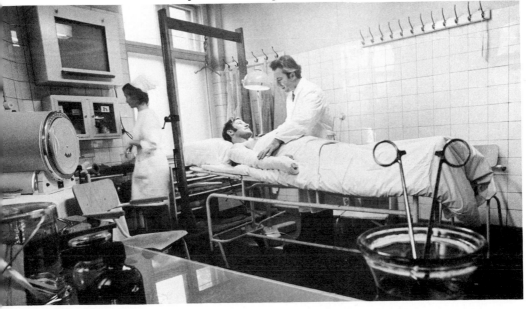

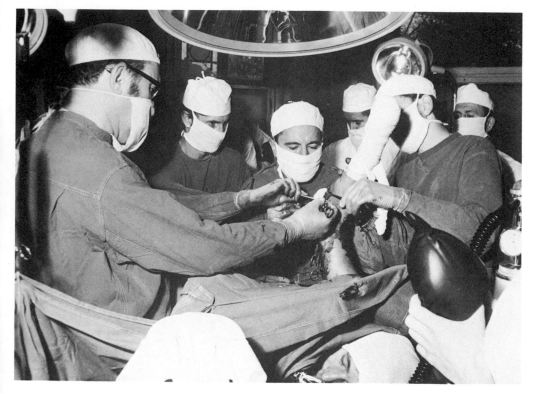

Performing the operation in East Germany, 1971.

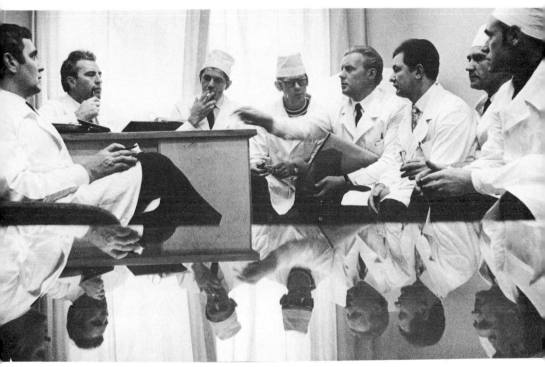

The author as director of the Department of Orthopedics, at a meeting with his staff, Moscow, 1973. *From left:* Dr. V. Mikhailenko, Dr. V. Golyakhovsky, Dr. N. Burlakov, Dr. G. Artemov, Dr. A. Pechonkin, Dr. G. Valentzev, Dr. V. Lukin, Dr. V. Kosmatov.

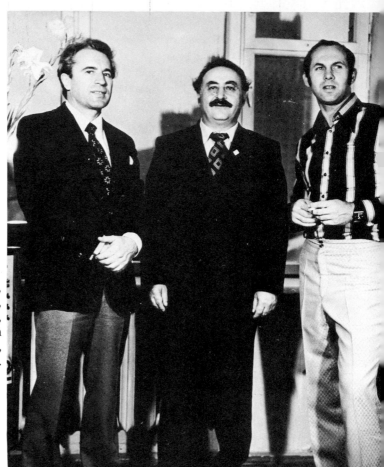

The author,
Dr. Ilizarov,
and V. Brumel,
Olympic champion
in the high jump,
Moscow, 1974.

With medical students, Moscow, 1976.

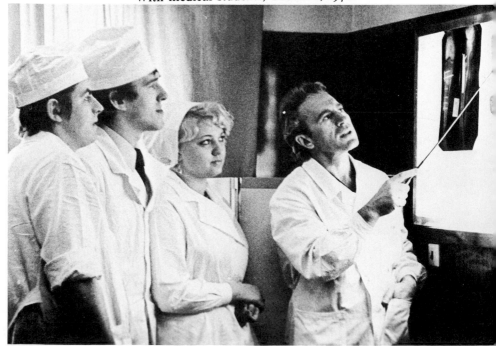

had been supplied to the store, how much had been sold, how much money had been supplied to the store, how much money there was in the cash register. But the upshot of such raids was always the same: Slavka would pass around bribes, ply the enforcement officers with vodka, and send them away with packages containing choice cuts of meat.

Our Dutch guests always praised Irina's cooking and remarked in particular that Russian meat was very good. They did not know that the meat they enjoyed so much was obtained at the price of waiting at the back door of the store and hobnobbing with the boisterous Slavka; that those pieces were selected from a mound of third-grade frozen meat; and that hundreds of people waited patiently for hours for a chance to grab the rejects.

Finally, I told my friend Lev how I procured the meat. He answered, "You know, if you told it to my countrymen, they wouldn't believe you. Meat is so plentiful in Holland that it's beyond them to imagine that buying it can be such a taxing endeavor, involving so much humiliation, particularly for a doctor. No, it's a special feature of you Russians. You have too many complexes, of which masochism holds pride of place."

To a certain extent he was right; Russian history is that of a people who have suffered continuously for centuries and suffer to this day without ever having done anything to end their ordeal.

There was much in life that challenged my imagination and provoked my thought. Finally I decided to put down my observations and ideas in writing. In this way I started my diary. At the end of each day, late at night or sometimes early in the morning, I wrote down my impressions for the day past. It has become my lifelong habit. When I read my diary for the first year, I was surprised to find out how bitterly anti-Soviet it was. I did not stop my diary, but I learned to hide it.

31

Dr. Lev Landau, the renowned Jewish Soviet scientist, winner of the 1962 Nobel Prize, member of the academies of sciences of many countries, including the U.S. and the U.S.S.R., was badly hurt in an automobile accident in Moscow on January 7, 1962. As a result he had a very complicated fracture of the pelvis bones and lost a lot of blood.

The ambulance brought the injured man to the emergency department of Hospital #50 housed in Building #3, a newly built eight-story edifice. The ambulance did not carry special anti-shock equipment; it was not a "resuscomobile" with a crew of resuscitation specialists. Dr. Landau was simply laid on a stretcher inside the car and given shots of cardiac drugs—Cardiamine and Strophanthin. That was the extent of the first aid he received though he urgently needed specific shock treatment; his life hung in the balance.

The required therapy could only be provided by a hospital equipped with the latest in medical technology. At that time, Hospital #50 was regarded as among the best of new medical institutions in Moscow; all its facilities were brand new. I knew the hospital well and visited it on many occasions, for my father was chief surgeon at it's Building #2.

And yet, the hospital had no resuscitation department, no life-support equipment. All it had was a multitude of plain rooms with uncomfortable iron beds devoid of even backrest boards, let alone devices for controlling the patient's position. There were no monitors, no breathing-control equipment. Many valuable hours and days were irretrievably lost while frantic efforts were mounted to provide proper medical care to Landau.

No sooner had Moscow's grapevine carried the news of who was dying than equipment started to flow to Hospital #50 from all over the city. Every hour a new apparatus arrived, but the patient's body was not fit to wait until proper conditions were in place to overcome the shock; it could not adapt itself to the vagaries of Soviet bureaucratic boondoggle. Landau was sinking by the hour.

I brought him the precious Swedish-made Engstrom breathing-control apparatus from our Botkin Hospital, possibly the only unit of its kind in Moscow (except, of course, in the Kremlin Hospital). The unit worked around the clock for three weeks, stabilizing Landau's tortured breathing.

I cannot give enough credit to Landau's colleagues, the physicists. From the start, all of them, led by Dr. Pyotr Kapitsa, realized what had to be done if their friend was to survive. So they combed Moscow for the precious equipment and pulled strings all over the world for the required medicines. They called all the luminaries of physics in America and Europe, beseeching them to send over the drugs that were simply unavailable at Moscow's hospitals and pharmacies. It is possible that such drugs were in stock at the Kremlin Pharmacy, but Dr. Landau received no help from that quarter. As soon as Landau's condition improved sufficiently to permit moving him, he was transferred to the Burdenko Institute of Neurosurgery. Physicians and physicists alike were concerned about Landau's brain. For a long time he had been unconscious, and then it took a longer time to regain his speech.

The right side of his pelvis was displaced, shortening his right leg. When he was started on a program to learn to walk again, the patient suffered excruciating difficulties; with each step he leaned too far to the right and literally lost his balance. He was supported by attendants, and custom-made orthopedic shoes were provided, but such measures helped hardly at all. Besides, due to the permanent displacement of the pelvic and abdominal organs, and above all the intestines, Landau suffered unrelenting stomachaches. The complaint "I've got a stomachache" dominated his conversations. Many surgeons examined him, but no one could alleviate the condition, which further damaged his psyche, already severely scarred by the accident.

Thus in the year he won the Nobel Prize, a lot of people thought privately that he was no longer normal. His "stomachache" refrain misled everybody. I treated him for several years and came to understand how extraordinarily difficult it was for him to endure such pain.

Lev Landau was truly a genius. Quite possibly, he was the only man of genius I have ever known. He was hospitalized in 1967 at the Central Institute of Traumatology and Orthopedics, where I worked at the time, and was entrusted to my care. I had many occasions to talk to the great man. Paradoxical though it may seem, many physicians and nurses thought he was deranged. He did seem abnormal because his mind was constantly immersed in a world totally beyond their ken. He stayed at our hospital for two months, paying little if any attention to the people around him—who needs better proof of imbecility? He was accommodated in a small room next to the chief physician's office where I kept my things. I, too, failed to elicit much of Landau's interest, but his occasional casual remarks clearly demonstrated his sanity and the remarkable depth of his vision. For instance, once I left for Tashkent for a short while to help the victims of an earthquake that devastated the city in June 1967. As soon as I returned to Moscow, I came to the hospital and dropped by to see Landau. He was poring over a book on himself in English and paid scant attention to me. He greeted me superficially and turned his attention back to the book. I sat down on his bed and told him that I had just returned from the nearly leveled city. Landau asked me, "Much destruction?"

"A lot," I said. "So many houses destroyed. . . ."

"Come to think of it," he said, "the earthquake measured eight on the Richter scale, which only runs to nine." He thought it over, came to some silent conclusion, and resumed his reading.

Dr. Kapitsa came to our institute several times and asked us to help him talk Landau into resuming his work. He had made several attempts, but Dau, as Landau was widely called, greeted all such requests with silence.

I tried to raise the question of work with Landau on several occasions. Not that I overrated the importance he would attach to my opinion, but I hoped that the peculiar patient-to-doctor relationship would make him hear my tiny squeak. Dau listened to me in silence.

"Lev Davidovich," I said, "your general condition will definitely improve if you resume work little by little. Why don't you start working right here, at the hospital. We'll provide a proper environment and allow all your assistants to visit you freely. Would you like that?"

"I can't," Dau replied.

"Why?"

"I've got a stomachache."

"We'll administer all necessary medication and you will see how much better you'll feel once you start working. . . ."

Apparently Dau got bored. All of a sudden, he laughed and asked me, "Have you heard this one? The boss is dictating a letter to his secretary: 'On Wednesday, we'll be holding . . .' when suddenly she asks him, 'How do you spell Wednesday? "Wensday" or "Wennsday"?' He mulls it over for a minute and then says: 'Make it Thursday.' "

My famous patient died on April 1, 1968, six years and four months after the accident. He was buried in Moscow in the Novodevichye Cemetery, where Russia has traditionally laid to rest its immortals. Landau's grave is very close to Khrushchev's, but a monument was not erected on the physicist's grave until seven years later—thanks largely to propitious circumstances.

32

In 1965, I was dispatched by the Ministry of Public Health to the Siberian town of Kurgan to investigate Dr. Gabriel Ilizarov, an orthopedic surgeon. In 1951 Dr. Ilizarov had pioneered the use of external fixation apparatus for treating bone fractures. He drove special pins through the bone and secured the pins at the ends with metal rings of his own design. Manipulating the rings, drawing apart and displacing them, Dr. Ilizarov aligned and immobilized the broken bone fragments. Using this technique he reported extraordinary results.

For over a decade, Dr. Ilizarov, a forty-year-old Tat (the Tats are a small group of Jews in the Caucasus) tried to prove that his apparatus and method were superior to the conventional techniques used in the country. But none of the Moscow professors deigned to listen to that insignificant physician from a tiny, provincial town. Undeterred, the Kurgan surgeon continued to pester bureaucrats at the Ministry and the management of our Orthopedics Institute. At last his perseverance bore fruit: a decision was made to send someone to Kurgan to see what that insistent Dr. Ilizarov was doing and check his results.

The trip to Kurgan fell to me. The institute bosses gave me this parting briefing: "Don't trust his stories one bit; he's a crook. Go to the hospital and personally examine every patient, writing down notes on each case. It's high time that con artist was exposed."

But Dr. Kaplan, my immediate superior, gave me different instructions: "You know what? That Ilizarov fellow is by no means the fool he's portrayed. Try to be objective. Who knows, maybe there's something of value in his method. But be careful: he is a Jew."

Kurgan was the place where the first Russian revolutionaries were exiled after the abortive December 1825 uprising. Over the ensuing 140 years, it had undergone little, if any, change and was still essentially a town of single-story log huts. Even the houses of the Decembrists were still standing, but now they served as museums.

The Kurgan airport was a vast meadow with a single-story log hut on its edge. It could only receive small planes. I was accompanied on my flight by several men on crutches—Dr. Ilizarov's patients. Over the years, his fame had spread, and patients from all over the country poured into Kurgan, seeking deliverance from their misery. They learned about the existence of Dr. Ilizarov only from the grapevine, swapping stories about the miracles performed by the "Magician from Kurgan." Dr. Ilizarov met me at the airport in his battered minicar and drove me to the four-story Moscow Hotel, the only new building in the town. Almost half the guests were his patients, who either waited for their turn to be hospitalized or wore corrective contraptions and were waiting for them to be removed.

For a month I worked side by side with Dr. Ilizarov in his tiny hospital. The "Hospital for War Invalids," as it was known officially, was a two-story wooden house with stove heating, distinguished primarily by its cramped and indescribably awful conditions. The operating room was very small, dark, and hot. While we were operating, a woman nurse's aide would barge in, carrying a heap of logs. We cut and sewed while she knelt at the stove, wearing a soiled gown atop a parka, stoking the burning wood.

Ilizarov was an outstanding surgeon; he operated economically, briskly, and precisely. An osteotomy of the tibia with the application of an external fixation apparatus took him an incredibly short twenty minutes. I am sure only his brilliant surgical technique spared his patients the complications that were likely to develop under those horrible conditions. Apart from his fantastic surgical proficiency, everything else in the hospital was primitive in the extreme. The X-ray pictures were of such poor quality that quite often one could not even tell what it was they showed.

All the modifications of his apparatus were made for Dr. Ilizarov by his grateful patients at their factories and smuggled out a part at a time. Nothing of the requisite technology was manufactured by the medical industry. Naturally, he had to overcome many difficulties, but somehow or other he always managed to prevail.

The results of Dr. Ilizarov's method were as incredible as his surgical brilliance. He could stretch bones by as much as twenty-five centimeters! I personally checked all cases, examining the patients and measuring the fracture sites with a ruler, hardly able to believe my eyes. I was full of admiration for the "Magician from Kurgan" and did not try to hold my feelings back. Initially he treated me with suspicion, but finally he determined that I could be trusted; the ice melted and we became friends.

I brought back to Moscow my records of patient examinations and delivered a report on my impressions/findings. I showed sketches of some of Dr. Ilizarov's original methods and tried to persuade our brass that the Kurgan surgeon deserved all the help possible to develop his ideas. All was in vain. Instead of studying the sketches and listening to my explanations, they told me, "Are you crazy, talking about twelve-inch bone stretching? You should know better than to spread this nonsense. And in general, your judgment is faulty because, quite obviously, you lack objectivity in assessing that crook."

The only result was that I acquired powerful enemies at the institute for commending Dr. Ilizarov's work. I was even punished by demotion to a much more humble position, that of a consulting surgeon at an outpatient department.

Dr. Kaplan once called me into his office, carefully shut the door, and told me: "You know what? That Ilizarov fellow will get what he wants, you mark my word. They'll all be jealous of him yet. Yes, yes. Because he's a very persistent guy."

At that time, Valery Brumel, a professional high-jumper, was the world's premier athlete, an Olympic champion, a world champion, even a U.S. national champion, for it was in America that he had established his record of two meters twenty-eight centimeters, considered then nothing short of phenomenal.

One night in the summer of 1967, Valery Brumel rode a motorcycle driven by a friend. An accident occurred and his right foot was run over by the motorcycle. He sustained open fractures of both shinbones, the wound was contaminated, the bones were crushed to a pulp. I was called at home by Tanya Katkovsky, my old friend. She was Brumel's girlfriend and planned to marry him. Tanya sought my advice: Valery was dissatisfied with the treatment he was getting but didn't know what to do. I told her, "He should go to the town of Kurgan to seek out Dr. Ilizarov. He is the only one who can save Valery's leg."

Brumel complied with my counsel and went to Ilizarov. The Kurgan surgeon performed a brilliant operation and a year later Brumel could clear two meters.

That success catapulted Ilizarov to national prominence. Sports journalists started to write about Brumel's miraculous recovery and about his savior, the surgeon from Kurgan. Soon Ilizarov's fame eclipsed that of Brumel himself. Celebrities came in a stream to Kurgan. When General of the Army Beloborodov, Commander of the Moscow Military District and one of the most powerful Soviet soldiers, sustained a hip fracture in an auto accident, he was taken to Dr. Ilizarov. Soon thereafter Politburo member Alexander Shelepin called the Minister of Health and ordered him to implement Ilizarov's method of fracture treatment by use of external fixation apparatus. In his turn, the Minister called Dr. M. Volkov, director of our institute, and the next morning the frightened Dr. Volkov came to me and told me to start using Ilizarov's procedures right away since, having been taught by Ilizarov himself, I was the only one who could do it.

"I'm surprised you've procrastinated so long in introducing this advanced technique at our institute," the director reproved me.

I stood speechless: wasn't I the one who had been punished for praising Ilizarov's work? How in hell could I have implemented his method against the wishes of the management?

My friendship with Ilizarov remained firm. Sometimes I would refer patients to him; at other times he would call me from Kurgan with a request to operate on someone or other. Thus, he referred to me a young navy lieutenant named Pestrikov with a chronic shoulder dislocation who had undergone two unsuccessful operations at the Kremlin Hospital. Ilizarov told me: "You're better than I am at such operations. Try to help the young sailor stay in the navy. His dad's a big shot who would be of use to you."

I succeeded where the Kremlin surgeons had failed. Lieutenant Pestrikov's "big-shot dad" personally came to express his gratitude and assured me that he would always be at my service.

In the meantime Ilizarov acquired yet another celebrity patient. The composer Dmitri Shostakovich now came to Kurgan at regular intervals. He suffered severe backaches and Ilizarov was the only doctor who was able to alleviate the pain, if only for a time. The surgeon and the composer became friends. They had several things in common: both were outstanding personalities, and both had had to pay a high price for success.

Ilizarov introduced me to Shostakovich. I judged him to be a very complicated man. He spoke sparingly and nervously, swallowing words and coming alive only on the subject of soccer, of which he was a fervent fan.

I stared at Shostakovich in awe; for me he was a living miracle. Since early adolescence I have adored classical music more than any other form of art. Aside from love, music has always been my greatest passion. I knew that sitting next to me was a great composer. I always tried to sneak to the premieres of his new symphonies. Each of them, as a rule, was the only performance, because practically all his compositions were promptly banned by the powers that be. Shostakovich attained extraordinary depth and expressiveness in enunciating, through music, a humanity that was at variance with communist ideology but in complete harmony with the emotions of the Russian intellectual. That is why Shostakovich has always been *the* composer of Russia, just as Boris Pasternak was the country's true poet.

In the eyes of Stalin and his cohorts and successors, even those who, like Nikita Khrushchev or Leonid Brezhnev, were not made in Stalin's mold, the only function of art was singing praise to the state. As far as they were concerned, the great composer was bound to sing in unison with them. Thus, the only creation by Shostakovich upon which official recognition was bestowed was his Seventh (Leningrad) Symphony, which reflected the composer's patriotic feelings during the fight against the Nazis.

I felt like kneeling before Shostakovich. Instead I could not help thinking that he himself had been forced to crawl before the dictators all his life. His career had unfolded before my eyes; I had listened to his new compositions and read the scathing criticisms in reviews issued by the Central Committee of the Communist Party that took aim not only at his music but at his very soul. In this respect the fate of Shostakovich closely paralleled that of Pasternak: both were persecuted, hounded, and humiliated; both suffered, but both loved Russia more than themselves and declined to leave it.

By the end of his life the authorities finally relented and acknowledged the composer's greatness. He was showered with the highest awards and decorations and allowed to take an imposing managerial position at the Composers' Union; strange as it may seem, Shostakovich craved positions of responsibility. He was made chairman of the Composers' Union of the Russian Federation.

In fact Shostakovich was not much more than a figurehead because Tikhon Khrennikov, another composer, who was a member of the Central Committee and the Supreme Soviet, wielded all real power. A power struggle between them ensued. But it was no contest; a member of the ruling elite, Khrennikov was by far the stronger. Shostakovich garnered little if any advantage from his official position; as before, his new symphonies were allowed just one performance.

In the late sixties and early seventies, with the help of Dr. Ilizarov, Shostakovich managed to hold his ground against severe pain in his lower back and legs. But finally the composer's health collapsed. On the rare occasions that I met him I never failed to notice that he had increasing difficulty in keeping his body upright and walking; he was almost always propped up by his young wife. At last he found walking so difficult and experienced such excruciating pain that he could no longer leave his apartment in the musicians' cooperative building on Ogaryova Street. His disease of the spinal nerves was a systematic affliction. I am convinced that his ailment must have been exacerbated by the enormously painful ordeal he had been made to suffer all through his life.

33

In 1965, my boss gave me the subject for a D.Sc. (Doctor of Science) thesis. I had long besieged him with requests for a scientific project until one day he summoned me into his presence.

"Do you want to hear something?" he asked.

"Of course."

"Elbow joint."

"What about elbow joint?"

"Your subject for a thesis."

"Thanks. But what exactly should I study about the elbow joint?"

"Injuries."

"Which ones? There are so many varieties: dislocations, fractures of all sorts . . . !"

"All of them!"

To tell the truth, the subject was overwhelming. Orthopedists know that elbow joint injuries are extremely varied and sometimes very complicated. Elbow joint surgery almost always presents a tough challenge to the surgeon because all arm nerves and blood vessels are densely packed over a limited area, like sardines in a tin. Moreover, it is never easy to predict the outcome of such an operation; physiologically, the elbow joint is a complex piece of machinery, actually a combination of three joints: humerus-ulna, humerus-radius, and radius-ulna. Frankly, I would have preferred a smaller field, concentrating on just one kind of injury. However, I was in no position to be argumentative, for Dr. Kaplan was an eminent professor, an author, and my scientific supervisor into the bargain. Besides, his idea was tempting as a challenge: what if I really tackled the whole gamut of injuries and then followed up the thesis with a textbook? A rough estimate indicated that a project of such magnitude would take at least five years—assuming I worked nonstop.

From time to time, I showed him my patients and reported on the clinical results, not infrequently coming in for severe criticism. It hurt because I was really trying my best. He was particularly critical (and so was I) of the outcomes of severe comminuted fractures of the elbow. I tried all known treatment strategies, but in almost all cases I could not achieve a significant improvement in elbow mobility and many patients left the hospital crippled. Unfortunately, we did not have a standard Association of Orthopedists set of plates and screws, which was developed in the late fifties by the Swiss orthopedist Dr. Maurice Muller. Only Russian orthopedists have to make do without them. I was aware of the existence of these instruments from European and American publications and dreamed of laying my hands on them. On more than one occasion, I pleaded with the director of the Institute of Orthopedics and the Ministry hierarchy, trying to talk them into buying the AO instruments—only to hear them reply, "The Ministry is short of hard currency."

A smelting factory, Poldy, in Kladno, a township near Prague in Czechoslovakia, began manufacturing excellent replicas of the AO set. Several times the Czechs approached us with offers to sell their quality instruments, but they were turned down by our pig-headed medical bureaucrats.

"We're going to manufacture our own instruments," they said.

But their promises remained just that—promises. And little wonder: there was no Vitallium metal, no production technology or know-how, no competent experts—in short, nothing to develop the needed technology.

Russia's backwardness in the area of medical technology is simply stupefying; I am confident that in this respect the country is at least forty to fifty years behind the industrialized world. All Russian technical capability and resources are dedicated to the war effort. Medicine has to be content with mere crumbs.

What was I supposed to do, particularly in cases of severe elbow injuries? Willy-nilly, I had to try an alternative approach: prosthetic replacement of injured elbow joints. Endoprosthetic operations of this kind were unknown in Russia, and only a handful were described in the West. Consequently I had no prototype of the prosthesis I had in mind.

Now each night, while my family was asleep, I worked at my desk, drawing sketches of my prosthesis.

Initially, I planned to reproduce in my design the basic elements of the natural joint. However, I realized pretty soon that modern technology was so far behind nature that duplication was impossible. In a fit of desperation, I would brush the umpteenth sketch aside, grab a fresh sheet of paper, and take up work on my poems. Since they were earmarked for children, I had my work cut out for me, for kids perceive nature in a special way even though their vocabulary is bone dry. In rough translation one poem went: A path runs through the woods / Narrow as a gossamer. / Anyone who finds it / Is led straight to the lake. / There, willow trees / Bend their heads over clear waters. / And in the glare of day / Shy deer came out to drink from the lake.

The poems were to be bare of details, and so, too, was to be the prosthesis design. I would shove the poems aside and attack the artificial joint once again. My goal was to design a joint that would be capable of performing the basic functions of the natural joint— just as natural descriptions in verse evoke images but stop short of presenting the full picture.

I spent the long winter nights racking my brain in search of an optimum design. At long last, by the spring of 1968, I was done: both the final sketch of my artificial elbow joint and the finalized version of the book sat on my desk. I took the poems to the publishing house, but where was I supposed to take the sketch? I had worked on the design in secret lest my colleagues learn about it.

One of my patients, Vitaly Isaev, was an engineer and supervisor of the tool shop at Avangard Factory. He was a pleasant, simple man of about fifty, whose leg I had operated on for a fracture he sustained on the job. Out of gratitude he sometimes supplied me with custom-made metal tools. The factory turned out rocket equipment and was accordingly classified as top secret, so he had a hard time smuggling my tools through the closely guarded checkpoint at the exit. But many workers were adept at fooling the guards and managed to take just about anything out of the factory.

I showed my sketch to Isaev; it took him a while to grasp the queer idea of replacing elbow joints. Still, I managed to engage him in a technical discussion. Finding himself on familiar ground, he brightened and attacked the problem vigorously.

"Can you make a prototype?" I asked.

"No problem. But I'll need technical drawings and some assistants."

He brought to me two other engineers and blue-collar workers. I put a bottle of cognac on the table and we discussed technical details. None of them was familiar with medical technology and consequently they found the idea outlandish. Finally we struck a deal: they undertook to make the prototype without charge, except that I had to provide free alcohol for the machinists involved. It would cost me a substantial sum, exactly half my monthly earnings. Providentially, my wife had been saving money to buy herself a new coat for 160 rubles. I went to the kitchen and explained to her in a whisper, "You must try to understand that it's an important achievement to develop a new elbow prosthesis. I've had the idea for months and worked hard on the sketch; it looks like it will work. But first I must have a prototype and try it on a cadaver. Isaev agreed to make the prosthesis free, but he can't make the drawings himself, so we have to find a way of paying. . . ."

Irina brought her coat money to the kitchen. I kissed her and paid the engineers. When they left, I launched into a long-winded lecture, explaining to Irina the value of replacing a fractured elbow joint with a man-made prosthesis. She listened appreciatively, but I was sure that she could lecture me on the importance of replacing her old, worn coat with a new one.

The whole thing weighed heavily on my conscience. It was over ten years since our wedding and I was still unable to provide amply for my family. We barely made ends meet, and now I had deprived her of both a needed piece of clothing and of the joy of anticipating it. I suffered pangs of conscience for two weeks and then I took my treasured Winchester to a pawn shop, sold it for 160 rubles, and paid the debt to Irina.

Finally, the day came when I was to receive my prosthesis. I stood behind the corner of the tall brick wall surrounding the factory, at a safe distance from the checkpoint through which workers left the building. Two of them, Sergei and Pavel, were to smuggle out my prosthesis broken down into components.

My pocket bulged with a bottle of 192-proof medical-grade alcohol—my payment for the order. I had wangled it out of the matron on the pretext that I needed alcohol to mix an herbal tincture. I held my bulging pocket with my hand, anxiously casting glances from around the corner: what happens if they fail to carry my prosthesis safely past the guards? Then all my work would be for nothing! I was sure they could smuggle out an entire rocket. Still. . . . At last my fears were dissipated by their appearance. They approached, their pockets bulging with cargo just like mine was. Pavel, an inveterate alcoholic, was consumed by desire for a drink.

"Have you brought the alcohol?" he asked.

"You bet," I replied, furtively glancing around.

Like thieves, we walked away from the factory. As soon as we approached the nearest park, filled with strolling mothers and their playing kids, Pavel said impatiently, "Let's see the bottle."

An exchange took place. They produced the components of my prosthesis wrapped in soiled rags. Sergei proceeded to put them together, explaining the procedure to me, while Pavel tugged at his sleeve.

Spring was in full bloom, birds were chirping, children were playing. One of the mothers was reading aloud a poem from my latest book: "A path runs through the woods, narrow as a gossamer. . . ." I listened to my poem and admired my prosthesis. It was unadulterated happiness.

Now that I had the prototype of my elbow joint prosthesis, I decided to go public with it at the institute; at that stage the idea could no longer be stolen. My colleagues, particularly the older ones, were skeptical. They would examine the prosthesis, ask a couple of questions, and voice their doubts as to the feasibility of such an operation. Undeterred, I went right ahead experimenting. Now I spent evenings at the morgue, developing the implantation technique on cadavers. I did not need the relatives' permission to experiment on cadavers; all it took was an offering of alcohol to the morgue attendant. In exchange for free libation he took out of the freezer and laid on the autopsy table any cadaver I needed—male, female, old or young.

In the course of experimentation I refined the technique of future elbow replacement procedures and explored the prosthesis for defects. In this way summer passed. On several occasions I returned the prosthesis to Isaev for design modification, and each time thereafter I stood, bottle in pocket, at the wall of Avangard Factory, waiting for the machinists Sergei and Pavel.

As always, we would walk to our park to exchange the contents of our respective pockets. The mothers who patronized the park learned that at a certain point in our transaction a bottle would appear, and they regarded us as bums, shepherding their kids away when we approached.

Finally, the day came when I decided that the preliminary experimentation stage was over and clinical trials were now needed. I had to find a suitable patient, but I had no intention of going through official channels and applying to the Ministry for permission to perform the first operation—it would have taken years.

My potential patient was to meet two criteria: a debilitating loss of elbow movement and an adequate level of intelligence to be amenable to my persuasion. I did not intend to make the patient pay for the operation, but I felt duty bound to explain to the subject that he or she was the first to undergo an entirely new surgical procedure. Finally, I chanced upon an artist and engraver named Victor Vurlakov, thirty, who two years previously had fallen from wood scaffolding in a church not far from Moscow where he was painting the ceiling. The fall resulted in immobility of the right elbow. He suffered enormously, the more so since he could not work and thus had no means of subsistence. I asked him why he had taken the church assignment.

"I was moonlighting and so all the risk was mine," he replied. "The prior promised to pay me well, but I was constantly on the alert for the police, who could chase me away. When I fell down, I could not claim any compensation because the job was not sanctioned officially."

I liked him and his way of reasoning. One day I offered him a chance to have his ankylosed elbow replaced with an artificial metal elbow joint.

He showed interest. I discussed the project with him several times until at last he made up his mind and declared that he was ready to submit to my procedure. Still, I delayed surgery for another two months to let him cement his resolve. His determination remained unshakable.

I obtained permission from Dr. Volkov, director of our institute, and on October 2, 1968, performed my first elbow replacement operation. The procedure lasted almost five hours, because I was very agitated and had to restrain myself; besides, a friend of mine, an amateur cameraman, was filming the operation.

That night I was on duty at the institute and at frequent intervals visited my patient to check the condition of his arm. Everything was normal. Three weeks later I started the patient on a rehabilitation program, personally assisting and teaching him. Since his muscles had weakened considerably over the two years of forced inaction, the rehabilitation process progressed slowly—but progress it did.

Two months after the operation I demonstrated my patient at a morning conference to all our orthopedists. The patient had regained mobility of the repaired elbow almost completely and even resumed working. My colleagues looked at him with surprise, at me with distaste. But Professor Max Michelman, a noted orthopedist, came forward and said: "Frankly, I was a disbeliever, but now I must admit I was wrong. We owe Dr. Golyakhovsky congratulations for developing a new surgical procedure and a new prosthesis. He also deserves praise for the success of his first clinical trial." He started applauding. The rest of the surgeons joined in, though with noticeable lack of enthusiasm. I bowed awkwardly, as all people with no stage experience do.

I was extremely proud of my success, though I tried hard not to let my pride show. Be that as it may, I knew that others would perform the operation according to my method and using my prosthesis; that for years to come they would cite me in their papers and lectures. The operation marked my transition from a performer to a creator.

34

The first half of 1968 was dominated by the events in Czechoslovakia, a country I held dear to my heart. The "Prague Spring" bolstered hopes for freedom not only among the Czechs and Slovaks, but in Russia as well, particularly in intellectual circles. By that time Leonid Brezhnev had been in power for merely three and a half years, and we still hoped he would launch some sort of democratic reform. Our hopes were given a powerful lift by Alexander Dubček who, together with a group of vigorous, like-minded confederates, set about instituting democratic reforms very quickly and effectively. We all watched the developments anxiously, conjecturing whether Brezhnev would allow Dubček to go on or would suppress the democratic process in Czechoslovakia. Had Brezhnev adopted a hands-off posture, we would all have been affected inevitably, for the communist camp is a single monolith: a single political system and an integrated economy. Many Russians were in sympathy with Dubček's idea; some of us even subscribed to a Prague newspaper, the *Rude Pravo,* to enjoy its bold and perky political articles.

On the morning of August 21, 1968, I was getting set to leave for work while Irina was in the kitchen, cooking breakfast. We kept a radio there and every morning both of us listened—perfunctorily—to the news and—very attentively—to the weather forecast. All of a sudden, I heard Irina's hysterical outcry:

"Scoundrels! Lousy bums!"

Taken aback and a little frightened, I rushed to the kitchen. She stood at the radio, tears welling in her eyes. "Those damned bastards, they've invaded Czechoslovakia!"

So, that's what it was! . . . The news hit me hard. I immediately realized that all hopes were in vain—there would be no change for the better.

I had a friend in enslaved Czechoslovakia. He was a slave now, captive of the victors. I could easily imagine his feelings of impotent rage and hatred for the Russians. Would he hate me, too? I was overcome by an irresistible impulse to somehow let Miloš know my true attitude toward the invasion and tell him that I was with him, that I joined his protest. But how? It was out of the question to try to call him; all telephone lines, except government lines, were cut off. I sat down at the table and drafted a cable: "Dear Miloš, my dear friend, I want you to know that I am wholeheartedly with you. I love your country and hope for a better future for all of us."

I was afraid the post office would refuse to accept such an outspoken cable. Surprisingly, though, the clerk at the post office, where I went before going to the Institute of Orthopedics, indifferently read the message, counted the words, told me how much it cost, and issued a receipt.

Very soon we found out from Soviet newspapers that "the entire population of Czechoslovakia to a man supports the decision to introduce troops in their country," while the Voice of America and the BBC, whose broadcasts were jammed particularly intensely in those days, told us that almost all the 14 million Czechs and Slovaks protested against the invasion and tried to resist. Moscow wits came up with a new joke: "What is the population of Czechoslovakia?—28 million, because 14 million are in favor of the invasion and 14 million are against it."

On the directive of the Central Committee of the Communist Party public meetings were held at all factories, plants, institutes, and even schools to express popular support for the invasion. The speakers at such gatherings spared no invective for Dubček and praised the "wisdom" of Brezhnev.

I refused to attend the meeting at our institute. I did not have the courage to emulate the open protest of a group of dissidents headed by Pavel Litvinov who paid for their valor with exile. But neither did I want to be among those who spoke in support of the invasion. Thank God, at least I could afford that mild form of protest because I was not a Party member.

After I performed my first original surgical procedure, the elbow joint replacement, I grew in stature and my practice increased. Together with Dr. A. Kazmin, deputy director of the Institute of Orthopedics, I performed several major operations. One of our patients was the stepdaughter of Minister of Culture Yekaterina Furtseva, the only woman ever to sit on the Politburo. She was entitled to medical treatment at the exclusive Kremlin Hospital, but her stepmother personally approached us with a request to operate on the young lady. The operation was a success.

In October 1968, while Dr. Kazmin and I were discussing the condition of that postoperative patient, an American orthopedic surgeon, Dr. K. from Milwaukee, Wisconsin, came to see Dr. Kazmin. A squat, balding man, somewhat sluggish and very quiet, he was not the typical American of my naive musings (tall and virile—like John Wayne). Dr. K. came on a private visit. He did not represent anything or anybody; he merely spent his vacation in Moscow. This meant that he was nobody as far as our institute was concerned and as such was not to be accorded the VIP treatment due official foreign guests. For this reason Dr. Kazim gave me the privilege of taking care of him—an unprecedented honor.

Dr. Elliot K. spoke some Russian, which was a major relief for I spoke no English. He told me he was on his fourth visit to Russia and that he kept coming to our country simply because he liked it here. I found his peculiar interest strange but refrained from questions.

I offered to drive him around Moscow and show him some interesting sights. He agreed with obvious pleasure. Generally speaking, in order to give him a tour of Moscow I was supposed to apply for permission to Department #1 or obtain a director's order. But in this instance I felt that as long as I had been officially charged with the task of entertaining the guest, no one would find fault with my taking him home in my car . . . and, of course, I was within my rights to show him some sights on the way. We strolled through the city for about two hours, and I was increasingly consumed by a desire to ask him about America. So I braced myself and invited him over to dinner. It was strictly forbidden and I risked grave consequences if anyone found out, but I knew already that the American surgeon was about to leave Moscow and had no intention of coming back to our institute. So he would not be in a position to let it be known— out of naiveté and ignorance of the way things were in Russia—that he had visited me at my home, while I was unwilling to warn him that I invited him secretly and at great peril to myself. He accepted the invitation gladly. He brought a bottle of whiskey and a handful of Parker pens. Irina cooked a light supper.

I spent the evening peppering him with questions about the state of medicine in the United States. Irina talked to him in English and I swelled with pride: see the kind of wife I had! We had a nice time; I learned a lot of things entirely new to me: the structure of American medicine, the state of medical technology, the level of doctors' remuneration. We were surgeons of approximately equal stature, but while my annual income was 4,000 rubles ($6,000) he earned some $80,000—a thirteen-fold difference!

At this time my infatuation with America was growing steadily. Far from being a practical interest, it was just an innocent desire to learn more about a strange country, a strange society, a different way of life. My interest was all the more acute because after the recent invasion of Czechoslovakia I had lost all hope for even token democratization of my country. I idealized America—the logical outcome of years of listening to the Voice of America, reading the

Russian-language *America* magazine, and hearing the stories told by my lucky acquaintances who had been there. I liked all things American I had a chance to see or hear. I liked the information content of American radio broadcasts; the democratic mindset of Americans; the fantastic quality of American printed matter, particularly the color photographs in the *America*. I spent a lot of time perusing those photographs whether they depicted architectural monuments, new machinery, or the latest in fashion. Occasionally I saw an American car in the streets of Moscow, and the sight would repeatedly drive home its message of the enormous technological gap between America and my country.

My American aunt, Lyuba Churchin, came every other year to visit my father and the rest of her siblings. I loved to hear her stories about New York City, about America. Unfortunately she knew very little of the medical field, except that treatment was very expensive.

I realized that America also had its problems, but they were of no concern to me. I thought of America as one thinks of a beautiful woman: one remains enraptured in spite of her drawbacks.

35

In December 1969, Bolshoi Ballet prima ballerina Maya Plysetskaya ripped her left calf muscle during a rehearsal. She fell to the floor, crying in agony. Nikolay Fadeyichev, who had been dancing with her, picked her up and carried her off the stage as the others stared in helpless shock.

Since the Bolshoi Theater had no medical trainer for its 250 dancers, Fadeyichev carried Plysetskaya to Zhenka, the masseur. Zhenka, a short, hard-drinking man, poured three flasks of chloretil, a chilling solution, over her calf to numb the pain, but she just cried more.

By the time Plysetskaya arrived at our institute, the pain had grown worse because her calf muscle had torn even more. Dr. Z. Mironova covered her whole leg, from hip to toe, with a plaster cast without first placing some stockinet or absorbent cotton or even some vaseline on her skin. Since her skin was still frozen from the chloretil and since the plaster was coarse and made of caustic calcium salts, the cast soon began to burn and rub her skin.

Plysetskaya cried and begged for three days for a doctor to remove the cast. The institute gave her a separate room, and the institute director, Dr. Volkov, tried to calm her, but she kept pleading. Finally, Dr. Mironova cut the cast off and discovered that all the skin around her shin and calf had blistered so badly that it came right off with the plaster. When Plysetskaya saw her gory leg, she wept hysterically. She refused to stay at the institute any longer and immediately arranged for her husband to drive her home.

When they got home, Plysetskaya's husband, the well-known composer Rodion Shchedrin, called me.

"We'll be very grateful if you can examine her," Shchedrin said. His intonation meant they'd pay me well. Shchedrin and Plysetskaya were among the richest couples in the Soviet Union, and the rich usually paid for private house calls.

I hurried over. Shchedrin and Plysetskaya lived at 25 Gorky Street, on the sixth floor, in a large, luxurious, five-room apartment with two bathrooms and a maid's quarters. An apartment that size is a rare privilege in the Soviet Union.

Maya Plysetskaya, thin and fragile, gazed up at me with her huge, sad eyes from her king-size bed. She looked like a dying swan. I unwrapped the cloths and rags she and her maid Katya had tied around her leg. When I unwrapped the bottom layer, which was a piece of sheet smeared with some smelly ointment, I had to hide my surprise and disgust. Her whole calf was a running sore dotted with islands of black, dead skin. Through the surface, I could see the outline of the muscle tear. Her foot hung limp; she could barely move it.

"People have told me what miracles you've performed," she said in a small, hoarse voice. I paid no attention to this flattery, but was determined to impress her with calm, professional authority, because I already knew she was very independent, eccentric, manipulative, and distrustful. I sat silently for a long time and thought about how difficult it would be to heal the injury.

As I was leaving, Shchedrin tried to shove an envelope stuffed with rubles into my pocket. I was already familiar with this manner of payment. He looked off into space and pretended not to know what his hands were doing. I pushed his envelope back and said: "I won't accept any money from Maya Plysetskaya."

When I returned, I wrapped her leg in fibrin bandages coated with a Swiss preparation called Solkoseril and immobilized her leg from the front with a plaster brace. The American violinist Isaac Stern has aptly compared Maya's legs to two Stradivariuses. Her leg muscles are unusually thin and strong from hours of stretching, flexing, and leaping every day for years. I took more care than usual to help it heal properly.

Once or twice a day, I came to change her bandages, to check her progress, or to reassure her. Although she could see the gradual healing, she worried constantly. Between visits, she often called me with trivial questions about her treatment and progress. To facilitate my visits, she sent her chauffeur to pick me up in her Volga (she also owned a Citröen and a Landrover), and she ordered her maid Katya to cook me meals with food purchased in a restricted foreign-currency store. Rodion occasionally presented me bottles of fine foreign wine from the same store.

During these visits, Maya told me a lot about her family and career. She was born to a Moscow Jewish family in 1925. Her father, Mikhail Plysetsky, had been an engineer for a Swedish company and was therefore arrested by the communists in 1937 and perished without a trace.

Maya began to dance professionally in 1943 and soon became famous. She was invited to dance at Stalin's seventy-year celebration at the Kremlin Theater. Just before she went out onto the stage, she started for a corner where a box of colophony for her shoes lay.

"Where are you going?" demanded one of the guards. Armed soldiers stood guard everywhere backstage and throughout the theater.

"To colophony my shoes."

"Colophony them tomorrow!" he snapped.

While she was dancing, she felt Stalin's murderous eyes follow her and almost paralyze her movements. He sat in the front row, surrounded by his foreign toadies—Palmiro Togliatti, Moris Tores, Clement Gottward, Boleslaw Bierut, Wilhelm Pieck, Wylko Chervenkov, Petru Groza, and Mao Tse-tung.

"You can't imagine the sensation," she told me, "of dancing in front of the hideous, gloomy faces of those stupid, indifferent tyrants. I was terrified, because they could crush me like a louse at the slightest whim, but I forced myself to dance, to try to melt their hatred. When I finished and curtsied, Stalin clapped his hands over his head enthusiastically. The others immediately followed suit, and some even stood to applaud. Even the guards backstage met me with smiles and clapping."

Soon afterward, she received her first of many awards, Meritorious Artist. She has since won practically all possible Soviet awards for artists and become the Bolshoi's prima ballerina, eclipsing her great rival Galina Ulanova.

On New Year's Eve 1970, about twenty days after her injury, I removed the plaster brace. Maya looked anxiously at her leg as if it were a newborn baby. She still couldn't move her foot, and the skin was nearly transparent, but her leg seemed to have new life. I gave her a pair of crutches, and she hobbled around the room, holding her leg out forward. I told her to begin exercising her foot in a whirlpool she had. Since she couldn't get into the tub with the help of her crutches, I picked her up—she was very light—and set her in.

A few days later, she began to do ballet exercises, but in shoes instead of ballet slippers because her foot still needed support. She had a mirrored practice room in her apartment that she had only used previously as a storeroom. It was filled with piles of imported dance costumes, shoe boxes, record albums, autographed art books, and even included a white Steinway piano that the American impresario Sol Hurok had given her. Rodion and I pushed this stuff aside and set up a tape recorder for her. Rodion was too busy rehearsing his new cantata "Lenin in the Nation's Heart" with a couple of singers to play for Maya. She exercised her leg every day under my supervision.

Eventually, she began to attend rehearsals at the Bolshoi Theater again. She asked me to come along at least for the first few days to monitor her leg. The first rehearsal began at ten o'clock with an hour-long political lecture on the theme, "Together with the

Whole Nation We Greet the Twenty-fourth Congress of the Communist Party." The whole roomful of great Soviet ballet stars listened to the lecture with total indifference, but then livened up when the rehearsal actually began. Maya introduced me to her friends as her "savior" and they thanked me for bringing her back.

About three months after her injury, Maya returned to the stage in *Carmen*. She sent my wife and me front-row tickets, and her chauffeur delivered us to a private entrance on Petrovka Street for Party rulers, government ministers, leading academicians, and celebrated artists. The VIP cars ignored the No Stopping signs at this entrance and disgorged men in elegant suits and women in expensive furs and diamonds. My wife and I drew stares because of our plain clothes, and it even seemed that the doorman might block our way, but luckily Rodion Shchedrin ran up, greeted me loudly, and introduced us around.

The ballet began with a roll of drums as Maya stood on the stage. She posed with "our" left foot slightly behind her right foot. I held my breath, because I knew that she would step out sharply with her left foot as soon as the music started. She stepped out with no problem and danced the whole part magnificently. She received a standing ovation, and when she came out to acknowledge the bravos, she curtsied deeply and directly to me.

36

In 1968, I made the first attempt to treat bone fractures with the aid of magnetic fields. That attempt was the high point of over a decade of reflection on the external forces that could affect the knitting of broken bones. While all other tissues are replaced by scarry connective tissue, bone alone is capable of complete regeneration. This process has developed philogenetically over millions of years in evolution. It always passes through a fixed number of immutable stages and always proceeds very slowly: it takes at least four weeks, on the average, for a broken bone to knit—too slow by far to satisfy millions of patients suffering from bone fractures. Physicians had been searching for many years for ways to speed up the knitting process but never got anywhere, although they had their share of hopes, illusions, disappointments, and scientific frauds.

One day I examined a man of about forty who came to Moscow for a consultation from the Kursk area. He had a long, ugly, and dirty cast on his right leg. The patient told me he had suffered fractures of both bones of a shin a month previously while working in an underground mine. To prove the time of fracture and the diagnosis, he had a medical certificate issued by his area hospital. I decided to replace his poor cast with a new, more reliable, and better applied plaster cast. To this end, I first had to X-ray the fracture site. Examining the X rays, I was stupefied to see that the broken bones had completely healed within a mere month, although I could have sworn that a fracture of this gravity should have taken at least twice as long to heal. The cure was so complete that the patient no longer needed a cast of any kind. Puzzled, I proceeded to question him about his accident, trying various indirect methods to verify the date: after all, there could be dating errors both in his memory and in the hospital certificate. But no, everything indicated that there was no mistake: the fracture had occurred exactly one month previously. At the news of the happy outcome, the patient cheered up and a broad grin split his face.

"Shall I tell you my secret, Doctor?" he asked. "Do you want to know how I treated myself?"

"Of course," I said, though frankly, I was sure a layman would not be able to tell me anything of significance.

"I applied magnetized iron to my broken shin through the cast."

"*Why?*" I was openly surprised.

"To tell the truth, I don't know," he said in some embarrassment, "but I live within the boundaries of Kursk. Old people there tell a lot of interesting stories connected with magnetism. Miracles that you can neither account for nor believe. Now then, when I had that fracture in the mine and the doctor applied the cast, I asked him how long it would take for the bones to heal. He just shrugged and told me I would be lucky if the bones healed within three months but I should be prepared to wear the cast for six months."

"And he was right," I interjected.

"Maybe he was, but I had no intention of waiting that long. So I decided to try magnetic action. I took a simple lump of strongly magnetized iron, the kind they use in school demonstrations, wrapped it in a gauze bandage, and attached it to my cast next to the fracture. I only took it off when I set out for Moscow to see you. It was awkward and heavy; besides, I didn't know how you would react to the magnet."

What could I say? Absolutely nothing. I had never heard of such an unorthodox method of treatment.

At home that night I told Irina about the case. Preoccupied by her own affairs, she evinced little interest, but it was important for me to share the story anyway, for had I not told her, in all likelihood, I would have forgotten it. As it happened, however, the story stuck in my mind. The next day I pondered the likelihood that magnetic field could have any effect on live tissue. I had read in popular-science magazines that several biologists had recently begun research into the effect of magnetic field on animals. They found, for instance, that migratory birds used the Earth's magnetic field for navigation on their long journeys—it appeared birds had a kind of biological magnetic compass in their bodies. Apparently living organisms could sense magnetic field by means of a physiological mechanism containing metal ions.

I tried to engage physicist and biologist friends in conversations on the subject but found little enthusiasm on their part. I was alone in my deliberations. I started looking for research papers on the subject. There were no direct suggestions that magnetic field could affect the bone-healing process, but I found out that quite a few researchers had long been studying magnetism and the many ways it affected live tissues. Then I decided to join their ranks and become the first to study magnetism as applied to broken bones. After three years of research, in July 1971, I was granted a patent for a "Method of Accelerating Bone Healing in Fractures." I achieved excellent results by using magnetic field as a therapeutic tool.

Between the chance, empirical discovery by my patient and the day I received my patent lay hundreds of experiments on animals, difficulties, disappointments, despair, and delight. I had to conduct my experiments sub rosa, for they fell outside of the research plans approved by the institute directorate. I needed all kinds of magnets—weak, strong, large and small. One of my patients, an eminent Jewish physicist, kept me supplied with requisite magnets. He also helped me carry out measurements of the magnetic field intensities in his laboratory. I was totally ignorant in everything pertaining to physics and had to really apply myself to master the technique. Then I studied the effect of magnetic fields of varying intensity on rabbit bones over various lengths of time. I dragooned a pathologist friend of mine, and we spent nights and Sundays at the lab. We found that the best results were produced by a weak magnetic field applied permanently for an extensive period of time—between three and four weeks.

Now the question was, who would be my first subject? Again, it had to be done unofficially. There were no strict rules on the application of new treatment methods, but I bore a moral responsibility to the patient. Besides, were I to fail and the failure became known, the Ministry would be in a position to outlaw my technique altogether.

Since 1969, I had been treating forty-year-old Dr. Vladimir Struchkov, who held a Ph.D. degree in physiology. He had sustained a severe open fracture while defending a woman who was mugged at a railway station near Moscow. He had been operated on three times, but his fracture had not healed, and he had been forced to walk on crutches. I told him about my experiments. "I can use my method to treat your leg," I told him, "but without any guarantee of success. You're a physician yourself and should understand."

He agreed and I put two of my special magnets in his cast. Three months later my colleagues and I together with my patient had an occasion for celebration: the bone that had not responded to treatment for two years had healed perfectly. Victory!

37

On April 9, 1970, I defended a doctoral thesis and got a Doctor of Science degree. The scientific degree translates into a significant pay boost, and, more important still, clears the way toward the most prestigious and lucrative positions. Not surprisingly, there is a scramble for degrees. Many people go into science and aspire to research jobs for purely material reasons, like poor suitors beseiging a rich girl. But just as a rich girl chooses just one from among the throng of suitors, spurning the rest, so many physicians striving for a career in science are denied scientific degrees and hence a short-cut to well-paying jobs. A special administrative unit, the Supreme Certification Commission at the Council of Ministers, sees to it. All theses are subject to strict, confidential review and quite a few fall short of the mark.

Soon thereafter I was summoned by the director of the Skliffasovsky Emergency Aid Institute, Dr. Boris Komarov, with whom I had studied at medical school.

"Congratulations on your doctoral success," he said.

"Thanks."

"What are your plans now?"

"So far, nothing."

"Why don't you come to my institute? I'll appoint you director of the trauma and orthopedics department. Agreed?"

I was overjoyed. The Skliffasovsky Hospital, founded by Dr. Yudin, was one of Moscow's best. "It's a deal," I told him.

"One more thing," Komarov added. "You'll automatically become chief orthopedic surgeon of Moscow."

I stood as if struck by lightning; not even in my wildest dreams could I hope for such a huge stride forward.

"How long have you been in the Party?" he went on.

"How long? . . . As a matter of fact, I am not a Party member."

"What do you mean you are not a Party member?" He was incredulous. "How did the commission approve your thesis then?"

"They just did!" I said.

"Then you must join the Party immediately. The chief orthopedic surgeon position cannot be filled without the approval of the Moscow Municipal Party Committee. If you're not a communist, you'll never be approved. You still have two months to join. I'll be waiting for you to bring the card of a candidate [non-voting] member of the Party."

He did not doubt for a moment that I would comply. But I did have doubts, many of them. I had always stuck to my principle not to join the Party unless my life depended on it. "Well, so be it, an attractive job is not reason enough for becoming a Party member," I thought. Two months later I again entered Dr. Komarov's office.

"Show me the card," he demanded.

"I've got none, Boris."

"You must be crazy. Don't you realize the career opportunities? First of all, your salary will be five hundred rubles or maybe even six hundred a month; you'll get a free chauffeured car, a free government-allotted apartment, a special monthly bonus, and a lot of perks like access to exclusive stores and sanatoriums. Don't be a fool; apply for Party membership. I'm telling you this as a friend."

I never came back and soon he filled the vacant position with Dr. V. Okhotsky, a Party activist.

I was not in the least sorry, because not for a moment did I doubt that Party affiliation would destroy me. Had I complied, I would have had to vote with everybody else; speak at meetings like everybody else; even think like everybody else. I simply could not stomach such an awful prospect. True, even though I was not a Party member, I could not afford to speak up and vote against it, but at least I did not have to attend those idiotic meetings and could retain my inner freedom.

Irina concurred with my decision. No one in my family or hers belonged to the Party.

Luckily, a short while later a new chair of traumatology, orthopedics, and military surgery was set up at the Moscow Medical and Dentistry School, and a contest to head it was declared. That position attracted me even more than the one Dr. Komarov had dangled before me. As head of a chair I would have better opportunities to pursue my scientific interests than as chief orthopedic surgeon, a highly administrative job. So I applied; I was the sixth applicant behind five Party members. This competition put me in low spirits because I really wanted that position. To make matters worse, several of my rivals were orthopedists of considerable renown. My only advantage was my age—I was the youngest of the contestants.

I simply had to talk to Dr. Alexei Belousov, dean of the medical school. Handing in my application, I dropped in at his office. A short, portly man with a bulbous nose, he bore a striking resemblance to Nikita Khrushchev. Belousov was surrounded by people and barely had time to talk.

"There are quite a few applicants," he told me. "We'll decide together with the Party Committee and let you know."

Later I spent many hours in the anteroom of his office, but to no avail.

I wanted to have a substantive one-on-one talk with him to tell him of my work plans and, above all, to showcase myself and try to influence him in a personal way. It was almost impossible to do this because Belousov was always extremely busy, always mobbed by people, always in a hurry. But I found a way: my friend Dr. Georgadze and I invited the dean to a hunting expedition in the woods not far from Moscow.

It had been a long time since I had gone hunting. I did not even have a gun anymore. But the hunting preserve we went to had everything we needed, and then some: hunting gear, cognacs, game. It was an exclusive preserve of the Politburo and the government, located in Zavidovo, ninety miles northeast of Moscow, near the ancient city of Pereyaslavl-Zalessky. Dr. Georgadze, a nephew of Mikhail Georgadze, Secretary of the Presidium of the Supreme Soviet, managed to obtain a permit to shoot an elk through his influential uncle.

We set out on our expedition at night in two cars. There were six of us, including three physicians, the dean's sycophants. The trunks of our cars were packed with delicacies Dr. Georgadze, a Georgian, received from Tbilisi, the capital of the Georgian Republic. He was eager to ingratiate himself with Belousov at least as fervently as myself, because he, too, sought employment at Belousov's school. I brought vodka and cognac.

We passed Zagorsk and turned left, entering an exclusive highway under an Off Limits sign. It was a direct road to Zavidovo. Our cars were waved through. Belousov only wanted to hit the food and drink, and soon he asked for the cars to stop. We opened the trunks and took out the Georgian delicacies and several bottles of brandy.

I was amazed at the drinking capacity of my prospective boss; he emptied unassisted two bottles of a very strong brandy, downing it in tea glasses. Before long, he was very drunk. Others followed suit. All of them told dirty jokes, swore profusely, and fawned upon Belousov. Since I was one of the two drivers, I drank moderately. Even so, analysis would surely have revealed an illegal level of alcohol in my blood. But we were positive that no policeman would dare stop our cars on that highway.

We passed the Main Manor House, designed for Brezhnev, Kosygin, and other leaders, and drove deeper into the woods. Darkness fell when we arrived at our destination: a small hunting lodge/hotel. An old hunter and his wife welcomed us with a simple peasant-style dinner: borsht, a heap of boiled potatoes, sliced lard, and pickles. Once again, everybody got gloriously drunk. There was no way to talk business with Belousov.

Next morning at 4:00 A.M., while it was still dark, a Russian-made jeep came to pick us up. It brought all the hunting gear we needed. I selected an excellent Winchester that reminded me of my old rifle. We put on tall boots and windbreakers, and soon everyone looked like genuine hunters, although Belousov and his pals, who obviously needed the hair of the dog, presented a sorry spectacle.

Alyosha Georgadze whispered in my ear: "I'll ask the huntsman to drive the elk directly at Belousov. He's so drunk I doubt he'll be able to so much as pull the trigger. Watch carefully; if he fails to make the kill, you or I should shoot."

We were taken to the forest, where a band of about fifteen huntsmen, peasants from nearby villages, were awaiting us. They were part of a force of village folk paid for the sole duty of rousing and driving game toward rulers-turned-sportsmen. It was still dark. The chief huntsman told us that the night before a big bull elk had been spotted here. So it was a good place to hunt from. We would be positioned on special shooting towers.

"Where are you going to be?" I asked. "We don't want to shoot you by accident."

"About a hundred and fifty feet behind the elk. The trees will shield us. But since we're going to drive him in your direction, be careful anyway." He fell silent, then added: "Once a huntsman was killed under just such circumstances. A tragic accident."

I did not ask who had killed the huntsman. The answer was self-evident: one of the powers-that-be.

We walked through a clearing to the shooting towers, which were spaced about one hundred feet apart. Each one of us climbed into a separate tower. The clearing was fairly wide, so when the beast jumped out of the woods, he would be easily seen.

We had to wait for well over an hour. Finally we could hear the huntsmen setting up a clamor in the forest, trying to rouse the elk. The noise was getting near. We stood motionless. Suddenly I heard a loud snoring; it came from Belousov, soundly asleep and embracing his rifle. I looked at Georgadze; he motioned that he had heard the snoring, too. Needless to say, the elk would hear him also and surely turn away. What could be done? I climbed down from my tower and crept toward Belousov. I had to wake him up, but in such a way as to prevent him from making any noise. I climbed into his tower and pressed a palm to his mouth to stifle an outcry. He started and looked at me with fright and dumb surprise. I pressed a finger to my lips and signaled for him to keep silent. Finally his mind cleared and he nodded. I was about to sneak back to my own tower when I heard the crunching of twigs, the noise of powerful breathing, and a huge bull elk appeared from the thicket directly in front of us. A shrewd beast, he stopped at the edge of the clearing and looked left and right before rushing across. I nudged Belousov and we both raised our rifles. The gun held by the drowsy and still drunk Belousov shook uncertainly and drifted in all directions. We pulled the triggers simultaneously, but it was clear Belousov's shot had missed the target widely. The elk dropped dead.

"You've shot him!" I said. "Congratulations. A marvelous specimen."

The rest of the hunters climbed down from their towers and crowded around him, congratulating Belousov on his superior marksmanship: the bullet had struck the elk under the left shoulder blade, right into the heart. No one doubted that it was Belousov's shot that had mowed down the mighty beast, for everyone knew the rule of the "czar's hunt": only the "czar" has the right to claim triumph. Belousov was beside himself with joy; he eagerly accepted congratulations, kissed us one and all, and waved his short arms.

"I heard him well in advance," he told us excitedly. "I held my breath. All of a sudden he emerged from the woods. Boy, what a marvelous sight! No, you won't escape me, I thought, while he was turning his muzzle this way and that, getting set to jump the clearing. But I beat him to the jump and let him have it from both barrels!..."

He had a single-barrel gun. Nevertheless, everybody resumed the hugging and congratulating, vying with one another in flattery. I must admit that I added my voice to theirs.

A truck came to pick up the dead elk; the huntsmen hoisted it aboard and drove off for the lodge. We came back in the jeep and resumed the binge where we had left off the night before, drinking to Belousov, to his success, to his hunting talent. An hour later he could hardly stand on his feet, and I realized that my hope to have a talk with him was dashed once and for all.

Later, I approached Dr. Kapiton Lakin, vice-dean of Belousov's medical school and his closest aide. We had been schoolmates and Lakin had edited my first poems published by the students' newspaper.

"Listen, Kapiton, could you put in a word for me with Belousov?"

"I'll be honest with you," he replied. "I'll support you but only prior to the Party Committee session at which the applicants are going to be screened. I can't do more because you're not a Party member. And the choice will be made by the Party Committee."

To sum it up, the hunting expedition was for nought; I did not make my "killing." At least not yet.

38

In July 1971, the Ministry of Public Health of the German Democratic Republic invited me to perform a surgical elbow joint replacement, the first for that country. The Germans offered to pay all my expenses, but not a fee for the operation. I was to operate at the Orthopedic Surgery Hospital of the Greifswald University, in the north of East Germany. The hospital director was none other than my old Czech friend Professor Miloš Janeček, who worked there on a temporary contract. East Germany was short of skilled professionals. Many of them had fled to West Germany before the Berlin Wall was erected in 1961.

The Soviet Ministry took a good three months to process my papers. I had to fill out scores of questionnaires, obtain a reference from the District Party Committee (where I was hardly known), and get the approval of a special board at the Central Committee of the Communist Party. Dr. Oleg Shchepin, head of the Foreign Relations Department of the Ministry, was to represent me at the latter hearing. I filled out all the necessary papers, but the Protocol Department was in no hurry. Dr. Janeček called from Greifswald several times, asking what was happening. I explained that my case was hopelessly mired in red tape. Russian doctors were rarely if ever invited as guest surgeons to foreign countries. Consequently I was simply forgotten and my papers were gathering dust at the Ministry while my potential patient languished at a hospital a thousand miles away. All possible deadlines passed. Once I came to the Ministry to inquire, for the umpteenth time, as to the progress of my case. I found out nothing and stood crestfallen in the corridor, when I. Babanovsky, head of the Planning and Finance Department, happened to be passing by.

"Why so gloomy?" he asked.

"They won't let me go to East Germany to perform an operation, and the people there are tired of waiting."

"Who's paying for the trip?" he asked with professional interest.

"The Germans."

"There's no problem then. Come."

He took me to Dr. Shchepin and asked him to have my case attended to as soon as possible. Three days later I flew to East Berlin.

At Sheremetyevo Airport I was to undergo a customs inspection and I did not savor the prospect in the least. For one thing, I had several of my elbow prostheses in my baggage that were not covered by any documents. Those were my personal models made at the Avangard Factory by my patients. If I had tried to have them officially registered, there would have been a hell of a bureaucratic mess, for the models bore no trademark. Secondly, I was carrying a gold men's watch and a gold bracelet for Dr. Janeček, who had offered to pay me back in East German marks. According to regulations, all gold items had to be declared at customs, but if I did so,

I would have to bring the watch and bracelet back. I decided not to declare them, and was tormented by anxiety: what would happen if my prostheses and gold were seized? You never know what to expect from the customs officials in Moscow.

Thank God, I was spared; my valise was not opened. Finally I was past the Soviet border. I knew, of course, that I was not flying to a free country; still, it was my first trip abroad on official business. I carried a business traveler's passport and looked forward eagerly to a new experience. In East Berlin, I was issued expense money for a two-week stay.

A limousine was sent to fetch me from Berlin to Greifswald, a distance of about three hundred miles. It was fall, the days were cold. I rode through Germany, thinking: "Strange are the ways of Providence. Since childhood I've regarded Germany and the Germans as mortal enemies, and here I am traveling about Germany as an honored person. Wonderful highways they have in Germany; I wish we had such roads in Russia." I covered my legs with a plaid blanket ("excellent blanket, I must buy one, you can't get them in Moscow") and dozed off.

Greifswald was totally unscarred by World War Two. In the spring of 1945, the commander of its garrison, Colonel P. Petershagen, surrendered to Russian troops without a single shot. It was a university town, almost all surrounded by an ancient wall. Everything was neat and tidy in a classic German way. Shop windows exhibited foodstuff and consumer goods unavailable in Moscow.

I spoke enough German to understand and be understood. Dr. Janeček, with whom I communicated in Russian, helped me out as an interpreter. He met me as a long-lost brother. We had not seen each other for several years, during which time Russian troops had invaded his homeland. When we sat down at a table at the university club the first night, he told me, "You don't know what a treat it was for me to see your cable the day after the August invasion! At such trying times it's important to know you're not alone. I was moved to tears. All of us have lost all trust in Russia. But it would have been even more of a blow to me to know that politics had ruined our friendship."

My patient, a twenty-six-year-old factory worker, Wolfgang K., waited for me at the small ancient hospital. Three years before he had been involved in an auto accident. Since then his right elbow had ankylosed and crippled him. I was assisted during surgery by the hospital director, Professor Janeček; his son, a medical student; and a German doctor. Everything in the operating room was surprising to me, but the most striking feature was the abundance of equipment and surgical instruments. You could see that Germany was indeed a country of century-old technological culture.

Despite the fact that it was my twelfth such operation, I was exceedingly nervous, like an actor on his first tour abroad. University professors, orthopedic surgeons, and many medical students were in attendance to watch me at work, so my "audience" was like a musician's. None of the spectators had ever seen this kind of operation because there were no elbow prostheses in their country. Finally, after almost four hours of unrelenting pressure, I closed the elbow wound, applied a dressing, and went to the director's office to rest.

I was invited to speak that night at the professors' club of the university on the subject of Soviet-German friendship and on my inventions. I did not know what to tell them of friendship, so in my speech I confined myself to an expression of gratitude for their attention to me as a representative of all Russian doctors. The Germans awarded me with polite applause, and I was invited to a banquet. The banquet room contained a large table with easy chairs around it and Czech beer on it—one bottle per participant. That was the extent of the revelry. Accustomed to traditional Russian dinners with a superabundance of food and drink, I found the German banquet a little strange.

That night at Miloš's home I handed him the watch and the bracelet and he gave me the money. Irina had furnished me with a long list of prospective purchases: a coat, a sweater, shoes and boots for her, several items for our son and for myself; besides, I had to buy presents for my parents and in-laws.

The next morning I set out on a tour of the shops to see which of Irina's orders could be filled. The selection of merchandise was far greater than in Moscow and everything was laid out so beautifully that, unaccustomed to such opulence, I was dazzled. When I returned to the hospital to change the dressing for my patient, I found a crowd of reporters awaiting me. I was taken by surprise: in Moscow, I had performed operations of this kind for three years and, except for scientific journals, received no publicity at all. Here, apparently, I made quite a splash! So I had to answer questions, strike impressive poses, even change the dressing in the presence of reporters to let them photograph me with my patient. This kind of intercourse with newsmen was a novelty to me.

Then came a telephone call from the Orthopedic Hospital of Leipzig. Professor P. Matsen, a prominent orthopedic surgeon, invited me and Miloš to come to Leipzig and speak at a conference of orthopedists being held there at the time. Radio and TV had already carried news of my operation. I began to feel like a movie star.

In the beautiful city of Leipzig, we were put up in a first-rate hotel. That night we were invited to dinner at Professor Matsen's. German orthopedists were also present. Everybody asked me about my prosthesis, congratulated me on the first operation in Germany, and drank to my success. Indeed, I was becoming a celebrity.

The next morning we went to the conference where I was to give my paper. On the way I noticed a large high-class store, Exquisite, selling only the best of imports from West Germany, France, Spain, and Italy. Stores of this kind were nonexistent in Moscow, and I decided to visit Exquisite and buy everything on Irina's list there. My paper was scheduled to open the proceedings after the first intermission.

I had not more than an hour to complete the whole undertaking. Rather frantically and incoherently I tried to explain to a pretty salesgirl the kind of lady's garments and the size I needed. She listened patiently to my broken German and then asked to see Irina's note. After a look at the figures the salesgirl declared that they were her own size precisely. I was surprised; she did not look like Irina, but then no other woman is like your wife. I decided to take a gamble and asked her to try on the things I would be selecting, and then we would decide together whether or not to buy. The pleasant German girl agreed and we spent the hour playing that funny game. As a result, I bought two coats, an assortment of sweaters, dresses, shoes, and some other things. I barely had time to return when my paper was announced and I was called to the podium.

Almost all popular East German magazines printed articles about me and the operation. Miloš and I returned to Greifswald to find my patient recovering fast. For the first time in three years he could move his elbow. I had finished my business, bought all the things I was supposed to buy, and taken a little vacation on the Baltic coast near Rostock. Now it was time to go home.

After the East German media had given such attention to my operation, the *Vechernyaya Moskva* evening paper carried a tiny TASS (Telegraphic Agency of the Soviet Union) piece about me: "The orthopedist Vladimir Golyakhovsky, on a visit to the German Democratic Republic to take part in an international conference, performed the first surgical elbow joint replacement in that country."

39

I waited anxiously for the Scientific Council of the Medical and Dentistry School to determine the victor of the contest to fill the new position, but the voting was delayed time after time. Each Tuesday, the day the council sat in session, I came to the school to hear the news, but each time I was told that the question had not yet been discussed by the Party Committee, without whose recommendation the council could not make its choice. I tried to pump Dr. A. Belousov, but he was so busy that he merely waved at me and said, "You're still in the picture. Wait."

Being "still in the picture" meant I was not out of contention —not bad, but not good enough either. I approached several influential professors of my acquaintance and they all promised to put in a word for me at the dean's office. Two months passed, but the matter was still not resolved.

"You ought to soften Belousov with a present," my friend Dr. Georgadze advised me. "He likes presents, everybody knows it."

A present meant a bribe.

"What does he like best?"

"Anything will do, particularly money. But the best thing would be a diamond ring."

A bribe, pure and simple. I was averse to bribing Belousov. For one thing, I was afraid, because giving bribes was a crime punishable by law. Secondly, I did not regard myself so unworthy of the position as to buy it with a bribe. Finally, even if I bribed him, there was no iron-clad guarantee that the position would be mine. Belousov was a notorious grafter. At one point he had risen to become Deputy Minister of Public Health, Personnel; the peak of his career was in 1952–53, when he directed a campaign to purge Jews from good positions in medicine. After Stalin's death Belousov fell to insignificant administrative positions, but recently he had staged a comeback. He had many friends at the Central Committee of the Party, and they helped him upward again. Starved for power and money, he extorted large payoffs to make up for the lost time.

One Tuesday, when I came as usual to wait for word of the decision, I met my schoolmate Dr. V. Matveeyv, a psychiatrist.

"Congratulations, you've been passed by the Party Committee," he told me with a smile.

The Party Committee had voted for my nomination! Victory was now assured, for not a single professor on the Scientific Council would ever dare vote against the decision of the Party Committee.

And Dr. K. Lakin also told me, "You may consider yourself elected. The Professors' Council is still to vote, but it is a mere formality. Belousov supported you very strongly; without his support, you would never have made it."

So now I was head of the chair. I was overwhelmed by unexpected joy and emotion. I had craved that position so intensely and it meant so much for me that I could hardly believe my dream had finally come true. I immediately called Irina, but she was away. Then I called my mother-in-law and, restraining my emotions, told her with appropriate stolidity: "Please tell Irina I've been approved as head of the chair."

"I've always said you would become a big professor yet," mother-in-law replied, as if taking credit for my triumph. "You can see now I was right."

I had never heard statements to that effect from her.

Dr. Georgadze, with whom I killed a bottle of brandy to celebrate, asked me confidentially: "How much did you give Belousov?"

"Nothing at all."

"I don't believe it! Why then did he support you at the Party Committee?"

"How should I know?"

"Listen, don't make a mistake: even if you did not pay him before, you should pay him after. Otherwise he'll get angry and go after you. He's a past master at that."

I did not doubt that Belousov was an expert in making life miserable for those he hated, so I had to think of bribing him. It was a distasteful chore; I felt miserable. Why did I have to bribe him when in justice the position belonged to me? Justice? What did justice have to do with reality? I had been a physician for eighteen years, but I had rarely seen justice. If you are a Jew, even a half-Jew, and not a Party member to boot, you'd better not count on justice.

Those thoughts spoiled the joy of my victory. Still, I decided to give Belousov a gift—not too cheap, not overly expensive—something I had just brought in from East Germany.

At an opportune moment, when I found myself next to the dean and no one was around, I told him softly, "I'd like to visit you at home."

I had barely finished the phrase when he edged closer to me, looked warily around, and whispered back:

"As late as you can, not earlier than eleven or twelve."

Still feeling miserable, but dressed like a dandy in a new German overcoat, I went to him at midnight, carrying my new German briefcase packed with assorted gifts. He lived in a richly but tastelessly furnished spacious apartment in a big building on Lenin Prospect reserved for VIPs. Belousov himself opened the door. He wore slippers on bare feet and unbuttoned trousers.

Belousov was drunk. He embraced me right in the doorway, greedily eyeing my briefcase: "It's real nice on your part to come to see an old man. Congratulations on your election. It's a great success, yes, sir! Now you've got a brilliant career ahead of you. It's no joke to become head of a chair at a Moscow medical school at forty!"

"Thank you very much," I said. "I know you've done a lot for me."

"I sure did!"

"I brought presents from Germany. . . ."

"Hey, that's great! Real great! Let's see them!"

He dragged me by my sleeve to the kitchen. I took the gifts

out under his impatient eyes; he snatched and unwrapped each package. First there came a brand-new luxurious Braun electric shaver, which in Moscow cost at least 300 rubles—if you have the right connections. He liked it! Then I took out a pair of blue jeans.

He held them against his potbelly, but the jeans were obviously the wrong size (I had bought them for myself). However, at that time a pair of jeans cost at least 200 rubles in Moscow and Belousov welcomed them. Next came two bottles of liquor, English gin and Scotch whiskey, both beautifully packed. They induced particularly pleasant emotions in him. Foreign alcohol, too, was valuable merchandise in Moscow; each bottle could easily fetch 50 to 70 rubles on the black market. Then I took out a pretty tablecloth.

"That's for my wife," he said in a thrifty voice.

Then came several carved wooden articles from Yugoslavia followed by a few packets of chewing gum—a very rare commodity in Moscow.

"That's for your grandson," I told him.

When I emptied the briefcase, he peered inside to make sure nothing was left, and said, "I'll take the briefcase, too."

I was amazed at his greed. Come to think of it, though, there was nothing to be amazed at! "I am lucky he hasn't taken my coat off me," I thought.

Without further ado he poured two tea glasses of diluted alcohol. We drank them down and followed up with pickled mushrooms.

"I'm a heck of a worker," I told him. "You won't be sorry with your choice."

"Relax, I know everything about you worth knowing." He waved his short arm. "Don't forget I've worn out many pairs of pants on personnel chairs. Big people strongly recommended you, called me, came to see me personally. But let me tell you: the Party Committee objected very strongly to your candidacy. 'He's not a Party member, and he passes himself off as a Russian while his father is Jewish,' they said. I told them time and again that you were a leading specialist, an outstanding scientist with a brilliant career ahead of you, that at your tender age of forty you had more inventions than the rest of our professors put together. They wouldn't be moved. 'Yes, but still he is a Jew, still he is not a Party member.' Well, as for Jews, several of our professors are Jewish, so that's nothing new.

But all of them are Party members. Just to think of it: fifty chair heads, all Party members, except you. But I'm not sorry. I need a man of the world, a man with a good business sense, above all. Let's try your booze."

We opened the bottle of gin. Again we downed full tea glasses and followed up with mushrooms. I did not want to match him drink for drink, but neither did I want to fall conspicuously behind. I was a little giddy, while his speech was getting increasingly slurred. Still, he continued talking; as a Russian proverb says: what a sober man keeps to himself, a drunk pours forth. Belousov pulled me to the living room and showed me a head of an elk on a wall.

"Do you remember how you gave me this elk?" he asked.

"Well, your shot felled him." I tried to look innocent.

"Come on, I know it was your bullet. But I liked the way you presented him to me. And I thought right off: here's a guy who knows how to do business. And as for your father being Jewish, it's nothing to worry about. I remember him. He was deputy director of the Institute of Surgery and dean of the surgery department, wasn't he?"

Little wonder that Belousov remembered; it was on his orders that my father had been fired.

"First of all your internal passport says that you're Russian," he went on. "It means we'll not go over our quota of Jews and you won't mar our statistics as far as the District Party Committee is concerned. Besides, what's wrong with being Jewish? Personally I do not suffer from Jews."

I had to restrain myself not to shout: "But the Jews have suffered a lot from you!" But I had to hold my tongue.

"I have lots of Jewish friends, yes, sir! If I have to do business, Jews are the only people I can turn to. There! I like you and will always protect you. But let me give you a piece of advice: be very careful, there are so many scoundrels around, and all of them are at each other's throats. Do you know how many of them try to bring me down? They write denunciations every day. There's no way they'll get me, their arms are too short. But you must remember . . . remember . . ."

He dozed off, and I left still wondering what it was I had to remember.

I came home in a cab, rather drunk. Irina was awake, waiting for me.

"Where's your bag?" she asked with a smile. "Lost it while under the influence?"

"No, my new boss appropriated it for himself. You won't believe how utterly disgusting it was." I told her what had happened. My victory did not seem so wonderful anymore.

Early in the morning of November 1, 1971, I came for the first time to my new job at Basmannaya Hospital #6, in downtown Moscow. Peering through the cold morning fog, I saw that the hospital consisted of several two-story wooden barracks, old and dilapidated. I found out later they had been built a century before, during the Russo-Turkish War of 1873, as temporary quarters for soldiers felled by an epidemic of typhus. From outside the barracks in no way looked like a hospital. Inside, the resemblance was even more remote.

Behind the wire netting of a small cloakroom, an old Russian woman bundled up in a wraparound shawl was sound asleep. I woke her up gingerly.

She stared at me. "What do *you* want?"

"I'm sorry to have awakened you. I am Dr. Golyakhovsky, the new director. Good morning! I'd like to check in my coat and get a gown."

"No way," she said indifferently.

"Beg your pardon, you've probably misunderstood me. Today is my first day on the job as professor and director of this department."

"I don't give a damn who you are," she replied with a yawn. "If I get orders to issue you a gown, I will; if I don't, I won't."

Soon doctors started to come; they knew me and prevailed upon the old attendant to issue me a gray and wash-worn visitor's gown. I was about to start up the old, creaky, wooden stairs to the second floor when the door opposite me was flung open, a gust of cold air blew in, and two young physicians entered, carrying a patient on a wooden stretcher. They turned out to be orthopedic residents on duty, and they had carried the patient from the emergency room housed in another barracks in the yard, a distance of some 150 yards. They hauled the stretcher up the stairs, panting with effort as the patient was heavy and the stairs steep and narrow. At one point they nearly dumped him. I followed them upstairs and watched them put the stretcher on the floor in the corridor next to several other patients sprawled on mattresses and stretchers. A few more patients lay on collapsible beds.

"Why do you keep patients on the floor?" I asked the residents.

"No beds available, comrade professor. All the rooms are packed."

"Anything happened? A mass accident or something?"

"Nothing's happened, it's a usual thing for us. They'll have to stay on the floor for a couple of days, waiting for a bed in one of the rooms or the corridor to become vacant."

I had not seen such misery since I had worked seventeen years ago in Pudozh. "What happened to the elevator, why did you have to carry the patient in your arms?"

"The *elevator?*" They stared at me in disbelief. "There is no elevator here and there will never be. The building barely stands as it is."

We spent the first half of every day rearranging the patients, but some patients would remain in the same place on the floor for two or three days. The situation reminded me of the evacuation hospitals during World War Two, but this was thirty years later in Moscow, a "model communist city." Some doctors and nurses made a lot of money by charging the patients 10 rubles to put them in a bed ahead of the other patients. The patients gladly paid this money, since even the most crowded and stuffy room was better than the corridor floor.

The hospital was famous for the fact that its patients had to pay cash for every kind of medical care. The pharmacy didn't have enough medicines; the operating room didn't have enough instruments; the supply room didn't have enough linen; the X-ray room didn't have enough film; nobody had enough of anything until the patients paid, and then everything was suddenly available.

Just a few months ago a new department of intensive therapy had opened. This department had none of the medicines that it needed. The relatives of the patients were prepared to buy the necessary medicines at any price, but they didn't know where to find them. The chief of that department, Dr. Yuri Chub, had a supply of them he had obtained from acquaintances, paying for them out of his own pocket. Dr. Chub told the relatives of the patients that the necessary medicines were not available but that he might be able to convince "somebody" to sell them—for a high price. The relatives agreed, and he sold the medicines to them through a middle man. Most of the relatives were thankful, but one of them informed on Dr. Chub to the Department for the Struggle with the Theft of Socialist Property (OBKhSS). During the course of the next two years, the police tried to blame him for stealing. Although the medicine hadn't been formally stolen, Dr. Chub had to leave his position at the hospital. And what did the patients gain from this? Nothing. The mortality rate in the department rose sharply.

It would be easier for me to list the available medical equipment in the hospital than it would be to list the equipment that was not available.

Since the Russian medical industry doesn't produce disposable equipment, the nurses had to spend hours boiling syringes and needles, each of which is used hundreds of times. The syringes were never ready when the doctors needed them, so the doctors had to wait. I've held up an operation for as long as a half hour because a syringe was in the storeroom or was still being boiled or because the nurse had to run to the next department to borrow theirs.

Because of this rush, the syringes and needles were frequently boiled for too short a time and consequently spread diseases. This happened all the time.

The scalpels were so dull that they ripped the skin instead of cutting a fine, thin line. The dull scalpels weren't discarded, though. Instead, they were collected and sharpened on ordinary emery stones, which scratched the blades and eventually caused corrosion and rust.

Since X-ray film was also in chronically short supply, patients had to wait for months for an appointment to be X-rayed. In desperation, the patients traveled around to other hospitals and clinics, but there was no film anywhere.

The staff of physicians had been put together before my arrival. I found two old acquaintances among my assistants: Dr. Vladimir Mikhailenko and Dr. Anatoly Pechenkin. They greeted me with smiles:

"You've surely taken your time!"

I was not too glad to find them here, for I remembered that

when all three of us had worked at the Central Institute of Orthopedics in the 1960s, both devoted more time and energy to Party business than to medicine. However, I concealed my apprehension and greeted them cordially enough.

Dr. V. Mikhailenko was secretary of the Party Group of the department of which I was now director. Obviously proud of his lofty position, he told me right at the start: "Now you and I will manage the department together."

I had no intention of sharing managerial duties with him. "I'll manage," I replied. "And you will *help* me."

He turned perceptibly gloomier and averted his eyes.

Dr. A. Pechenkin stayed on the sidelines, shying away from Party positions. Very soon I found out that he assiduously shirked his medical duties, too; he was invariably the last to come to work and the first to be gone.

From the very first day, Mikhailenko went out of his way to demonstrate his loyalty. He reported to me on his colleagues and even criticized Pechenkin for loafing. He also liked to tell me of his work in Kuwait in 1969.

"So I was sent to that Kuwait," he began the story of his exploits abroad. "First, I sat through the various briefings and was then given a military rank of KGB captain in reserve. There were just three of us, but we obeyed iron discipline. We held Party meetings, kept our accounting in order, the works. As for the country, you wouldn't believe how loaded that Kuwait is. They've grown so fat on their oil that they produce nothing, just buy everything. For instance, all medical equipment, you name it, comes from the United States, West Germany, Japan. . . ."

"Are you saying their equipment is better than ours?" I asked.

"Am I saying it?"—he threw up his arms—"You can't imagine how much better! Just wink at the nurse and she'll bring it. And everything is disposable. Occasionally I even felt guilty for discarding such wonderful things. And their doctors earn far more than we do."

"How much did you earn?"

"We got a lot of money, but we had to surrender three-quarters of our earnings to our embassy to contribute to the state currency reserves. Even so, I earned enough for five or six years of good life. I bought myself a car and a two-bedroom cooperative apartment. Here in Moscow if I had stayed at home instead of going abroad, I would never have been able to save as much."

He strove to become my premier assistant, my right hand, doing his best to become indispensable. He accompanied me everywhere and forestalled my wishes. I did nothing to either encourage or discourage him, studying him all the while.

Once Nata Wolf, a twenty-four-year-old graduate coed, a Jewish girl, asked me when there was nobody around:

"Do you trust Dr. Mikhailenko?"

"Of course, he's my assistant, isn't he? Why?"

"Nothing . . . But I wouldn't trust him if I were you."

"Why shouldn't I?"

"Do you know what he did the last time I was on duty? Early in the morning when everybody fell asleep after night work, I dozed off in the X-ray room. He entered and crept to me. At first I feigned sleep, but when he lay on me I pushed him off. That's when he confided in me: 'Everybody says that you sleep with our new professor. I want him to trust me as much as possible. So I decided that if I make love to you, you'll help me influence him.' "

"I hope you've refuted his assumption."

"No, why should I?" She lowered her long eyelashes demurely.

Be that as it may, she confirmed what I had suspected all along: I had to be wary of Dr. Mikhailenko.

But I had to be even more circumspect with the other professors whom I met at weekly sessions of the Scientific Board or at the dean's office.

Party membership was the primary criterion for selection of the teaching staff for medical schools. I was a very rare exception. Over 80 percent of our faculty and all professors/directors, with one exception, were Party members. My observations showed that over half of them were incompetent in their respective fields of medicine and clung to their positions through mutual support.

In my department, there was not a single sound specialist; I had no one to rely upon. I knew quite a few orthopedic surgeons who could make wonderful tutors for our students; but almost all of them were Jews, did not belong to the Party or, worst of all, combined the two. I realized very soon that if my department was to meet a certain standard, I had to change several assistants. But I could not begin my reign by reshuffling personnel. First I had to solidify my own position among the professors.

Of course, there were a few distinguished scientists among the faculty, authors of textbooks. They differed from the rest of the crowd made up of Party upstarts. The renowned professors behaved more naturally and dressed better; their faces bespoke education and intellectual interests. But the rest of them were a gray mass of petty bureaucrats, resembling one another as if made in the same mold. They dressed uniformly in poorly cut and ill-fitting dark gray suits; their shirts were never fresh and their faces were stern, stolid, tersely serious and devoid of any glow of intellect, a far cry from what one would expect from medical school professors.

At one of the sessions of the Professors' Scientific Council, Dr. Vasily Rodionov, one of the Party crowd, delivered a long-winded report on the subject "Ideological Training of the Faculty." For two hours, never taking his eyes from a prepared text, he exhorted us to strengthen our ideology and morality, bombarding the audience with quotations from Marx and Lenin.

"All our professors and instructors should read the works of great Lenin every day!" he screamed—and paused.

Surprised in the midst of a whispered discussion, Dean Belousov, the secretary of the Party Committee, and the other members of the Presidium started and burst out in applause. All the professors followed suit. Trapped, I also had to clap a suitable couple of times. At that instant, Dr. Stepan Babichev, who sat next to me, bent toward me and said, all the while applauding:

"Hey, he's right! A very sound idea, so to say. . . . Yes, we must read Lenin every day. Well said, so to say. . . . Eh, what do you think?"

"Yes, I like his idea," I said, looking aside and thinking: "Both of you be damned!"

My parents rejoiced in my success and were very proud of me. Mother believed that I was going to be an important man in medicine. Father, who had retired but continued from time to time to consult with some patients in his former hospital, next questioned me.

"How's your department doing?"

"Everything's fine, thanks."

"And how do you feel in your new position?"

"Fine."

"You seem unwilling to discuss your work with me."

"I'm too busy; besides, I'm tired."

"All right, you'll tell me some other time."

Once, when I came to visit my parents, Father was out and Mother asked me: "Why are you so sad lately? Anything happened?"

"No. But I am not all that happy about my new job."

"Really? I thought you were satisfied."

"I was. But I find myself liking my job less and less. Well, maybe habit will bring love."

"You mean there's a spoonful of tar in your cask of honey?" Mother asked.

"Sometimes it seems it's a cask of tar with just a spoonful of honey," I replied.

40

As a department director I drew the top salary attainable by a physician, 500 rubles per month, and besides earned another couple of hundred rubles by consultations at several special outpatient hospitals. It was a decent income by Soviet standards and we could even afford to start a savings account at a state savings bank. An increasing number of private patients, enticed by my title, besieged me with requests for a consultation or operation—and were willing to pay for it.

For the first time Irina and I felt we were rich; for the first time we did not have to scrimp to get by. The circle of my connections at retail food stores and wholesale centers was expanding, and I no longer had to depend for my meat supplies on Slavka the butcher.

His place as my purveyor of provisions was taken by another patient, Gusman the Tatar, a storekeeper at the Ministry of Foreign Trade. Leonid Brezhnev's son Yuri was Deputy Minister of Foreign Trade. On his orders a special canteen was set up on the floor where his office was located. Brezhnev's canteen offered just about anything one could possibly fancy. Of course it was a far cry from a New York delicatessen, but in the Soviet Union it was a dream place. The canteen catered only to top-level functionaries, from the rank of Deputy Minister and up. The privileged few ordered provisions that were packed and delivered to their homes. My patient Gusman handled the orders and packed food, which gave him unobstructed access to the stock. He put my name on the list of permanent customers. I would call him on the phone and tell him what I needed: caviar —no problem; fresh filet mignon—no problem; any kind of fish—no problem; instant coffee (the rarest of rarities!)—no problem; salami from the special "Kremlin" shop of the Moscow meat-packing plant —no problem (the salami was fragrant and far tastier than the brands available at regular stores). He even dispensed olive oil, which was never sold anywhere, and delicious Pilsner beer from Czechoslovakia. The only inconvenience: at each delivery I had to loiter at the policeman's booth behind the Ministry, waiting for my package to be brought out, because I was not allowed inside.

While supplying big bosses, Gusman did a large private business and sold part of the provisions to a certain number of clients at twice or thrice the official price. Thus, with his profits he had more money than many big doctors and professors less affluent than he was.

Life was in full swing, and our financial situation improving. Then Irina decided to change her job, for she was having trouble with her boss, Dr. A. Adoh, and the psychological high of having just successfully defended a doctoral thesis made her think that she could rightfully claim a more respectable job. We both started looking around and soon she found a position at the Institute of Surgery. It was still headed by Dr. A. Vishnevsky.

Having made all arrangements with her new employer, she quit the allergological laboratory/stable. But then, when she brought her documents for registration at the new lab, she was told at the personnel department: "We can't accept your documents; the institute director has reversed his initial decision."

It was baffling. The director knew that Irina was his closest friend's daughter-in-law. He had known me since childhood and in general had been close to our family as long as I could remember. My father and I went to see Vishnevsky, who was a very influential and important figure, being a general, Chief Army Surgeon, and deputy of the Supreme Soviet.

He welcomed us cordially, embraced my father and me, and bombarded us with questions. After a few minutes of small talk, my father got to the point.

"Shura, what's happened? Why was Irina turned away? You promised, didn't you?"

"Listen," Dr. Vishnevsky said uneasily, "I feel so guilty, but I can't think of a way to get her in! You see, after I had promised her that position, a commission from the District Party Committee came to the institute. They checked all personnel and told me that I had too many Jews. It's true; you know yourself how many of my people are Jewish."

About 15 percent of the research staff at the institute were Jews. Dr. Vishnevsky himself was half-Jewish, on his mother's side, though officially he was considered to be a blue-blooded ethnic Russian.

"I gave them a promise not to employ any more Jews," he went on. "Alas, Irina was the first to come seeking employment the very next day. Well, personnel knew, of course, about my agreement with the Party Committee and refused to accept her documents, although personally I did not turn her down. Now we'll have to wait. As soon as one of my Jews quits, Irina will have priority claim."

Neither my father nor I liked that conversation. My wife was jobless for the sole reason of being Jewish! What was to be done?

I tried my best to cheer Irina. I took her to theaters, concerts, and shows; every Sunday we went on cross-country skiing expeditions in the Opalikha Forest near Moscow. We also increased the frequency of visits to friends, though neither Irina nor I fancied table-talk, that favorite pastime of intellectuals in Moscow.

Once we visited a patient-turned-friend, a Jewish lawyer named Mark Keller, who was well past fifty. Mark and his wife were intelligent people and I often sought his advice on various problems. This time I wanted to discuss Irina's situation with him and hear what he had to say.

The Kellers' only daughter, a recently married twenty-two-year-old, was a graduate of the languages department of the Moscow University. She had a great gift for languages and knew several Arabic dialects. We learned that several months previously Galya and her husband had emigrated to Israel. It was our first encounter with a concrete fact of someone from our circle having left Russia. We were both thunderstruck; it seemed to us so strange, so improbable. Galya's father Mark calmly told us the story.

"Galya graduated with honors, but being Jewish, no one wanted to hire her. She spent six months futilely looking for a job, but whenever her nationality came up she was invariably told no. Poor girl, she was utterly demoralized. Naturally, we did as much as we could to comfort her. She and her student husband lived with us and we totally supported them. Then one day she said: 'That's it! We're applying for emigration to Israel. I don't want to stay in this country!' What could we say? We appreciated her feelings."

From time to time I looked at Irina and watched her face as she heard details of Galya's story. Initially the authorities had refused to grant them exit visas. Many Jewish supporters from the United States visited them at home; several United States senators wrote letters on their behalf. At long last, they were allowed to go. Now they were in Israel, where they had found jobs immediately and enjoyed life.

Then Mark asked me a question: "Why don't you emigrate? Have you thought of it?"

I had not and neither had Irina. To us, the idea of leaving Russia belonged to the realm of fantasy. It acquired the flesh of reality in the early seventies when the United States Congress passed the Jackson-Vanick Amendment to the Russian trade bill, whereby the most favored nation status was to be denied Russia as long as the Russian government obstructed free emigration of Jews, Armenians, and Germans wishing to reunite with their relatives abroad. The first families started emigrating in the late sixties, and gradually more and more people were involved in the exodus. But I had not given any thought to it.

What was I to reply to Mark?

"You know," I mumbled uneasily, "I've just gotten a great new job. It's not all perfect, of course, but I am still full of plans and energy. I don't see any reason why I should leave."

That night, in my diary, I described that conversation. It stuck in my memory.

I finally succeeded in finding a job for Irina. As always, connections helped. She was hired at 200 rubles a month as a research associate at the Gamaleya Institute of Microbiology and Epidemiology.

Dr. D. Kaulen, a Finn, who had been my schoolmate in medical school, was deputy director there. We were friends and he prevailed on the director, Dr. O. Baroyan, to give Irina a chance considering that, aside from other qualifications, she spoke German and English. An Armenian, Dr. Baroyan was less bigoted than Russians toward Jews. For all his academic titles, he was no scientist. Many years ago he had been head doctor at the Soviet Hospital in Teheran and a master spy in the Orient. He was appointed to head the Institute of Epidemiology because it had secret laboratories developing bacteriological warfare agents. The laboratories were located deep in the large inner yard and were off limits even to most of the institute staff. But naturally enough, there was no dearth of rumors, and all employees knew very well indeed what their colleagues with special security passes were doing.

41

At the sight of a state-owned black Volga limousine with the license plates MAC-OO-II hurtling down the center lane of a Moscow street, traffic cops would hurriedly wave other traffic aside and snap to attention, hand at cap in a military salute. They knew the car belonged to General Igor Karpets, head of the Criminal Investigation Department of the Ministry of Internal Affairs.

I rode in that car on many occasions because General Karpets was a patient and a friend of mine. For a decade, from 1967 to 1977,

I moonlighted as a consulting surgeon at the Ministry of Internal Affairs Central Outpatient Clinic, at 25 Petrovka Street.

The criminal investigators annually uncover and investigate hundreds of thousands of crimes: murders, robberies, rapes, muggings, thefts, forgeries. All these crimes are indistinguishable from those that plague other countries, but there is one important difference: they are almost never reported by the media and most of them are adjudicated behind closed doors. Like the tip of an iceberg, visible crime is but a fraction of the reality, while the rest are securely hidden in the classified folders at the Criminal Investigation Department.

The new morality being crammed down the throats of the citizens of communist society runs counter to man's natural proclivities. The authoritarian system strives for 100 percent adherence to the law. But human vices are as old as humankind itself, and the art of mayhem is among the most refined of all human endeavors. To cover up their failure to stop crime and to create an impression of their omnipotence in controlling public morals, Soviet authorities have simply made criminal statistics a state secret. Neither newspapers and magazines, nor radio and TV broadcasts, nor books and movies are allowed to let slip news of crime. One reason for keeping the true crime picture hidden is to create an impression in the West that crime does not exist in the Soviet Union, that communist morality has triumphed where the free world has failed.

In the fall of 1976, General Karpets fell seriously ill. His ailment baffled experts: crazy temperature fluctuations, fever, aching joints and muscles all over his body. He was treated by the Special Unit of the Ministry of Internal Affairs Central Outpatient Clinic, but the doctors there failed to diagnose his disease. The general's condition followed an uneven course: occasionally he would feel better, only to revert to misery the next day. His case was taken over by the Kremlin Hospital physicians, but they could not lay their finger on the correct diagnosis either. General Karpets was examined at the Kremlin Hospital by Dr. V. Pokrovsky, a noted authority on carrier diseases, who decided that his patient suffered from a tropical fever. These diseases are commonplace in areas infested with tropical mosquitoes, but such insects are nowhere to be found in Moscow and the general had not left the Soviet capital in the previous months.

His condition steadily deteriorated; fits of fever followed one another in rapid succession; the patient swam in perspiration and was constantly in pain. Not surprisingly, he was extremely depressed. Once his wife, desperate for sound advice, called me for help. The next Sunday, my wife and I went to their state dacha. The entrance to the exclusive settlement was guarded by a militia patrol that turned away all traffic but waved the general's car through. We drove along empty streets flanked on both sides by tall fences, with militia guards at all intersections and KGB guards behind the fences. A tall gate opened to let us in to a huge wooded plot with a two-story log cabin in the far corner. The eight-room house came to the occupant fully furnished.

I found the general very weak from his ailment and completely baffled: how and where could he have contracted any infection? Out of professional habit he would analyze, time and again, all possibilities but invariably became discouraged. Though not equipped to treat carrier diseases, I found it strange that his disease had not been diagnosed. So I suggested that the first thing to do was to find out the kind of disease that had struck him. To this end, his blood sample was to be sent for serological tests to the N. Gamaleya Institute of Microbiology and Epidemiology. My wife worked there and knew many good specialists.

The woman doctor whom my wife asked to run a serological test on the general's blood sample peppered her with questions: when and how did he contract the disease? Then came the crucial question: "Does he live in Krasnaya Presnya?" (an area in Moscow).

The general did not. Yet his agglutination titer was extremely high; the test conclusively indicated that he was suffering from brucellosis, a highly dangerous carrier disease that cripples for life many of its victims. Brucellosis usually results from exposure to sick animals, above all cows, or from drinking nonpasteurized milk. Hence it rarely, if ever, occurs anywhere outside rural areas; nor is it transmitted from man to man. Brucellosis is very difficult to treat and it almost invariably has damaging aftereffects.

Having found out the diagnosis, I rushed to see Karpets again. To make sure it was brucellosis he had contracted, I proceeded to ask him whether he had drunk raw milk anywhere or come in contact with cows or other animals. He replied to all questions in the negative.

Then I asked him: "Did you happen to be in the Krasnaya Presnya area immediately prior to the onset of the disease?"

"Yes, but only once and for just a few minutes at that. I went to the Research Institute of Criminology, of whose Scientific Council I am a member. I was pressed for time and so I just took part in the voting on a thesis and left."

I returned to the Gamaleya Institute and told the woman serologist that the patient had indeed visited Krasnaya Presnya once before his affliction.

"But what's so important about that area?" I asked her. Then she told me that for several months she had conducted serological tests on hundreds of Krasnaya Presnya residents stricken en masse by a strange infectious disease similar to the general's. The disease was found to be brucellosis, but the diagnosis puzzled experts: there were no cows in the area, nor was raw milk on sale in Krasnaya Presnya stores. It was the first brucellosis epidemic in Moscow.

The mystery was dispelled by accident when it was learned from confidential sources about the existence in Krasnaya Presnya of a small, supersecret biological warfare laboratory where lethal infections, including brucellosis, were studied. The foul air with a high Brucella count from dangerous experiments, instead of being disposed of as required by safety regulations, was simply vented through a rubber tube sticking out of the window. As a result, such a high concentration of the germs built up in the environment that eventually residents of nearby buildings one after another came down with brucellosis. The Gamaleya researchers were speechless with amazement: hitherto, no one had suspected that brucellosis could be contracted by inhalation.

Told this detective story, Karpets flew into a rage. He thundered that the criminals would not go unpunished and began furiously dialing secret phone numbers to find out the whereabouts of the germ warfare lab.

Weeks later he told me (we were alone in the car), "I failed to get anywhere. I have no right to conduct an investigation in a military unit; they have their own investigators and their own regulations."

There the story ended. The general went on suffering from brucellosis.

The physicians of the outpatient clinics and small hospitals in the vicinity of the laboratory could not explain the origin or the nature of the strange disease that afflicted hundreds of their patients. They believed it was a modified form of flu. Many patients were in the dark as to the diagnosis of their illness because not all of them were subjected to serological tests. And none of them, except for the head of the Criminal Investigation Department, knew the source of the infection.

42

Among my staff at Basmannay Hospital #6 was a Jewish physician named Yakov Egalevich, a plain, unobtrusive man of fifty beaten down by daily hardships and the ever-present need to supplement his meager income by doubling at other jobs. When I came to the hospital I did not know him. At the end of my very first day on the job, he knocked timidly on the door of my tiny office. He entered and started bowing, rocking like a Jew in a synagogue.

"Take a seat," I said.

"You can't imagine how happy I am!" he exclaimed.

"What makes you so happy?"

"The fact that you'll be our director."

"Thank you. But you don't know me, do you?"

"Yes, I do. All our Jewish physicians know you. And we're all happy that you've come to us as our director. Your election is a victory for all Jews."

Personally, I did not think it was much of a victory for the Jewish cause, but I decided against letting the air out of his joy. It is a rare occasion indeed for Jews in Russia to have reason to be happy for one of their own.

Dr. Egalevich's only son was eighteen. The next year he applied for admission to our medical school. His father had been beside himself with anxiety the whole previous year, tormented by the question: will he be admitted or not? Any time he met me, he interrogated me with questions like these:

"What's the Jewish quota at your school?"

"I should grease a palm or two? I mean now; later I'll give more."

"They say your Belousov accepts bribes from entrants. I'd be glad to pay him, only how should I approach him?"

"Have you heard the rumor that this year the number of Jews among entrants dropped against the last year?"

In most cases I either could not or would not answer such questions. Parental hysteria accompanying high school graduates' attempts to get into college was nothing out of the ordinary. If a boy failed at his entrance exams, the next year he was up for a three-year draft. Therefore the parents of boys were more worried than those with daughters. And each summer I was besieged with questions and requests by scores of friends and friends of friends. Everybody hoped that I would be able to help in some way, if only by an introduction to one of the people having to do with admissions. But I followed a strict hands-off policy.

Still, I sympathized with Egalevich, and at least tried to calm him. "Why worry so much?" I said. "If your son gets passing grades at all four entrance exams, he'll be a medical student."

"Are you sure?" he exclaimed with enormous relief. "You forget we're Jewish, that's where the rub lies. . . ."

I understood his feelings. All my life I had hidden behind my mother's Russian blood, whereas he, with nothing to hide behind, had to endure.

One morning he burst into my office, beaming. "He's been admitted! My son is a student of medical school!" he shouted in jubilation. "Thank you, oh, thank you so much!"

"Congratulations, but your gratitude's misplaced," I said smiling. "I've done nothing to help your son. The credit for passing the exams is entirely his."

"You gave him your moral support, that's what I'm grateful for. I always told him: 'Professor Golyakhovsky feels that you'll pass the exams with flying colors.' And so he did!"

I decided not to argue my innocence.

A year later, Dr. Egalevich entered my office and heavily

slumped into a chair; so crestfallen was he that he forgot to say hello.

"They've kicked him out!" he said hoarsely. "My son has been expelled from the medical school. It's the end of everything. Now he'll never be able to get into college again. Then he'll be drafted into the army and—his life is ruined. Mine is, too. . . ."

"What happened?"

"A scandal. He had a row with Professor Vasily Rodionov, who lodged a complaint with the dean's office and the Party Committee. They've expelled him."

"Tell me calmly, without emotion."

"What are you saying? How can I be calm? Now you're our only hope. Please help! I'm pleading with you on my knees."

"If I can do anything, I will," I said reassuringly.

"Only you, only you can help. . . ."

After a while he regained his composure sufficiently to tell me what had happened. A group of students, including his son, had romped in the lobby of the lecture building, waiting for classes to begin. The students had come too early and whiled away the time, singing, making merry, joking with the girls, munching on sandwiches. Enter Professor V. Rodionov, a surgeon, whom they did not know because they had not yet taken up surgery. A rude and uncouth man, he began yelling at the students without preliminaries. Most of the boys were cowed, but several students, Egalevich Junior included, resented his manners. With youthful fervor, Egalevich entered into an argument with the unknown man. Rodionov immediately concentrated all his venom on the new adversary. The following dialogue ensued (as roughly related by Egalevich Senior):

"You have no place at the medical school!" bellowed Rodionov.

"Why do I have no place here?"

"You know very well why!"

"Because I'm Jewish?"

"I didn't say it, you did."

"But you said I have no place here and that I should know why. Explain what you mean."

"Lay off me," screamed Rodionov. "You don't know whom you're talking to."

"I don't give a damn who you are. But I do know that I'm talking to an anti-Semite," Egalevich replied. He edged closer to

Rodionov and threateningly grabbed the lapels of the professor's jacket.

He was expelled for amoral conduct.

During the two months that followed, I talked on many occasions to the dean, pleading with him to reinstate Egalevich Junior. I finally succeeded, but he exacted his pound of flesh: Junior was to work as a laborer on a construction site for six months and only then would he be readmitted to the medical school, busted back to freshman to boot. Still, he was extraordinarily lucky to get away with such a light penance.

Soon, however, I was to pay for having helped a Jewish student, even if indirectly (I would probably have had to pay even if I hadn't helped him). Dr. Lerman, a Jewish physician at the ophthalmology department, decided to emigrate with his family to Israel and applied for visas. Under the law he was within his rights and could not be obstructed officially, but the dean and the Party Committee called a special meeting of the faculty to pillory Dr. Lerman for his "crime." The goal of that auto-da-fé was not so much to condemn the "culprit" as to browbeat other Jews and half-Jews out of similar ideas.

Zhanna, the secretary, called me at the hospital. "The dean insists you attend the meeting and make a speech into the bargain," she said.

I decided to skip the gathering. But some time later Belousov himself called. "You must come to the meeting," he ordered. "Yes, and be sure to speak there."

Just before the meeting was scheduled to start, I was told to come to the dean's office. Entering the room, I saw several professors and the inevitable Secretary of the Party Committee. I looked around and realized that only Jews or half-Jews were in attendance: Professors V. Kurlyandsky, A. Mashkelleison, V. Orlov, and several others. They sat with uneasy expressions on their faces, listening to the dean.

"You must all speak at the meeting to condemn that louse and traitor who wants to leave our Motherland! A representative of the District Party Committee will be present and I warn you: you're holding your own fate in your hands. Your criticism must be strong enough to show your true attitude toward the scoundrel and to others of his ilk who stoop so low as to betray the Motherland that has given them everything: education, jobs, happiness. Do you understand me?"

Did we ever! Plainly speaking, we Jews were forced to scourge a Jew. It was impossible to avoid the humiliation, for refusal to participate, whatever the pretext, would be tantamount to a revolt and interpreted as such. The dilemma was very simple: speak up or ship out.

The auditorium was jam-packed; there were many more people than usual. The "condemnee" was absent. I did not know him personally, and at least his absence made the forthcoming ordeal a little bit easier.

First the dean and the Secretary of the Party Committee delivered highly emotional orations, heaping scores of epithets and defamations on Dr. Lerman. They incited the audience; people started to yell:

"It's true, he's a traitor!"

"He has betrayed his Motherland!"

"Down with scum like him!"

"The louse!"

Without looking, I recognized some of the voices; they belonged to physicians, professors of our school. I recalled similar meetings of Stalinist times and could not see any difference.

Then the floor was given to Professor V. Kurlyandsky, an eminent and widely respected sixty-five-year-old scientist, author of several textbooks on dentistry. A Party member of long standing, he had become inured to meetings of this sort. Therefore he had no trouble railing against his coreligionist in an unbridled manner ("principled criticism" in Party jargon), by and large repeating the gems of his predecessors. In fairness to Professor Kurlyandsky, the first two speakers had depleted the available stock of invective so thoroughly that little was left for his use.

My mind was racing feverishly: what should I say? I searched for such wording that would take a middle ground between condemnation and neutrality. Already Kurlyandsky was winding up. He ended his speech with a shout:

"And our comrades from the audience are absolutely right: there is no place for a traitor like him in our collective, in our country, among our Soviet people!"

The floor burst out in applause. Still desperately groping for the right turn of phrase, I thought: Incidentally, he himself decided to emigrate. Too late to shout he has no place here; he has figured it out himself. . . . At that instant I heard the dean calling out my name. I stood up and went to the podium. My feet did not obey me, and I stumbled. Trying to retain a dispassionate expression, I caught myself praying not to tell them what I really thought of the proceedings. I ascended the podium and bent to the microphone because all strength had suddenly drained out of my voice. I looked at the hundreds of faces in front of me. The dean, the Party Secretary, the District Committee man, all turned in my direction and stared at me, waiting for me to speak.

"Comrades, it is a very sad fact that the man has chosen not to attend our meeting," I began. The opening phrase meant nothing, but I had to fill the required three to four minutes with meaningless blabber.

"If he had come he would have been sitting among us, he would have been able to see his colleagues and hear us speak, and he would have been ashamed, comrades!"

Again my inner voice stepped forward and silently said: Because he would have seen the kind of scoundrels his colleagues are. I continued.

"The country he wants to go to [I did not want to name Israel] for many years now has caused concern among peaceful Arab inhabitants [My God, what nonsense I am saying, particularly that nightmarish "Arab inhabitants"]. She behaves aggressively [Can Israel behave otherwise, having known not a day of respite since the day it was founded?]. And yet he wants to go there! [Well, if he wants to go, let him; he is a grown man, it's up to him!] Every day we read in the newspapers and hear on the radio about the raids of the army and air force of that country against Arab inhabitants. [And they are perfectly justified. Or should they wait passively to be butchered by the Arabs?] It is impossible to imagine how much blood and tears are being shed in that part of the world, in the Middle East [including Jewish blood, including Jewish tears!]. Why would he want to go to that aggressive country? [Each day Israel is branded an aggressor in hundreds of articles; may the Lord absolve me for parroting this idiocy!]"

At that instant the dean interrupted: "What is your personal attitude to his deed?" he asked.

"I can't understand him."

"But do you condemn him?"

"Yes, of course, I do. [Damn them. *Damn them!*] I support what all those who spoke before me said. He has no place here."

And with that I stepped down from the podium. As I remember, there was no applause. Anyway my head throbbed so loudly I could hear nothing.

I came home totally exhausted and told Irina everything. I drank vodka, I smoked, I lay down, I jumped up. I recalled all the times I had to lie publicly by word or silence. I recalled a student meeting at which we had condemned a religious coed and a meeting where student Rivkin had been accused of being a "Zionist" and an "agent of Zionism." How long had I lied? How long?—all my life!

In the middle of the night I woke up in a cold sweat. Irina was awake, looking up at me anxiously.

"Don't tell my father about that meeting," I begged her.

Over the years, Father had aged, weakened, and his temper had gone sour. I did not want to give him any further trouble. He felt enough pain from the fact that his son did not bear his name or his ethnic identity to have to suffer an additional disgrace of knowing that his son condemned Jews and Israel at a public forum!

I pressed against Irina and fell asleep for a brief spell.

43

Of all my professor's duties, the one I enjoyed most was dialogue with my students. It really was a source of great pleasure for me. As a children's poet and father of an adolescent boy I always sought ways to do something for the youngsters. I felt sorry for those boys and girls, acutely aware of the hardships that awaited them— hardships in everyday life and professional activities alike, marked by back-breaking work and meager remuneration. For these reasons

I tried not to wall myself off from the students. I tried to treat them in a simple and courteous manner, as naturally as I could never behave toward my colleagues.

Unaccustomed to pampering by the faculty, our students disliked most of the professors. Thus they found it unusual to be able to talk to me during intermissions; to be invited to my office after lectures and be treated to coffee with cookies; to be allowed to smoke, and in general feel at home. The student body of our medical school soon drew a line between me and the rest of the faculty. I could clearly see the change of attitude in their trustingness, smiles, and discussions.

Their questions followed a pattern:

"What future do we face upon graduation? Are we going to be paupers?"

"I, too, had to start at a very low pay," I told them. "Yet, as you can see, I managed to survive."

"But not everyone is destined to become a leading physician."

"True, but there are other jobs paying as well or better."

They rejoined: "In order to attain such jobs, one must join the Party earlier than medical school, and devote more time to political functions than to medicine. In such cases, one counts on eventually becoming a big shot and earning good money. An ordinary physician is doomed to a life of poverty. There are many parents who send their child to medical school with the words, 'Remember, dear son, if you study well you'll become a doctor; but if you study poorly you'll be a head doctor.'

They understood everything and their assessments were right on target. I did not object and they felt my agreement. Other professors engaged in such propaganda and were heartily disliked by students who with typical youthful frankness mocked them and gave them unflattering nicknames.

Once they asked me, "Why is it that the American surgeon Michael DeBakey was summoned to operate on Mstislav Keldysh, President of the Academy of Sciences and member of the Central Committee Party? Don't we have surgeons capable of performing that job? Was it a special operation or a special patient?"

I groped for an answer. It was a tough question. It was hard to keep from disclosing the whole truth—and the truth was not flattering to the Russian medical establishment. The Soviet government was afraid to operate on one of its own in 1972 because Russian surgeons could not rival the Americans in terms of experience, technical proficiency, or equipment. By that time, Dr. DeBakey had operated on thousands of patients with vascular disorders and replaced hundreds of aortas with brilliant success, whereas the entire collective experience of the Russian surgeons amounted to a paltry few score such operations with poor results due to the dearth of experience, poor operating technique, and dire lack of good instruments. It was a favorite topic of conversation among Moscow's physicians. With quite a bit of malicious joy, they whispered to one another that in the game of oneupmanship, Dr. DeBakey bested our Minister Dr. Boris Petrovsky, himself a surgeon. A lot of details were revealed. Everybody was amused when Dr. DeBakey ordered his patient to get up and walk the day following surgery; Russian patients are kept in bed for weeks after aortal replacement. No less striking was the array of instruments the American doctor employed, or the breathtaking dexterity of the nurse who accompanied Dr. DeBakey. In short, everything about that famous operation was an eye-opener. But since Dr. DeBakey's visit and his operation on Academician Keldysh was officially treated as a secret matter, people talked about it in whispers. Now I had to answer before a whole group of students. To make matters worse, several of my assistants were in the room; they were clearly intrigued and eagerly waited for me to wriggle out of my predicament.

The last thing I wanted was to make a fool of myself in front of the students; besides, I was sure they knew the truth. Therefore I told them everything the way it really was, but added that I had not been present at the operation and my information was secondhand. I tried not to emphasize the Russian backwardness, but did not gloss over it either.

By the look on the face of my assistant Dr. Mikhailenko, secretary of the Party Committee, I saw he was not delighted with my reply. He did not try to interrupt me but he was watching the proceedings with obvious distaste.

For their part, the students loved the explanation.

"We've already asked the same question of Professor Rodionov," they told me. "Guess what he told us: he hadn't heard of Dr. DeBakey's visit and didn't regard American surgery as superior to ours. He lied, of course; not only did he know of the American's arrival, but he was even present at the operation. We asked another professor of surgery, Dr. Babichev. He scolded us severely and told us that it was all malicious gossip; that the operation had been performed by Minister Petrovsky; and that he had seen it with his own eyes. And yes, he added that American medicine could not hold a candle to our Russian science."

We were talking in a decrepit log house that abutted Basmannaya Hospital #6. All around us were poverty, cramped quarters, oppressive air. It took little imagination or fantasy to see how terrible it was.

After the students were gone, Dr. Mikhailenko lingered in my office.

"I feel uncomfortable about that conversation," he said.

"What's wrong with it?"

"Of course I know it was the American who operated on Keldysh, and I also know that American surgical instruments are better than ours. I worked for a year in Kuwait on a government mission and we only used American instruments in the operating room. Wonderful instruments, no question about it. But we're mature men capable of critically evaluating facts in terms of the Party moral standards. Those students, though, are still wet behind the ears; they're too young to understand such things. That's why other professors dodged their questions—all for the sake of proper moral education. You, too, shouldn't have answered them."

"I don't agree that deceit and evasion, as you put it, constitute the right approach to medical students," I said haughtily.

"You're entitled to your opinion, of course, but the youngsters are bound to spread it around and the Party Committee is likely to hear about it. As secretary, I feel duty bound to warn you."

I thanked him drily and cut the talk short.

Political indoctrination of the medical students was regarded as even more important than teaching medicine. Since my student days, some two decades before, the number of political-education chairs had proliferated. In my time we had just three chairs: Marxism-Leninism, philosophy, and political economy. Today, besides the three staple chairs, there are a slew of new ones: history of the Communist Party, scientific communism, historical materialism, dialectical materialism. No less than one-third of the academic curriculum is devoted to political subjects.

Our students came to medical school brimming with enthusiasm and hope, and gazing idealistically at everything around them: the medical profession, their medical school, their professors. Over the six-year course of study, however, most of them were, bit by bit, transformed into skeptics by everyday exposure to the facts of life. And the greatest casualty of all was their trust in their teachers.

During the fifth year of their studies, the students spent half of their class time learning how to perform surgery in regimental medical points (PMP), in medical battalions (MB), in independent companies of medical reinforcement (ORMU), in army mobile hospitals (APG), and in hospitals for light casualties (GLR). My assistants and I were subordinate to the Ministry of Public Health for general medical instruction and to the Main Medical Directorate of the Ministry of Defense for military medical instruction. Because of this, we teachers also had to take special military update courses every other year.

Every May we conducted a two-day exercise in a wooded area on the territory of the Moscow Military District's hospital, which was located near the Voykovskaya subway station. We set up PMP and MB tents and all of the associated equipment and ran around like the doctors in the American television show "MASH." Some of the participants pretended to be wounded, and then we had to divide them into groups of the seriously, moderately, and lightly injured, who were then given appropriate priorities of treatment. These exercises were supervised by a group of professional military surgeons headed by the chief surgeon of the Moscow Military District, Colonel Dr. Miliy Anichkov. The military surgeons timed and evaluated our performance. The Ministry of Defense had the authority to fire all of us from the school if we did not meet standards, so we took these exercises very seriously.

Fortunately, though, Colonel Dr. Anichkov was an old friend of my father's and a good acquaintance of mine. After the exercise, I usually treated him to dinner in a restaurant, where we drank and spoke frankly. He had served on the front during the war and was a very experienced military surgeon. He was able to give us good criticisms of our performance, but never gave us a bad grade.

Our medical students had to complete 276 hours in basic military medical training, military surgery, military therapy, and military epidemiology and toxology. In addition, the male students had to attend a summer camp.

After graduation from medical school, all new male doctors had to serve at least two years as doctors with the rank of lieutenant in the military.

More than two thousand professors teach military medicine at civilian medical schools in the Soviet Union. In addition, another two thousand professors teach military medicine at special military medical academies in Leningrad, Moscow, Gorkiy, Saratov, and Kuybyshev. These latter schools graduate more than three thousand professional military doctors a year.

If war starts tomorrow (as the popular Russian song goes), the Soviet Union will not only have millions of well-trained soldiers, but also tens of thousands of well-trained military doctors.

The coeds, who accounted for almost half of the student body, showed little interest in my subjects: orthopedics and, in particular, military surgery. Still, typically female diligence compelled them to study well.

One of the girls, named Lena Shalaeva, developed a great interest in orthopedics and often attended my operations. Petite, snub-nosed, with luxurious auburn hair, she was very attractive. But I pretended not to notice her. I knew from the bitter experience of others that any romance involving a professor and a coed was bound to end up in a major scandal. The Party Committee laid the strictest of interdictions on such liaisons.

Once she called me at home late at night, on the eve of an exam, and told me she had a bad case of asthma and consequently could not study for the exam. What was I to do? Maybe she was really ill, but it was also quite likely that she planned to maneuver me into a liaison, thus assuring her a passing grade.

The next morning she turned up at the exam looking for all the world like a dying swan, but thoroughly coiffed and made-up. I turned her over to my colleague; he gave her a good grade.

Lena stubbornly pursued me. She insisted on an internship in my department with a view to becoming a surgeon. But she was in no way suited to be a surgeon. So I blew my top and told her directly, "Forget about surgery. Neither your physical condition nor your personal qualities qualify you for a surgical career, so you'd better get yourself transferred to some other program."

Lena threw a tantrum in the physicians' room across the corridor from my office. I heard her screaming that I was out to ruin her life and that I was taking revenge on her. Finally, Lena swallowed the insult and left us, angry.

A large-scale international exhibition, "Medicine-74," was held in Moscow's Sokolniki Park, in several huge pavilions built for the 1959 U.S. exhibition. There was hardly a physician, nurse, or medical technician in Russia who did not yearn to go and learn at first hand the true state of the art.

Even before I went to Sokolniki I had heard the impressions of many of my colleagues, all of whom, without exception, had been dazzled by the Western equipment.

True to themselves, during the first days visitors stole a myriad of small exhibits either for their personal use or at least to show to their less fortunate colleagues unable to procure entrance tickets. Wise to this Russian propensity, the experienced organizers later nailed all exhibits to the display stands.

I went to the exhibition inured, I thought, by the many enthusiastic reports I had heard. But even though prepared, I was stunned by the incredibly advanced state of medicine that served the people in industrialized countries. It became painfully clear that Russian medicine lagged half a century behind, its level comparable to the state of medicine in the United States and Western Europe in the 1920s. And since there was no hope of development, the gap could only continue to grow.

My counterparts from Czechoslovakia introduced me to representatives of the Swiss section, who showed me video recordings of orthopedic operations by Dr. Maurice Muller. I had never seen such technical perfection. A courteous Swiss exhibitor brought me coffee and cigarettes and put me in an easy chair in front of a TV set. Then he took several cassettes from his pocket, inserted a cassette into the unit with a flick of his hand, and I saw an impeccably performed operation accompanied by detailed explanations.

I watched the screen, thinking, "Good God, he holds in his pocket several cassettes that show and explain everything far better than could all six of my assistants combined! How gladly would I trade my semiliterate aides for such cassettes! My students would only stand to gain from such an exchange."

Then I inspected laboratory equipment, watching with delight and astonishment a clever machine analyze a blood sample and spew out an answer in a matter of seconds. In our hospitals, everywhere except the Kremlin Clinic, doctors had to wait three or four days for similar results. And no machine of this sort was even on the drawing boards in Russia.

Automatic development of X-ray film drove me to particular ecstasy. Instead of tiredly stooping for long periods of time in a dark room, dipping the film in solutions, as absolutely all Russian X-ray technicians had to do, I saw the entire process proceed unattended in automatic machines in just a few minutes. And the film emerged from the machine dry, whereas in our laboratories each night wet film was hung on clotheslines across the room like washing left to dry.

But I was particularly impressed, of course, with orthopedic instruments that I had hitherto seen only in catalogs—and not all of them at that. I admired the instruments; I stroked them; I could not force myself to part with them. My Czech friends at the exhibition knew that I had wasted much time and energy trying to talk my bosses into buying their instruments.

But a pleasant surprise awaited me at the exhibition: a personal gift from the Czechs in the form of a complete set of instruments in two large metal boxes. The instruments were expensive— a truly princely present. And the ceremony at which the gift was presented to me was royal: a small reception/cocktail party at the Czechoslovak Embassy on Fuczik Street. The Czechs made speeches extolling the friendship of the Russian and Czechoslovak peoples (just six years after the 1968 invasion!) whereupon, in token of that friendship, the gift was formally presented.

The dean of my medical school, Dr. A. Belousov, still gave me staunch support in all my undertakings. When he learned that I had built myself a department to treat injured alcoholics in the basement of the hospital, he came to inspect it and was delighted. And when he was told that I had obtained a set of first-class instruments, he went as far as to rise at a session of the Scientific Council and say: "As I recall, there was some resistance to the election of Dr. Golyakhovsky as head of the chair. Yes, comrades, it did happen, and I had to twist some arms to convince you that Golyakhovksy was qualified to work here, even though he is not a Party member. And look how right I was: Golyakhovsky has found a beautiful new base for his chair and made major reconstructions there. And now he has even equipped it with the latest in foreign technology! So you see that I was right."

Many of the Party Committee members and other professors, my colleagues, heard those compliments with ill-concealed displeasure. But they were afraid to contradict the dean and had to put up with my existence.

Shortly after that public approbation Dean Belousov died at a meeting, in the midst of a speech. His death deprived me of an important protector, though by that time I believed that my position had become strong enough.

Soon afterward I had a talk with General Igor Karpets, head of the Criminal Investigation Department.

"Your dean had a great sense of timing," he told me. "We had him under investigation for corruption, and had he not died, by now my assistants would have nabbed him. Many of your professors were Belousov's accomplices in a bribery scheme. The dean extorted admission bribes at the rate of five thousand rubles per college entrant, while professors aspiring to positions at your school were charged payments in the form of diamonds worth ten thousand to fifteen thousand rubles. Your name doesn't show on the list, though."

Well, I, too, had to pay a bribe, but on a much less exorbitant scale: a state-provided elk shot on a hunting expedition and an assortment of pretty gifts. The only thing I regretted was the loss of my briefcase.

Soon after, I succeeded in moving my department out of the wooden barracks of the old hospital. A new Hospital #36 was built in southeast Moscow on the foundation of the old Blagushinskaya Hospital, and I managed to snatch half of a large seven-story building with sunlit and clean rooms. Compared to the barracks, the new building looked palatial. Of course, it had construction flaws, and there was no better equipment than in the old, but the new environment was far more congenial. For the first time I had my own respectable office. Through my patients, workers at factories in the neighborhood, I procured wood panels and furniture. Other professors came to admire.

"How did you manage to get hold of all this splendor?" they asked.

"Connections," I answered. I had acquired some experience and knew where and how to obtain what I needed for free. That was the only possible way of procuring things.

We had a lot of drunk patients injured because of alcohol problems, so we doctors decided to build a special drunk ward ourselves in the basement of the hospital. We made arrangements through some of our patients to acquire bricks, plaster, paint, wire, and the other materials we needed. Every day, during regular working hours, two or three of us changed into overalls and worked on the project, which we called "Building Communism." I personally spent about a third of my time on it. We knocked out sections of walls to make doors, bricked up some existing doors, plastered and then painted the walls. We surprised ourselves with our own abilities. When we finished, we were relieved that the hospital administration, which had neither authorized nor paid for our work, allowed us to keep the new ward and even praised our initiative.

The drunks didn't like the special ward, though. It looked to them like a dungeon. The walls were thick, the windows were locked, and the doors had peepholes and were bolted. But even worse was that the drunks we now charged for their treatment thought that medical care should be free for them in communism. One drunk even philosophized to me that in communism barrels of vodka with ladles chained to them would stand on every street corner. When I asked him why the ladles would be chained, he answered that the chains would prevent people from stealing the ladles. A good communist's understanding!

Since the doctors received a 15 percent bonus for the time they worked in the drunk ward, many of them worked there overtime night after night. The drunks also had to pay for a young and strong policeman assigned to the ward from the Moscow city police force.

One day in the fall of 1975, the policeman came up to my office with a problem. At first he was embarrassed because of my female secretary, but then he properly reported: "*Tovarishck* [comrade]

Professor, the doctor on duty in our special trauma ward requests your advice on what to do with a wedding ring on a drunk patient's sexual organ."

I went down to the drunk ward to investigate. The patient, a man who looked about sixty (he turned out to be forty-five) was lying on a table in the bandaging room naked from the waist down. He was muttering incoherently and waving his arms in pain. His penis was blue and swollen to the size of a pear but appeared to be tied up with something at its base. The duty doctor silently pulled back the skin to show me a large, thick wedding ring.

"How did that happen?" I asked.

"He's too drunk to tell us."

"What have you decided to do?"

"I've decided to ask you what we should do."

The policeman suggested smilingly, "Cut his prick off. He probably doesn't need it anymore anyway. And you can save the ring."

We certainly had to do something quickly to prevent the bladder from exploding or the penis from developing gangrene. We decided to cut the ring off with a very small saw that looked like serrated wire. We cut the ring from the inside out, placing a flat blade between the ring and the skin, and held both ends of this blade to the ring with Koher clamps. The gold was soft, but it took us about an hour to cut it through. Then we clasped the cut ends of the ring with clamps and carefully bent the ring back and off the penis. In the course of a few seconds, the penis partially unswelled and then started to spray urine all over the room like a loose hose. We all jumped into the corners to get away. Finally, the duty doctor bravely jumped back, grabbed the penis, and pointed it in a safe direction until the fountain subsided.

After the operation, we doctors wrote the case history, which was probably unique in medical history, and the policeman wrote a protocol that explained why we had destroyed the gold ring.

The next morning, awake and sober, the patient urinated normally and the danger of gangrene passed. We asked him how the ring had gotten stuck on his penis, but he just turned away and muttered that he didn't remember. The policeman threatened to hold him in custody until he explained.

A little later the patient's wife came to the hospital. She was a huge, fat woman, twice as large as her husband. I explained what had happened and quickly assured her that her husband was still whole. She was not interested in that, though.

"What about my ring?" she screamed.

"Oh, so it was your ring?" I asked.

"Of course it was. The damned drunk stole it from me. He steals everything he can out of the house to pay for his damned vodka. I was washing the floor, so I had taken my ring off and put it on the table. When he left the house, I searched him like I always do. I even searched him in the mouth, because I've caught him taking things out of the house that way, but I didn't think to search his prick. It wasn't until later that I noticed that he had somehow snuck the ring out of the house."

The policeman brought in the patient, staggering and gingerly holding his sore member, which was wrapped in gauze.

His wife put her huge fist up to his head and yelled: "You goddamn dried-up little shrimp! What do you think you're doing putting my ring on your dick?!"

The husband stared down at the floor and pondered his situation.

"Well, answer me!" his wife demanded. Her fist was almost as large as his head.

He turned to me. "It's the only way I could get it out of the house. She feels me all over before I leave. She hadn't ever reached for my dick, though, so I decided to put the ring on it. It got stuck, and I couldn't get it off. So I drank a half-liter with the guys anyway, and after that I don't remember anything."

The policeman pulled the sawed and bent-up ring out of a cupboard and handed it to the woman. In tears, she signed for it and then grabbed her husband by the collar and dragged him out the door. After they were gone, the policeman looked at us for a moment.

"She'll cut off his dick for sure," he said. "I told you we should have done it ourselves and at least saved the ring."

In my opinion, alcoholism is a phenomenon of physiological preconditions on a background of social conditions. Alcoholism is an individual illness, but in certain social conditions it becomes a mass phenomenon, a national epidemic.

The roots of the tendency toward alcoholism have their beginning for Russians in their wild forefathers, the Scyths. We know from ancient history that the Scythian tribes who populated southern Russia and the Ukraine more than one thousand years ago were all uncontrollable in everything. They were subject to a passion for alcoholic drinks, and this passion was combined with the wildness of mass orgies. For example, they turned the funerals of their leaders into general drinking bouts. The whole tribe would get drunk, and then all of the men would make love with the leader's wives, after which these wives would be killed and buried with the leader.

During the course of ten centuries of Christianity in Russia and the Ukraine, these closely related nations were distinguished by their immoderate consumption of alcohol. The peasants in the villages always drank moonshine, and when the working class began to form in the eighteenth century, almost all of the workers were drunkards from the very beginning.

The famous Russian czars Ivan the Terrible and Peter the Great were alcoholics, and all of their noble court constantly participated in royal orgies. Many great people of Russia were chronic alcoholics and died prematurely from alcoholism.

The three most numerous groups of alcoholics in Russia are the factory workers, the village peasants, and the military officers. Alcoholism is less developed among the intellectuals in general, but there are a lot of alcoholics in the arts—actors, painters, writers, and musicians. Among the 129 Soviet nationalities, three—the Russians, Byelorussians, and Ukrainians—are the most vulnerable. These three nationalities have a common ethnic background. There are also a lot of alcoholics among the Latvians, Lithuanians, and Estonians. The fewest are among the Moslem nationalities—the Tadzhiks, Uzbeks, Kirgiz, Tatars, and Turkmen—because of the tradition of the Koran, which forbids alcohol, but gradually many of them are also turning to drink. As a rule, this happens under the influence of Russian friends.

Nobody knows how many alcoholics there are in the Soviet Union, but according to the most modest calculations, they include half of the adult male population and a fifth of the adult female population, which adds up to at least 50 million people. Two factors in the life of Soviet society contribute to such a mass spread of alcoholism—economic difficulties and moral depression caused by propaganda. The low average wage (150 rubles, or about $225 a month), the high cost of absolutely all goods, and the inadequate quantity of goods chronically undermines the material position of the average family. As a result, people develop a chronic dissatisfaction with their daily lives. The desire "to drink from sorrow" appears more and more often. To this is added the depression from the influence of ceaseless propaganda in the newspapers, radio, and television, in the movies and in the magazines, in the books and theaters. The whole population has to occupy itself with the study of Marxism-Leninism and listen to political lectures at work and participate in meetings every week. Under the influence of this unbearable, boring propaganda, against which people cannot object because they are afraid of political accusations, they become angry and find their only diversion in alcohol.

The Soviet rulers do not do anything to cut down the alcoholism in the country. To the contrary, through their domestic policies, they increase it all the time. Premier Nikita Krushchev and the President Leonid Brezhnev themselves were chronic alcoholics. I saw with my own eyes how they drank cognac from large glasses when I had dinner with them. Almost all the other members of the Politburo are also alcoholics. Even the single woman among them, the Minister of Culture, Yekaterina Furtseva, was a chronic drunk.

Occasionally, the government begins a campaign against drunkenness and the newspapers publish long directives that nobody reads. The lines in front of the vodka stores do not get any shorter because of these directives.

44

That fall I was subpoenaed as a witness by the Pervomaisky District Court. The courthouse was located close to the Yelokhovskaya Church, Moscow's Orthodox Cathedral, in a dilapidated three-story wooden mansion that must have been reconstructed and repainted at least a dozen times in a century of existence. The stairs were narrow, steep, and very dingy; dirty spots were visible even in the dim light of a foggy autumn morning. The air was oppressively stuffy. Court employees with briefcases and folders darted up and down the stairs. All doors in the corridor were wide open. A crowd of smokers milled on the landing; the smoke was billowing upward, irritating the eyes. Everybody was waiting. A nauseating stench of low-quality fresh paint wafted in the corridor. The odors of cigarette smoke, paint, and crowded humanity mixed up in the dimly lit corridor, epitomizing *the court.*

I was waiting for my turn to be called into the courtroom, uneasily aware of a feeling that the surroundings and the people in the building seemed familiar. Surely I had never been there before. . . . Why should I have that impression? Yet, an acute feeling that the surroundings and the case were illustrations of something that I knew very well would not leave me. Illustrations of what? The case I was to testify in involved murder. A man murdered his mother—and not just killed her, but beat her to death. The murderer's name was Dr. Nikolai (Kolya) Levitsky. Some time before he had been a staff surgeon at a department of which I was director. Now I was to testify at his closed trial and my testimony was expected to help the prosecution to depict him as a vicious, blood-stained criminal capable of matricide, the most monstrous crime imaginable. So, while waiting in the corridor I was wondering why I had never suspected that the quiet, intellectual Dr. Kolya had a streak of violence in him. Only two alternatives seemed plausible: either it was a case of accidental murder, or all of us ordinary folk are potential killers.

All of a sudden, I realized with a start the reason for my déjà vu feeling: the case bore a striking resemblance to the plot of Feodor Dostoyevsky's novel *Crime and Punishment,* and the perpetrator, Dr. Nikolai Levitsky, strongly resembled the novel's protagonist, Radion Raskolnikov. I was amazed to find how little the Russians and their way of life had changed over one hundred years.

Kolya was a young ethnic Russian, only twenty-nine, not a Communist Party member. He had been married for five years to a Jewish schoolteacher ten years his senior for whom he had an abiding love and respect. They had no children and in fact could not afford them because they were dirt poor: as a laboratory physician he drew a piddling salary of 100 rubles per month; she was paid even less. They had no apartment of their own and for several years had lived in a single room together with Kolya's parents, but then constant friction with the old couple forced them to move and rent a handkerchief-sized room in the outskirts of Moscow, beyond the Sokolniki Park. Kolya's wife applied for a one-bedroom cooperative apartment at her place of employment. Though tiny, the apartment cost the equivalent of their combined ten-year income. To scrape together the down payment, they saved every kopeck, denying themselves the bare necessities. Kolya's clothes were little more than rags; he went hungry all the time and constantly cast about in search of ways to earn a little more money. He eagerly grabbed at any chance of extra night work and thus managed to augment his meager income by another 50 to 60 rubles a month.

He was recommended to me by my assistant Dr. V. Kosmatov, whom I had helped write a Ph.D. thesis. I saw Kolya for the first time in my office three years before the trial. He was very tall and very thin, soft-spoken and exceedingly shy. Self-conscious in the presence of a professor and director, he fidgeted nervously, trying to look smaller and to hide his long arms and legs—a typical intellectual gawk and bungler. His speech, too, was typically soft, self-conscious, and hesitant. Yet he commanded an extensive vocabulary, betraying a well-read, erudite, and intelligent person. He told me he had been a military medic, then he had set his mind on becoming a physician and had completed the course of medical school two years previously. While we talked, I fleetingly discerned in him a morbid element, a barely visible streak of tamed savagery. But that was only a vague impression. I needed an intellectual for an aide, for the surgeons at my clinic were almost to a man lowbrows, all Party hacks. And so I did hire Dr. Kolya, though it was not easy to wangle a new staff position for him. We often had heart-to-heart talks; he hated the Soviet system, loved to tell jokes about Soviet rulers, and was crazy about forbidden poets like Mandelstam.

The whole time he worked at my department, Dr. Kolya tried to show me how interested in orthopedic surgery he was. We performed several operations together and jointly published a research paper. Kolya was happy and I was happy for him. To be frank he was not made to be a surgeon, lacking as he did the necessary faculties: efficiency, decisiveness, quickness of mind and hand. Neither was he educated enough to write scientific papers yet. But I wanted to instill confidence in him and help him overcome that morbid, tamed wildness.

On one occasion, Dr. Kolya lost his 100-ruble pay—a huge loss for him. He desperately roamed the hospital, looking for his money on the floor and in all corners. He was so pitiful that I stealthily put 100 rubles of my own money in a dark corner, called a nurse as a witness, and then summoned Kolya to show him my "find." He rejoiced like a child.

Finally the cooperative building was completed, and in a month's time Kolya and his wife were to move into their apartment. At the lottery arranged to distribute the apartments among the cooperative members, Kolya as always had a stroke of bad luck, drawing a ground-floor apartment, one of the worst in the building. But he was happy nonetheless. Kolya had a strange dream of keeping pickled cucumbers in a cask on his balcony, happily sharing it with all who cared to listen. Smiling dreamily, he would tell us how nice it would be at his house-warming party: when all the guests were assembled, he would put vodka on the table and fetch pickled cucumbers right from his own balcony. . . .

The fact is that the quiet, intellectual Dr. Kolya was a hereditary alcoholic with a history of treatment for alcoholism at a psychiatric hospital. I learned about his affliction accidentally, when it transpired that at the end of the day Kolya was often seen drunk. The hospital personnel had long covered up for him.

Then one day misfortune struck: on a drunken stroll through Gorky Park, Kolya was mugged and severely beaten. He was brought to our hospital with a basilar skull fracture.

He stayed at the hospital for six months. Kolya grew very weak, pale, and listless. He lost much of his capacity for work and had frequent memory lapses. To recover completely, he was to undergo treatment for at least two years and, above all, forget about vodka, as I always pointed out to him. He understood perfectly—he was still the intelligent man of old, but brains alone are not enough to follow through on a good idea. Kolya was aware that he had to forego drinking, but he was unable to decline an offer of vodka. Even had he been unwilling to drink he was too shy to turn down such an offer—no one refuses to drink in Russia, the proverbial Russian "generous nature" needs a vodka-induced high—but he was willing,

he could not help yearning for a drink. Though not cured of alcoholism and not yet fully recovered from a concussion, Kolya resumed
drinking. Finally I had enough and asked him to resign. Polite as
ever, Dr. Kolya thanked me for all I had done for him, said good-bye,
and was gone.

Six months later he killed his mother. Kolya's father had died
from alcoholic cirrhosis and his mother lived alone. She, too, was an
alcoholic, known in the whole neighborhood for her violent behavior
when drunk, which was quite often: she would scream, yell, swear,
rush outdoors stark naked. Repellent and bothersome, she got on her
son's nerves, let alone his wife's.

That day, Kolya's mother paid a visit to her son's new apartment. As was customary with her, she drank herself into a boisterous
mood and accosted her Jewish daughter-in-law, heaping abuse on
her in the choicest of Russian invective. Kolya flew into a rage, but
his mother was too drunk to be simply asked to leave. So Kolya
called for a cab and took his mother home. On the way, they bought
some more vodka. When they arrived at his mother's, they resumed
drinking, chasing a serious familial conversation with alcohol. The
son was accusing the mother, the mother the son; both were yelling
at the tops of their voices. Though inured by habit to noisy squabbles
in the old woman's room, her neighbors could hardly wait for the
noise to stop. Close to the end of the scene, the neighbors recalled
hearing blows and moans, but that was nothing new either. Finally
the ruckus ended and all was quiet. Kolya stayed the night because
he was too drunk to return home. In the morning, he dashed out of
the room, shaking with terror: his mother was dead, her cold body
bearing traces of brutal beating. It was difficult to determine the
exact cause of death, alcoholic poisoning or battery. Most likely, it
was a combination of both.

We were struck speechless to learn of the tragedy. Kolya
himself was at a loss to explain how he had committed a crime that
terrible. Blood has always been gushing in the world like a waterfall,
like wine; many of the official killers have been glorified for their
bloody deeds and declared benefactors of mankind. For all that
tolerance of bloodshed, however, spilling one's mother's blood has
always been and will always be regarded as a crime before man,
before the law, before God. . . .

In the semi-dark room, where I was summoned after a two-hour wait, I saw Kolya guarded by a policeman. He averted his gaze, but when he looked up I saw in his eyes the terror of an animal at bay. He refused to deny his guilt, though the woman lawyer dutifully quoted medical certificates listing his mother's many diseases, any one of which could have killed her at a moment's notice. There is no denying that Kolya's mother was a sick, bad-tempered, disgusting woman. But what made him do it? I was looking at his hands, the hands I had tried to teach the art of surgery. Surgery, not murder . . .

He was sentenced to twelve years' confinement. Kolya will be set free in 1987 at age forty-five. I am convinced he will go on obeying the dictates of the subconscious, hidden, intellectual killer that lurked in his soul—and that was described so masterfully by Dostoyevsky.

The environment has failed to modify the Russians' national character. It still abides, though its manifestations have been shaped by the changes in Russia's social and political system. It was not the courthouse stairs nor the corridors reeking of paint and stale tobacco, but the very Russian national spirit, the characteristic irrationality of action devoid of all logic, the madness leading to horrible crimes that seem to be totally at variance with the criminal's nature, that seemed so familiar to me in that story.

Should I add that not a word of the crime was ever printed? It is as if it had never happened.

45

Irina, our son, and I spent many of our vacations during this period traveling by car across East Europe. I had connections at the OVIR (Visa and Registration Department of the Ministry of Internal Affairs) who helped my family obtain permission for such trips as individual tourists, not as part of an organized tourist group.

The head of the Moscow OVIR, Colonel E. Smirnov, and his female assistant, Lieutenant Marina Duravko, knew that I was a consulting surgeon at the Police Hospital and expedited the procedure for me. Bulgaria, Hungary, Rumania, Czechoslovakia, Poland, and East Germany were far more interesting for us than the few old and boring Russian resorts. After we had crisscrossed the entire communist empire, we wanted to peek outside the Iron Curtain. But I was not allowed to go there. Two of my father's cousins from Antwerp, Belgium, sent Irina and me an officially registered invitation to visit with them, but the OVIR refused to let us go. It was useless to ask "why"; trips to the West were controlled by the KGB.

We wanted to go to Yugoslavia, a country half Russian satellite and half member of the free world. To go to Yugoslavia as a tourist, one has to undergo the same complex and lengthy procedure, the same security check, as it takes to go to the West—all because Yugoslavia lies beyond the Iron Curtain and can easily be used as a springboard for defection.

We had friends in Zagreb, Vlatko and Olga P., who had been in Moscow on business several times. Each time we entertained them at home, took them to the Bolshoi, and gave them car tours of Moscow's beautiful environs. And each time they would tell us, "Now it's your turn to be our guests. When are you coming to Yugoslavia?"

I asked them to send all three of us official invitations in the summer of 1974. When the letter came, I took the invitations to the OVIR, but Lieutenant Duravko told me: "We allow people to go to Yugoslavia only on the invitation of close relatives: parents, children, siblings. These people, who are they to you?"

"Our good friends."

"Then the answer is no. We're not allowed to prepare documents for trips to Yugoslavia on the invitation of friends."

Now I had to start looking for a way to get permission to use those invitations. By that time I had learned that blind alleys were a figment of imagination, that there was always a way out, particularly in the realm of public regulations.

I had a patient, Yuvenaly Polyakov, a high official at the Ministry of Foreign Affairs. Before entering the diplomatic service, he had spent several years in France as a correspondent. Polyakov was a nice fellow and I decided to talk to him about my prospective trip. As it happened, he turned out to be a close friend of General Verein, head of the national OVIR service. He immediately called Verein on the special Kremlin telephone link known as *vertushka* that interconnects all big shots in Moscow. The general promised to help me and I cheered up. But two weeks later he made it known that he did not have enough authority to allow me to go to Yugoslavia with my family.

"I'll be able to help you if I have authorization from Nikolai Shchelokov, Minister of Internal Affairs, or at least one of his deputies," he told me. "Can you get that authorization?"

It was all but impossible to be granted an audience with the Minister or his deputy, but even had I succeeded in gaining access to them my request would almost certainly have been turned down, acting as I was without a push. But apparently fate decreed I go to Yugoslavia, because literally the very next day a woman was brought to me with a dislocated shoulder and a concussion. She turned out to be Minister Shchelokov's personal secretary. I set the bone and treated her for concussion.

"Please do me a favor and arrange a ten-minute audience with the Minister concerning a trip to Yugoslavia," I asked her after she had recovered.

She obliged and I received an invitation to come to the Ministry. I was escorted by a police lieutenant to a second-floor waiting room with walls completely mirrored over. The Minister had been urgently summoned to the Central Committee. I had to wait for three hours. Finally I passed through the assistants' room and the secretary's room into the Minister's sanctum, accompanied by his chief of staff, a colonel who had been fully briefed about my request. I had treated the colonel's wife and he was eager to help.

"Be sure to bring a petition with your request in writing and hand it over to the Minister for his instructions," he had warned me.

I walked through the rooms, thinking that I was about to talk to Leonid Brezhnev's closet crony. When Brezhnev was First Party Secretary of the Moldavian Republic on the Rumanian border, in the 1950s, Shchelokov headed the Moldavian police. According to reliable rumors, Brezhnev had conducted himself in Moldavia as a real satrap, drinking, whoring, extorting bribes, and violating all kinds of laws, while Shchelokov faithfully covered up for him. But Brezhnev's excesses were so outrageous that he was demoted and exiled to

Kazakhstan as Second Party Secretary. When his star rose again, he summoned his friend to Moscow in 1966 and made him Minister of Internal Affairs and an army general with a marshal's star on his shoulder straps. Brezhnev even gave him a residence next to his own: each of them occupied a floor in a building on Kutuzovsky Prospect in downtown Moscow. The third floor belonged to KGB boss Yuri Andropov, also a general and Politburo member. Shchelokov's wife, Svetlana, was a physician, an ENT specialist. She worked at the same medical school as I, and I knew her quite well.

The Minister was a man of small stature, so small in fact that it was easy to overlook him in the huge office. Smiling, he shook my hand.

"Have a seat and tell me how I can help you," he said.

I had never talked to such a man of my personal affairs. At first somewhat uneasily, but calming down as I went on, I told him that I wanted to spend my vacation with my family in Yugoslavia.

"What do our relevant laws say?" the Minister asked his chief of staff.

"Trips to Yugoslavia are only allowed on the invitation of close relatives, Comrade Minister."

"You see," Shchelokov muttered, "we can't violate the law. But why do you want to go there on an invitation?" the Minister continued, warming up to the subject. "Why don't you go with a tourist group? It's much more interesting. Last year my wife and I spent our vacation in Italy. Later, when we returned, friends of ours who had been in Italy on an organized tour told us what they had seen. Believe me they had a far more meaningful vacation than we had."

An uneasy silence fell; we had nothing more to discuss. Then I took my last chance and told Shchelokov, "General Verein told me he'd be able to allow me the trip if he had your okay."

Too late it occurred to me that maybe I had just put Verein on the spot. Contrary to my fears, though, the Minister was obviously delighted. He beamed. "In that case let's give Verein his instructions."

He drew my petition toward him and wrote in the top left-hand corner: "To Comrade Verein: Review the problem and resolve it at your discretion. Shchelokov."

When I left the office, the colonel, who trailed me, said:

"Congratulations. Now that the Minister has failed to give him a definitive directive, Verein is free to act as he pleases. You know, no one wants to take personal responsibility in such matters, not even the Minister."

A month later I went to the Moscow OVIR to collect our passports. But to my surprise only two passports were issued: for Irina and myself. I asked the chief, Colonel Smirnov, "Why two passports? I want my son to come with us."

"Not allowed," he replied gently.

When we left the office, I asked Lieutenant Duravko: "What's happened? Is my son to stay here as a hostage?"

She nodded silently.

Needless to say, our sixteen-year-old son was disappointed, but he reconciled himself to the prospect of staying home on condition that we bring him a Japanese cassette player by way of compensation. Even more distressed, we were ready to promise him anything he wished.

We were only allowed to exchange rubles in the amount of $5 per day per person. Since we were to go to Yugoslavia by car, gas money was to come from that same measly sum. But I figured to fill up my tank in Hungary on the Yugoslav border. That would last me four hundred kilometers, and I also planned to fill another two canisters equivalent to a tankful of gas and take them along, stretching my budget a bit. Besides, we packed the trunk with canned food to save meal money and took a tent to save on hotels.

I bought an auto insurance policy for Yugoslavia, was issued special foreign license plates to put on the car instead of my permanent Russian plates, and we started for Yugoslavia via Kiev.

At the border checkpoint in Chop we were stopped and told that we could not go further by car.

"What do you mean? We have insurance papers and a special permit signed by the Minister of Internal Affairs!"

"I don't know nothing," the border patrol chief, a captain, told me. "We have a standing order not to let anyone go to Yugoslavia by car. You can go there by train; leave your car in the parking lot and pick it up when you return."

Sullen and confused, we went to the railway station to inquire about the train schedule. While we were wandering from one booth to another, we saw a baffling scene: a huge room was filled with long tables heaped high with household utensils, clothes, etc. People thronged about the tables, and here and there I could see the uniform of a customs official. The din was deafening: people were shouting, crying, arguing. The scene looked like a veritable pogrom. As a matter of fact that is exactly what it was: the passengers in the room were Jews leaving Russia for Israel. The officials inspected the emigrants' baggage down to the last spool of thread and confiscated many of their personal possessions. That was the reason for the noise, tears, and shouts. We stood flabbergasted and disgusted: God, what mockery of justice, what humiliation!

When we left the terminal, a big Jewish man followed us to the square in front of the station, carrying a large TV set in his hands. He looked around and shouted loudly:

"Are there any Jews here?"

No one responded. He shouted once again, even louder:

"I'm asking you: anybody Jewish here?"

The crowd was silent. Then the man raised his set and smashed it on the pavement. I realized that Customs had not allowed him to take his TV set and he had wanted to leave it to a coreligionist.

I decided to make one last try to obtain permission to go by car; without the car we would not take all our canned food and would have to stay in hotels. And we had too little money for that.

With great difficulty I prevailed on Lieutenant-Colonel V. Blokhin, commander of the border post, to call the commander of the Ukrainian border troops in Kiev. After lengthy negotiations the commander made an exception in our case and allowed us to proceed to Yugoslavia in our car. I spent half a day on the phone. The border guards were so astonished at my success that they just stamped our passports, raised the barrier, and waved us into Hungary without so much as a glance at our baggage. "I wish the others Jews could be so lucky!" I thought, driving over the border.

Yugoslavia welcomed us with a blast of heat. Everything seemed to us wonderful and exotic, but the biggest shock awaited us in the Zagreb open-air market. For the first time in our lives Irina and I saw more fresh meat than we had seen in all our lives. And no lines, not a single man or woman waiting! We froze before the mountains of meat as if in a spell; we could not tear our eyes from the wonderful novel sight. Nothing like this was remotely possible in Russia. Even in East European countries, which were better supplied with food than Russia, we had not seen such plenitude. Each time we saw counters bending under mounds of meat in Yugoslavia we unfailingly experienced the same shock at the sight of abundance. No question about it, life there was different!

Along with the astounding cornucopia in the stores, we were amazed at the many elements of freedom that we had not seen before either. Western newspapers and magazines were sold on every corner; Western movies ran in theaters. We went to see *Last Tango in Paris*, starring Marlon Brando and Maria Schneider. That movie received scathing critical reviews in the Russian press, though it was never shown on the screens. By the beautiful Adriatic Sea we saw nudist beaches. And the sea was dotted with private yachts of exquisite elegance. Thousands of Italians and West Germans spent their vacations on the Adriatic shore. During our stops at campsites, where we put up our tent, we talked to Britons, Germans, Swiss, and Swedes. Upon learning our identity, they all showed surprise because Russians never came to Yugoslavia as individual tourists; those who did come walked in groups and kept to themselves. We had to answer many questions about ourselves and Russia. Whenever our companions learned that I was a professor of orthopedic surgery, they invariably showed me signs of respect. For the first time in our lives we found it exceedingly easy to talk to strangers in a strange language, far easier in fact than to talk in Russia to acquaintances in our mother language. It was freedom of communication hitherto unknown to us. It struck us even more strongly than the abundance of meat.

I understood that Yugoslavia was in no way the epitome of freedom and democracy. Yet it contained far more of both than we could imagine. If things were that way in Yugoslavia, what would they be like in the West! Our friends in Zagreb, then later in Makoscica, near Dubrovnic, heatedly criticized the economy and political system of their country. They were angry with a lot of things: "Everything is lousy and getting worse and worse," they said.

"You have no idea of what it is like when things are really bad," I told them. "You would, if you lived for a while in Russia."

That month in Yugoslavia was a fairytale come true for Irina and myself. The trip awoke in us a desire to see more of the world. We knew it was fantasy, but still we dreamed.

We brought our son the promised Japanese cassette player.

But we also brought from Yugoslavia a budding idea: we had to leave Russia. We did not know yet when, or how, we were going to do it. But we already knew two crucial things: we should leave Russia, and we should go to America.

Soon after we returned, I made the following entry in my diary:

"This morning Irina and I finally made up our minds that we must leave Russia. It is going to be a long and tortuous path, but we are bent on embarking upon it."

46

In 1975, the Ministry and the Academy of Medical Sciences elected me to the Scientific Council of Surgery at the First Moscow Medical School—respectively, the most authoritative scientific council and the most prestigious medical school in the country. Only seventeen surgeons, of whom just three were orthopedists, sat on the council. All the members boasted big names and lofty positions, including the Minister, the vice-president of the academy, the director of the Institute of Surgery, the Dean of the First Medical School, and the like. All were highly decorated; some even sported the gold star of Hero of Socialist Labor (the highest civilian decoration of the country); all were sixty or older.

I was the only member not affiliated with the Communist Party. When I attended my first session of the council, all the sixteen already chosen knew one another, but only a few knew who I was.

Our function consisted of discussing and approving surgical theses and plans. Actually, thanks to its exceptionally authoritative membership, our council set the tone for all other councils and thereby exerted effective control over the surgical science in the country.

Needless to say, I was glad to have been elected. It added

nothing to my income, but a lot to my prestige. Frankly, I had not dreamed of such a huge leap forward and the honor came as a pleasant surprise. Although by that time I had almost one hundred scientific publications to my credit; held twelve patents for inventions in Russia, the United States, Great Britain, and Italy; and sat on numerous councils, committees, presidiums, commissions, and boards; I still did not feel the equal of the rest of the council members.

But I quickly discovered their true nature and laughed at their ostentation and puffed-up airs, at the decorations they proudly wore on coat lapels, and at the profound poses they assumed while dozing off at the sessions. Their stupid speeches exasperated me. All of them had three common passions: (a) to let only their personal protégés advance in the world; (b) to give a leg up to Party members, preferably of pure ethnic Russian origin; and (c) to block the careers of Jews and non-Party people. Guided by these three principles, their speeches reeked of politics and intrigue, with lavish praise heaped on inferior theses and criticism directed at excellent works. Since all decisions were passed by secret ballot and the ballots required no signature, I almost invariably voted against their decisions. And so a pattern emerged: it was either sixteen yes votes against one no or the other way round, sixteen no's and one yes.

I was amazed to find how willful and quite often incompetent those "eminent scientists" really were and I wondered how they had been able to attain such heights in the world of medical science. But one day the enigma was solved. Dr. Kovanov, vice-president of the Academy of Medical Sciences, said in his speech: ". . . When Dr. Struchkov (scientific secretary of the academy), Dr. Shabanov (dean of the First Medical School and First Deputy Minister), and I worked together at the Central Committee of the Party . . ."

At this juncture, they all started to nod and launched into reminiscences about the Central Committee. Now I got it! They had advanced in the world not by brainpower but rather by dint of wearing out the seats of their pants against Central Committee chairs. Of the seventeen members of the council more than half had built careers in science purely on their background as Party apparatchiks.

Damn them all, I decided. It was far more important and interesting to me to see my plans implemented than to waste energy on thinking about and debating those pompous asses. So I kept to myself. Still, my elevation instilled added confidence and the heady feeling of power in me. And I was ready to pursue my plan to shake up my staff of assistants, ousting several pieces of deadwood and replacing them with people of higher caliber from the list I had compiled.

Each time I replaced someone, the others were likely to wonder when their turn would come. With this in mind, I tried to set the stage for my coup in advance by talking to those of my assistants who were not targeted for removal.

We all knew that Dr. Anatoly Pechenkin was a substandard teacher and an inferior surgeon as well as a lazy, stupid, and functionally illiterate man. Many of his colleagues openly put him down, students mocked him, yet, for all his many drawbacks, one circumstance made his position well-nigh unassailable: he was a card-carrying Party hack. When I discussed with other assistants, also Party members, my intention to block Dr. Pechenkin's reelection for a new five-year term, they sighed, dropped their heads, agreed and disagreed with me. Dr. Mikhailenko told me directly, "First you get rid of Pechenkin and then it will be our turn to go."

I did not wield enough power to carry out a radical reform; but to replace this one assistant was an absolute must as far as I was concerned. For one thing, he was out of place in the lecture room; secondly, I was intent on demonstrating to others that I was capable of setting myself a goal and achieving it in order to keep them on their toes.

I had a talk with Dr. Kornienko, a secretary of the Party Committee. "You're a professor in good standing and all of us on the Party Committee are bound to listen to you and respect your opinion," he told me. "I agree that Dr. Pechenkin could work better—"

"He's an incompetent oaf and should be booted out," I interjected.

"Maybe you're right, but remember he's a Party member. The District Committee would never support us if we proceed to fire a communist."

I appreciated the seriousness of his warning. The Party had a standard set of rounded formulas: "support," "not to support," "recommend," "not to recommend" . . . devised as a guise to conceal plain dictatorial rule. Still I believed I could take them on and win.

I called a meeting of all my assistants in an official setting, complete with minutes. Dr. Pechenkin read a written report of his activities over the previous five years. The report was extremely weak and took just a few minutes to read, because in actuality he had done absolutely nothing during the period in question. I criticized the report and suggested that others come forward with their opinions. But other assistants spoke with a patent lack of enthusiasm. They reluctantly agreed with my criticism, but invariably added that it was not too late for Dr. Pechenkin to mend his ways. Good Lord! He was past forty! An opportune age to reform, no doubt! The majority refused to vote for his dismissal. Well, I lost the opening round, but the battle was not over yet.

In the meantime I made up my mind to do something more pleasant: ponder the plan of my future book. With this in mind, I took a month of vacation due me from the previous year, and in January 1976 I went to a sanatorium in Kislovodsk for a communion with nature, a rest, and work on my next book. Irina was to join me a fortnight later for a couple of weeks so we could ski and stroll in the mountains together. Life was in full swing, and occasionally we felt the need to relax and take a rest.

I was invited to the Kislovodsk sanatorium by Dr. Mikhail Pestrikov, the father of one of my patients, after I had succeeded in restoring movement to the shoulder joint of his son. Pestrikov Senior was in charge of the network of exclusive sanatoriums belonging to the Central Committee of the Communist Party, a physician in a managerial position. He promised me a fairytale of a vacation. Reality surpassed my expectations: the minute I landed in Kislovodsk it was as if I had stepped right through the door of a dream kingdom. I was brought to the "De Luxe" building of the "October 10" Sanatorium. My suite consisted of two vast rooms with a luxurious bathroom and a spacious balcony offering a magnificent view of the mountains. Everything around me was clean and tidy, far more so than in any sanatorium I had ever visited. The furnishings, too, were far richer than I could imagine: carpets, paintings, crystal bowls piled high with fruit. A nurse stayed on duty at the door of my suite around the clock (God knows why), and I was assigned a personal physician, a communist lady charged with the task of keeping me healthy. She was more servile than competent, but that was no surprise—servility is part and parcel of the qualifications of any physician in the Kremlin health system.

The air in Kislovodsk was gorgeous—crystal clear and laden with the smell of flowers. After the oppressive streets of Moscow I keenly enjoyed strolls in the mountains and gulped down the salubrious Caucasian air. The snow-capped peak of Mount Elbrus, the highest peak of the mountain range, could be seen in the distance. I pondered my affairs, staring at the stately mountain. The Caucasus had been a source of inspiration for the greatest of Russian writers: Alexander Pushkin, Mikhail Lermontov, and Leo Tolstoy. What a marvelous place indeed!

I never got used to the luxury of the sanatorium that had overwhelmed me at first sight. Every morning I swam in the gigantic pool, usually alone, for there were just a handful of clients on hand. We all got together in the dining hall. The denizens of the sanatorium shocked me with their looks. They were middle-level Party apparatchiks who behaved in the dining hall of the sanatorium as if they were at a Party meeting. They invariably turned up in the accepted Party "uniform": dark, poorly cut, Soviet-made suits, sporting obligatory medals or ribbons. Women, too, wore dark and poorly designed clothes, also adorned with decorations. All of them were gloomy, kept to themselves, and scrupulously observed the rules of Party subordination.

Since I alone wore multicolored sport sweaters and imported sport pants and since I was the only one residing at the "De Luxe" building reserved only for the top Party brass, my neighbors cast curious glances in my direction, apprehensively trying to figure me out. My neighbor at the dinner table, Tanya, a handsome forty-year-old Minister of Education of the tiny Republic of Abkhazia and the sole tastefully dressed woman in the room, was the only person I communicated with. She told me laughingly how baffled at my identity our dreary co-vacationers were. Some whispered that I was a top-flight atomic physicist in an extremely sensitive position; others got wind of the fact that I was a surgeon and spread rumors that I was a court physician to the highest of the Kremlin bosses. They all said their greetings very, very carefully.

The sanatorium had a sauna. I wanted to steam myself but it was a bore to go to the sauna alone. Fortunately, I met my old acquaintance and colleague, Dr. Yuri Lopukhin, dean of the Second Moscow Medical School. He was staying at a neighboring sumptuous sanatorium, also an exclusive institution. We arranged to go to our sauna together that night. I warned my nurse that I would miss supper and asked to be issued my rations; after the steaming session we planned to have a bash. The nurse looked at me in surprise and said:

"What do you need provisions for? You'll have all you can eat right there, in the sauna."

Still, not knowing what to expect, I took a food package with me to be on the safe side.

No sooner had we entered the anteroom of the sauna than we saw a table set for two and laden with caviar, exquisite fish, and many, many other delicacies. Embarrassed at my poor foresight, I secreted my food package in the corner, trying to hide it from another nurse who was waiting for us. She greeted us courteously and showed us all the sauna rooms and the swimming pool.

"How long can we stay here?" I asked.

"As long as you please. You can steam yourselves, swim in the pool, and enjoy yourselves at the table the whole night and morning, if you wish. All this is just for the two of you. I will be next door; all you have to do if you need anything is call me on the intercom. I, too, will inquire about your condition from time to time."

Dr. Lopukhin and I took our fill at the sumptuous table, reclining on soft Caucasian sofas under rich terry towels—the picture of feasting Roman patricians. From time to time, we steamed ourselves in the sauna, swam in the small pool, and again lounged on the sofas at the table. And each time we found new dishes. It was a real feast: the best of Caucasian cuisine—soups, shish kabobs, calzones, and, needless to say, the choicest of cognacs. We grew languid from steam, water, food, and drink; we spent the whole night there, breaking up the meeting at three in the morning.

Dr. Lopukhin and I had plenty to talk and reminisce about. We recalled the sad story of our common teacher, Professor A. Gesselevich, victimized by the anti-Semitic campaign in the guise of "struggle against cosmopolitanism," and recalled other purges in the scientific world. Dr. Lopukhin told me how he toiled to preserve Lenin's mummy and how there was in fact nothing to preserve. We conversed softly, in semi-whispers, lest the nurse overhear us. Besides, we were not sure the room was free of listening devices.

I was not required to pay anything for that exorbitant feast à la ancient Rome. Everything was courtesy of the house; by the most conservative estimate it must have cost at least 200 rubles. On the way out I unobtrusively scooped up my food package so as not to betray my outrageous naiveté.

Irina joined me for a fortnight's stay, also free. Her arrival dealt a final blow to the communists; only the highest brass—of the rank of secretary of a regional committee or secretary of the Central Committee—were entitled to vacation in the company of wives. Now they stood at attention to greet me. I gaily waved at them all.

A state-provided limousine with government-rank license plates and a chauffeur was assigned to me. When Irina came, we took short trips, staying for the night at similar exclusive sanatoriums in Pyatigorsk, Zheleznovodsk, or Yessentuki. All it took to arrange such a trip was to relate our desire to my personal nurse. Our wishes were accommodated with lightning speed. Everywhere we went we were accorded ostentatious hospitality, put up in special suites, and wined and dined in special dining halls. In the Pyatigorsk sanatorium, we found ourselves sharing the table with the wife and daughter of Yuri Andropov, the KGB Minister and eventually Brezhnev's successor. They took their meals separately from the other vacationers as befitted their exalted station in life. Yet they had to share the amenities with us, though it happened by accident. Somehow we managed to suffer each other's presence.

I wanted to go to Dombai, a distance of one hundred miles in the heart of the mountain range. Dombai boasted a famous ski slope much talked about in the whole of Russia. I had to delay my trip for a week because the mountain passes were blocked with snow. Finally we set out. Having developed a habit of getting VIP treatment wherever we went, we were not in the least concerned about accommodation. In Dombai we passed a seven-story hotel and the two-story log cabin of an old tourist camp, then we turned to the left and through a tall gate entered a closed lot. In the back stood a beautiful three-story palace of wood and glass. We did not know what it was, but a delegation of seven domestic servants rushed out of the house to greet us, looking for all the world like loyal servants hailing their returning master at his castle. Still unaware of the identity of the palace, we graciously returned the servants' greetings and entered the mansion. Even compared to our magnificent sanatorium, this place was a palace of wealth and luxury. We were escorted across a huge hall, whose floor was covered with expensive rugs and walls hung with paintings and ancient weapons, and up a wide flight of stairs into another beautiful hall with a roomy suite on either side. The maid declared that the suites were called "Large De Luxe" and "Small De Luxe." The latter, where we were put up, was thoroughly prepared for our arrival. Belying the adjective in its name, the suite contained a large bedroom with an opulent bathroom, a library, and a parlor. The walls and ceilings were completely paneled over. I have always been partial to wood-paneled walls, and these were made of some special varieties of timber skillfully matched in pattern and wood grain. The furniture, polished and very comfortable, was beautiful. Everything around us clearly bore the mark "imported."

Several minutes later the maid called on the intercom and inquired when we desired to have lunch. "Any time." "Then come down, please." The ground floor consisted of several living rooms and dining rooms and a library, as well as the hall we had already seen. We were ushered into a small dining room. One of its walls was a glazed French window affording a breathtaking view of the mountains. The table was set for two: at least fifteen different dishes sat on a snow-white, stiffly starched cloth. The maid and a female cook waited on us, oozing diffidence. I suggested that our driver be invited to the table. The servants were thunderstruck by my words, but immediately rushed to summon him on the phone from another building housing a garage and drivers' quarters.

After lunch we wandered about the huge estate, taking stock of its wonders. The housekeeper asked if we desired to watch a movie. Yes, but when and what? Any time, and whatever you choose. She gave us a long list of available movies. For starters, we chose a documentary about the Caucasus. We were escorted to the pool room on the second floor, which was furnished sparsely with an ancient pool table and a few armchairs. As soon as we were seated, the curtains on one of the walls drew aside, revealing a screen. For the first time in our lives a movie was being shown just for the two of us. It turned out that we could watch a movie any time, for the projectionist was at our service around the clock.

I asked if the amenities included a sauna. "But of course!

When do you prefer to use it?" "Well, let's say in an hour, after a stroll." "Whatever you say!" We wandered a little about the tidy paths of a small plot surrounded by a tall fence. It was the first time we had found ourselves inside a government-rank dacha; hitherto we had seen such fences only from the outside. Then we strolled along the long second-story balcony, enjoying the beautiful sunset.

After the sauna, the first time we had steamed ourselves together, we were treated to Pilsner beer and local hors d'oeuvres. We were then asked what we wanted to eat and informed that dinner would be served in the large dining room, with late supper in the hunting room. A little tired and all but stupefied by the novelty of our experience, we retired to the bedroom for a nap. The beds were large and comfortable: elegant bedding, wonderfully light and cozy blankets. Who was this luxury for?

After dinner, composed of a wide variety of delicacies and magnificient Caucasian chamois steak, I asked the young maid, "How long do you stay on the job?"

"Until you retire after supper."

"Would you like to call it a day right now?"

She blushed with the suddenly surfacing wild desire to be set free.

"Well, why don't you go," I said. "We'll manage to eat our supper without you in attendance."

"Thank you! Thank you so much!" she murmured breathlessly and was gone in a flash.

That night we ate late supper in the hunting room decorated with boar and deer heads hung on the walls and furnished with a table and chairs made in a pseudo-primitive style. Our lady cook told us that the maid was engaged to be married and her fiancé always waited for her at night beyond the gate—he was not allowed inside. The old lady was visibly glad for the young people. Sipping wine, I engaged her in a conversation.

The palace was officially called a state dacha for the Politburo members, she told me. It had been designed several years previously by Finnish architects and built from special varieties of wood in a mere six months, also by Finns. The house was totally concealed from the outside, but the view from inside included the entire panorama of the mountain range. All Politburo members came to vacation here, but of them Alexei Kosygin, Chairman of the Council of

Ministers, was the most zealous patron. Accordingly, people called the palace "Kosygin's lodge." Just a few days ago, Kosygin had vacationed here in the company of Finland's President Urhho Kekkonen. Delayed by heavy snowfall, they spent two weeks at the palace. Then a helicopter came to fetch them, but both the Russian Premier and the Finnish President expressed a desire to traverse the mountain pass under their own steam, on skis. The guards ran around them while the helicopter hovered overhead. Kosygin usually stayed at the "Small De Luxe," preferring it to the other suite, though the only difference between the two was in the style of furnishings. The cook, an ethnic Russian, had lived here all her life and mastered the secrets of the local Karachaev cuisine. She told me she liked us because we were simple, unpretentious folk: we had invited the driver to share our table and let the maid go home early. She did not ask us who we were. The government servants know that everything is a secret and never ask questions.

So that's what it was! Not only did Irina and I come close to the highest peak of the Caucasus, but we also found ourselves at the very peak of life Politburo-style. We slept in Kosygin's beds, ate from his plates, and were taken care of by his seven servants: a major-domo, a housekeeper, a cook, a maid, a projectionist, a driver, and a guard. In addition, there were outside guards whom we never saw.

Sometime during the night I was awakened in Kosygin's bed by a strange noise. I got up and went to the living room to investigate. It was water seeping through the ceiling and dripping on the refrigerator in the corner. I decided against bothering the domestics, took a huge fruit bowl from the table, and started toward the corner to place it under the waterfall. At that instant Irina woke up. She saw me in pajamas carrying a crystal bowl, and momentarily thought I had gone off my rocker under the flood of impressions. We both burst out laughing. Kosygin had a wonderful bed!

In the morning we went to examine the famous ski slope, accompanied by the guard. We were already approaching the chalet, a mere half-mile from the palace, when I discovered that I had left my camera behind. I told the guard I would walk back to fetch it, but the guard placed a phone call and the driver brought my camera, driving specifically to save me a half-mile walk! Entering the ski-lift to ascend the mountain, I wanted to pay for the ride (one ticket cost a mere 50 kopecks), but the guard told me there was no need to pay —everything had been taken care of.

The mountain and the terraced slopes were wonderful. All the skiing equipment had been laid ready for us, and again everything was free. Unfortunately, Irina and I are poor downhill skiers.

On the way back we dropped in at the only public hotel of Dombai. Though built fairly recently, it already exhibited early signs of decrepitude. Each room contained four, six, or eight beds arranged in double bunks. The hotel was seven stories high and was built over exactly seven years—one story per year. I asked why it had taken so long to build it and was told that lack of access roads was the reason. I wondered how Kosygin's lodge, almost half the hotel in size, had been built so fast. The hotel cafeteria offered a very meager selection of dishes; the entire menu occupied just a few lines: canned fish, hot dogs, one brand of stale cheese, coffee, tea, bread, and cookies. The difference in the standard of life was several hundredfold.

At the tourist camp conditions were even worse. Skiers slept everywhere, even on the floor; it was incredibly dirty; the air was oppressive; the cafeteria was empty. And the price of a vacation pass to the tourist camp was 140 rubles for a two-week stay, almost the national average monthly income!

We returned to our palace and were again treated to dinner in the large dining room and supper in the stylized hunting lodge. Irina and I watched the procession of heavily laden plates across the table and exchanged sad glances, recalling the way things were beyond the tall fence.

I laid out my papers on Kosygin's desk in the office and prepared to work on the notes for my book. Irina sat down on the chair arm and embraced me.

"You know what," she said suddenly, "let's leave. I don't like this place."

To tell the truth, I shared her feelings. The cook was very surprised at our decision.

"I hoped you would stay for at least a week," she said.

"Business, my dear, business," I explained.

47

After Irina left Kislovodsk, I stayed another week, working on the book, then went home.

That Saturday two of my former students who were now in the first year of residency in my department, Victor and Igor, called me early in the afternoon and asked for permission to see me. I liked the boys, they were businesslike, energetic, knowledgeable, and possessed a lot of drive. They had visited me at home on several occasions, so I was not overly surprised at the call. But this time both were obviously uneasy.

"We've come straight from the Party meeting of the department staff [both were Party members]," they told me. "You were the subject of discussion at the meeting. . . ."

"Are you serious?"

"Yes. They wrote a letter of denunciation to the Party Committee."

"What does the letter say?"

"It contains many accusations, but the most damaging is the charge that you educate our students in the Western spirit. A case in point, the letter says, is your propagandistic paeans to American medicine at the time Dr. DeBakey came to operate on Academician Keldysh. You also allegedly sang praise to American instruments and heaped scorn on Soviet medical technology—so much so that your students were outraged."

"But it's not true!" I exclaimed.

"Of course; we know it's all a pack of lies. Both of us defended you at the meeting. But your assistants were in the majority and they prevailed on the meeting to write that letter to the Party Committee."

"What else does it say?"

"That you treat the collective with disdain, that you like to push people around and disregard the opinions of Party members and heap undeserved insults on them, that you are out to oust them from their positions. They also wrote that you have an unbelievably bad temper, and called on the Party Committee to take steps to bring you back to your senses."

"What do they want, my resignation?"

"We don't know. We debated for a long time whether or not to tell you of the meeting. But we consider ourselves to be in your debt; besides, we disagree with the letter. For these reasons we decided to break the Party rules of discipline and come here to tell you everything so you could prepare your defense."

"Thanks, boys." I knew the risk they were taking, and was immeasurably grateful.

"One more thing: don't tell anybody we've been to your home."

"Of course not."

Well, it did come as a surprise, but I had some previous practice fighting back absurd charges. The worst of it was that now I would have to put my book aside and immerse myself in intrigue. But it had to be done. So I sat down at the phone and started calling the administrators at our medical school to ask what was going on. Nobody had heard anything so far.

Next morning, my first post-vacation day on the job, I called a meeting of my assistants and told them I knew about their letter to the Party Committee.

"How do you know?" Dr. Mikhailenko asked, astonished.

"I even know that it was you who authored the snide story of the way I talked about Dr. DeBakey."

"What do you know! So we have treacherous vermin in our Party ranks. Who could that be?"

I told them I was not going to modify my behavior to suit their tastes and would stick to my line at the department. I was intent on demonstrating my firmness right from the start. They were gloomy and averted their eyes.

Within a short time, a committee of inquiry appointed by the dean's office and the Party Committee started checking the activities of my chair—a routine response of management to any complaint. Professors of my acquaintance, appointed to sit on the commission, would come to my office, sift through papers, drink coffee and tell me about their own troubles. Almost every one of them had had to confront a similar situation: someone would write a complaint that would trigger an investigation.

"Tough luck!" they said. "Those assistants of yours are definitely out to get you. If only you were a Party member, you could fight them off much easier. But don't worry, you'll come out on top. We will write a favorable report."

And so they did. For three months one commission followed another, but ultimately I was exonerated. Finally, I thought, I had reason to calm down: the storm had blown over and I was still in one piece.

But more and more I was determined to leave Russia.

It was one thing to make an inner resolve to emigrate, but quite another matter to implement the decision. In a common human frailty, one rarely takes decisive action unless pressured by extraneous circumstances. And my situation after the inquiry did not compel me to follow up on my decision. Quite the contrary, with every passing day my position was getting progressively stronger.

I was already a little spoiled by being invited with increasing frequency to sit in the presidia of various conferences; by state-provided chauffeured limousines waiting for me on more and more occasions; by having little trouble procuring just about anything I wanted for myself or my family in consumer goods or foodstuffs.

Our son planned to enroll in medical school. He chose a medical career of his own accord—partly out of deference to the family tradition, partly because he knew that his father would help him get into and go through medical school. So now I had to make arrangements to make sure he would be admitted to college.

Books of my children's poems came off the presses almost every year now and total sales reached two million copies. My poems were printed in magazines, read on the radio and TV. I became a widely read and popular children's poet.

I continued churning out new inventions; I pioneered new surgical procedures: shoulder joint and wrist joint replacements using prostheses of my original design, made by the selfsame drunken machinists at the Avangard factory. Thanks to my ideas, they had become expert prosthesis-makers; thanks to my alcohol offerings, their drinking problems had become irremediable.

Patents for my inventions started to pour in from foreign countries: the United States, Britain, Italy, and Japan. The patent papers were processed officially through the Committee of Inventions and Discoveries, but actually I had to prepare all the documents and conduct all patent correspondence myself. I was very busy with my new inventions and a great deal more had yet to be done.

Still another factor contributed to my indecision—my old parents. Both of them were past seventy and in increasingly frail health. I could not leave them behind. But how could I dare suggest that they accompany us abroad; at their advanced age such a drastic upheaval might kill them. Besides, how could I explain to them, particularly to my now near-senile father, why I had decided to leave at the very pinnacle of my career? Surely they would never understand.

So from time to time I said at home: "We must leave, we must definitely go!" but never attempted to translate words into action. In 1973, I joined the Soviet Writers' Union, an influential organization offering its members important privileges. Soon afterward, I was made a member of the Literary Foundation Managing Board and, being a physician as well as a writer, charged with the responsibility for watching after the health of Moscow writers. Not only did the honor not give me any satisfaction, but it added disagreeable concerns to my busy schedule. Now I had to heed invitations to meetings of the Writers' Union.

Once I sat at a meeting at the Men-of-Letters House on Herzen Street, listening to a speech delivered by Felix Kuznetsov, first secretary of the Moscow Branch of the union, on the subject: "On Ideological Education of Writers." The speaker glibly quoted lengthy memorized passages from Marx and Lenin and made numerous reverent references to Brezhnev's works. I was torn between laughter and disgust because I had already heard an absolutely identical speech at the session of the Scientific Council at my medical school. The only difference was that Kuznetsov addressed his listeners as "writers," "poets," and "critics," whereas Dr. V. Rodionov, never raising his eyes from a prepared text, had appealed to "professors," "members of the faculty," and "physicians." I dozed off in my chair when Kuznetsov suddenly awoke me with a piercing scream from the podium:

"All our writers, poets, and critics ought to read the works of Great Lenin every day!"

Unable to stand it any longer, I stood up and left in the midst of an ovation without waiting for someone to ask my opinion on Kuznetsov's suggestion.

Before my son was to apply for admission to the medical school where I worked, I had a talk with the new dean, my one-time schoolmate Dr. K. Lakin.

"Okay, he can apply," the dean said.

It meant that my son was as good as admitted. In spite of the competitive exams, the dean kept his own secret list of entrants known as just that—"the dean's list"; all kids entered on the list were assured of admission regardless of how they did on the exams. They were mostly the children of big bosses, celebrities (actors, writers, academicians), and school staff members.

Meanwhile, my inner anxiety steadily grew worse. I could not explain it, but the gnawing feeling made me irritable and I developed what I termed "heart fatigue." I can find no other words to describe that condition. I had no medically certifiable cardiac trouble, neither shortness of breath nor arrhythmia, but a burden never left my heart. I even began toying with the idea of quitting medicine altogether and living by my pen once my son became a doctor. I did not go beyond the inception phase of the plan, but it clearly reflected my yearning to cut the moorings that bound me to the world where I was forever doomed to act against my will.

Although my son made it into medical school, after he passed the four oral entrance exams he had to put in two weeks of free work as a laborer's helper on the construction site of a new school building. It was a precondition for any freshman to be allowed to attend classes. This illegal practice had been in force for years, but no one dared object for the writ had been handed down by the Party Committee. Some farsighted freshmen-to-be tried extra hard on the construction site to attract the benevolent attention of the Party bosses. And thereafter, all through the course of study, such students devoted more time and energy to Komsomol duties than to academic endeavors.

Listening to my son's stories and watching him begin his student life, I was struck by how little things had changed over the twenty-two years since I had been a medical student. In some respects present-day students had it even harder than I had.

After his first day in school, I asked my son: "What have you learned from your debut?"

"Nothing," he replied.

"What do you mean, nothing?"

"Very simple: our first lecture was in Marxist philosophy. The students talked, getting to know each other, and no one listened to the professor. He muttered inaudibly from his lectern, from time to time making feeble attempts to keep us quiet. The lecture was followed by a meeting at which the secretary of the Party Committee talked at length and very boringly, exhorting us to be worthy of the lofty titles of Soviet students and future physicians. After he was done, another meeting was called for us to elect Komsomol secretaries, and then we were told that each year we would be required to put in a month-long stint on a collective farm, helping harvest the potato crop. Then we were broken down into groups and again had to spend some time electing group leaders and Komsomol secretaries. Some elections, indeed—all the secretaries had been appointed in advance by the Party Committee. And that about sums up the extent of what I learned during my first day."

Not much. Even less than I had learned during my first day in medical school back in 1947.

"And what group have you been assigned to?" I continued.

"The Jewish one," he smiled wryly.

"What does it mean?"

"It means this: all Jewish and half-Jewish boys and girls of the freshman class were brought together into one group, Number Thirteen. I, too, landed there. But don't worry: both the group leader and the Komsomol secretary in our group are Russians of pure ethnic stock—to watch us and squeal."

While he was speaking, I watched the steely glint in his eyes. I knew it was an ill omen; all my ethnic conflicts had begun in exactly the same way. Since the day I had had his birth certificate issued at the Registration Bureau in 1958, I had tried my best to shield him from suffering on account of the Jewish portion of his blood. But society with its customs and traditions was stronger than my guardianship.

After our talk my spirits fell and again I felt a gnawing pain in my heart. Nothing could alleviate the burden on my tired heart; even joy was adulterated with sorrow.

There were great kids in his Group 13. In no time they were good friends and started to come to my house. I always tried to feed them well because almost invariably they were hungry; the school had just one small cafeteria, dingy and cold, with long waiting lines and a meager selection of food. Besides, the kids had tremendous appetites.

Once they barged in even more noisy and joyous than usual. I brought them Czech beer and Czech sausages procured at the buffet of Brezhnev Junior. The rare treats added to the kids' merriment.

"Why so happy?" I asked them.

"The whole group went to the movies instead of taking a test."

"Good cause for merriment, no question . . . but what about that test?"

"That's the whole point: we passed the test, the whole group did."

"Where? In the cinema?"

"No, we simply bribed the professor. . . ."

"And he paid us back by giving the test credit to all of us. . . ."

"Not even bothering to ask a single question. . . ."

I really got interested. "Wait, wait. I still can't piece this thing together: what has the bribe to do with the movies?"

They launched into the story, interrupting one another in their eagerness. The professor of Marxist philosophy was an inveterate alcoholic, so the upperclassmen told them. The freshmen were advised to bribe the professor with a bottle of brandy, disguising the bribe as a gift for some suitable occasion. Successive generations of students had resorted to this unfailingly successful ploy. In exchange for the bottle, the professor had given credits to all students without asking them any questions in his subject. That is exactly what they did; they pooled their resources and invested 25 rubles in a bottle of expensive brandy. When the professor entered to conduct the test, eyeing his prey menacingly, the students solemnly presented him with the bottle, saying it was an advance gift for the Soviet Army Day—almost three months away (brandy doesn't get stale, does it?).

The alcoholic pounced on the bottle and darted out of the room, telling the students to wait for him. A few minutes later he returned, reeking of brandy. No longer bellicose, he simply put "credit" against each student's name in his log, whereupon the group was free to go to the movies.

I felt like a jester in a dunce hat in front of the students; after all, I was also a professor at the same school and could not but feel embarrassed on account of my colleague. Meanwhile, the students kept telling me one story after another: who of the professors was on the take and how much a credit at a test or a good grade at an oral exam was worth. As it happened, an average test cost 50 rubles, while a final exam was a more expensive item, costing as much as 150 rubles. The kids laughed uproariously, telling me their stories. They wangled bribe money out of their parents; some gave readily, others grumbled at the expense. . . .

I had to laugh with them, but when they left, my tired heart again started to ache. I was thinking of the kind of society I had to live in: professors extorting bribes from their medical students; parents allotting graft money; everybody knowing about it and not giving a shit. . . . I, too, was bound to keep quiet. I could not betray my young friends. Besides, what was the point of tilting at windmills?

48

On Monday, April 26, 1976, I returned from a two-day business trip to Ivanovo, a town 170 miles east of Moscow. At 8:00 P.M., somebody rang at the door and an agitated girl, my sixth-floor neighbor, panted:

"Please, Doctor, hurry . . . our neighbor, Kostya Bogatyrev . . . He's been murdered. . . ."

I rushed from my eighth-floor apartment to the fifth, where Kostya lived. My son followed me closely. Running past the elevator door on the fifth floor, I saw a large pool of fresh, uncongealed blood on the landing. Large fragments of broken bottle could be seen in the pool. The neighbors had already dragged Kostya into his apartment. His mother, an old woman, was confused and depressed, and she had obviously not yet perceived the meaning of what had happened. Kostya was lying on the floor of his library, next to the sofa. His head was tossed back at an unnatural angle, a death rattle escaped from his mouth.

Cautiously, trying not to cause any further harm, I turned his head to prevent him from choking on his own blood. The first neurological symptom I saw, fixation of the pupils to light and loss of oculovestibular reflexes, indicated a severe brain injury. I examined and felt the wound in the back of of his head. It was a massive depressed skull fracture of the kind that cannot be sustained by simply falling on the floor. It could only result from a strong, straight blow with a heavy object. "A bottle?" I thought. My son brought bandages and I applied a dressing to the bleeding wound. Then I tried to find out what had happened.

Several terrified neighbors from the fifth and sixth floors told me they had seen nothing, but had heard a noise on the landing, followed by the crash of a falling body and the sound of running feet. Someone was obviously running away. The neighbors opened their doors and saw Kostya swimming in blood. They were so taken aback that nobody thought of rushing down to try to get a glimpse of the escaping man. Besides, they were afraid. The elevator attendant, a seventy-year-old crippled woman, who usually stayed on duty at the entrance door, had been out for dinner.

There could be no doubt that someone had tried to kill Kostya. Years ago, he had served almost ten years in concentration camps on trumped-up charges of plotting to assassinate Stalin. And now he himself became the victim of an assassination attempt. His injury was extremely dangerous, maybe fatal. Who had attacked Kostya and why? There was nothing to indicate robbery as a motive; we found more than 50 rubles in his pockets; his watch and wallet were intact. He had been returning home alone when it was still light. There was no evidence of struggle, nothing to show that Kostya had put up a fight: no bruises, abrasions, scratches. It was clear that the attacker had ambushed Kostya beside the elevator shaft; perhaps Kostya had not even seen the attack coming. When he collapsed the killer rushed down on foot, though the elevator was still on the fifth floor.

Within fifteen minutes two patrolmen arrived on the scene. They started by asking whether Kostya was drunk. But I had previously smelled Kostya's breath and found no traces of liquor. I forced the policemen to smell his breath too. Taken aback, they obeyed, though they clearly resented it, and then entered the finding into their report. While the policemen were composing the report, an ambulance came.

The ambulance physician heard my story, thanked me, and took Kostya to Hospital #67 on Khoroshevskoye Highway. The hospital had a neurosurgery department headed by a good friend of mine. Both patrolmen intended to accompany the ambulance to the hospital, but all of a sudden the police captain in charge of our beat materialized. He knew Kostya well. The captain quickly questioned me and the policemen and declared that he himself would go to the hospital to make sure they took good care of the patient. What exactly did he want to watch? And for what reason? However, in the confusion of the moment I paid no attention to the captain's activity: if he wanted to go, it was up to him.

I waited the two hours that I figured it would take to get the patient to the hospital and put him through all necessary admission procedures. Then I called my friend, Professor George Yumashev, director of the department.

"George, a neighbor and good friend of mine has been taken to you—"

"I know," Dr. Yumashev interjected. "You mean that wino Bogatyrev, don't you?"

"George, he's not a drunkard; I myself administered first aid to him and he was not drunk. Why don't you check the police report, two cops were writing it in my presence."

"You must be kidding," he said reprovingly. "My doctors found alcohol in his blood. Besides, the police report states that he had a fall in a state of intoxication."

"What?" I exclaimed in disbelief. It could only mean that they plied him with vodka in the ambulance on the way to the hospital. Besides, it is crystal clear that one cannot sustain such a fracture as a result of a fall. It was a blow-induced fracture.

"What I do know is that he was dead drunk on admission here. In my view, he's beyond hope," he replied.

"Please, George," I pleaded desperately. "Do whatever you can for him."

"Don't you see he can't be helped?" the professor replied.

Kostya Bogatyrev stayed for ten days in Dr. Yumashev's hospital virtually unattended. He developed an abscess of the brain. Of course, the severe injury was partly to blame, but the hospital physicians did nothing to help the patient and administered no antibiotics to him. Kostya's second wife, Lena, finally succeeded in having her husband transferred to the Burdenko Institute of Neurosurgery, but it was too late. Two weeks later Kostya Bogatyrev died.

His murderer was not found, which is hardly surprising. The case was exceptional in itself—a murder in the writers' building, which was carefully watched and guarded by the police—but the sleuths made no attempt to determine the motive for the attack. I was questioned several times, both at home and at the Moscow Criminal Investigation Department, and each time the investigators did their best to make me say that Bogatyrev had been drunk. I firmly denied it. I called my patient and friend General Igor Karpets, and asked him to find out what he could. He told me later, "The KGB took over the case; it was handled by their investigators. Apparently there was a political side to the murder."

It was indeed a political murder, and the KGB took over the case lest criminal investigators find out the truth. And then an absurd rumor was started that Kostya had had an affair with a young woman, the mistress of a professional criminal, who killed his rival out of jealousy. I had known Kostya too well to believe that absurdity. But the police captain who supervised our building once said to me: "What do you say of Bogatyrev, you know, the guy from the fifth floor, apartment number forty-eight. Seemed such a quiet guy and here he's had this affair with a young chick. That's what he was killed for."

I am sure the captain had a lot to do with Kostya's death; he was certain to inform the KGB on Bogatyrev's foreign visitors and there is little doubt it was he who had forged the policemen's report.

The sad news that Kostya was dead spread first throughout the world. His friend Heinrich Boll wrote a very emotional obituary that I heard on the Voice of America. Dr. Andrei Sakharov, the leader of the dissidents, characterized Kostya's death as a great personal blow and a tragedy for the dissident movement of Moscow. His death was reported by all the radio stations and newspapers of the world—except the Soviet media.

I often recalled my neighbor and friend Kostya Bogatyrev. And I never failed to think: "Lord, what a horrible country! What a horrible time!"

49

I do not dabble in space medicine, but as an orthopedist I knew that lengthy exposure to outer space causes "bone softening" and calcium depletion. The first of the cosmonauts to spend a considerable amount of time in orbit (three weeks in 1964), General Adrian Nikolaev, could hardly stand unsupported upon landing. Outer space is devoid of Earth-generated magnetism, whereas our bodies are conditioned by constant exposure to a weak permanent magnetic field. My method of speeding up the healing of fractured bones by use of a permanent magnetic field boosted the microcirculation of the tissues, precisely what the cosmonauts needed to prevent the loss of calcium from their bones.

After prolonged negotiations, I was allowed to assemble a research group and conduct experiments on animals and clinical observations of patients during the 1974–75 period. All my findings were to be passed to the laboratory of Dr. Boris Yegorov, the only physician who had ever been to outer space, who studied the effects of prolonged exposure of man to outer space conditions. I was not given permission to come close to space vehicles, but it suited me perfectly, for the only thing that really interested me was further research into the ways magnetic field affected broken bones.

I was given a grant of 10,000 rubles—not much, but still better than nothing. Of this sum, 2,400 rubles were earmarked as my remuneration; the rest was to be spent on hiring assistants and buying equipment. In Russia, grants are known as "economic project agreements." They are a recent innovation in the field of scientific research and not many people are familiar with them.

I planned the project in such a way that my assistants could be given a share. For one thing, I wanted everybody in my department to take part in the project; besides, it was a good way for my assistants to earn a little extra money. We distributed and defined our respective functions at several meetings. Secretary of the Party Dr. Mikhailenko and trade-union leader Dr. Kosmatov were in on the project and solidly behind me. We agreed to allot 15 percent of our money to hire the needed workers who could not be put on the official payroll. I insisted that Dr. Kosmatov, rather than myself, be elected treasurer of the research group. Finally, the formalities were behind and work was underway. We conducted hundreds of experiments on rats and rabbits, and then were able to step up considerably the use of magnetic field for the bone-knitting process. We also collected valuable data on the concomitant improvement in tissue microcirculation.

My assistants exhibited little enthusiasm and worked sluggishly, requiring constant prodding. As a result, there was a lot of friction, but it was nothing compared to the money-sharing problem when we were paid, which happened once every six months. Contrary to our agreement and despite their meager contribution to the project, my assistants were reluctant to give the agreed-upon 15 percent of their pay to the people who had really applied themselves. I was aware of their sentiments but was not worried because we had an excellent internal bookkeeping system: each ruble was accounted for by receipts and progress reports from the recepients of the money.

Still, in the spring of 1976, Drs. Mikhailenko, Kosmatov, and Burlakov, all Party members, denounced me to the Economic Crime Unit of the Ministry of Internal Affairs. In their report, they wrote that I had embezzled 20,000 rubles of state money from the grant issued to me by a space research institution, and that I had deceived the grant donor by having accomplished nothing. They presented a falsified report of my activities.

I learned about the denunciation accidentally from Professor Alexander Kizmichev, a surgeon. "Your Assistant Burlakov is spreading rumors that you've stolen twenty thousand rubles from state funds," he told me. "Be careful with him."

"What twenty thousand rubles?" I asked in amazement.

"Grant money."

"Oh, I see. . . ."

I summoned the squealers to my office. "What's the purpose of this filth?" I asked.

They were silent, eyeing me with hatred. I was still their boss and there was no saying just yet who would prevail in the struggle.

"You know very well indeed that my report was accepted by the Institute of Medico-Biological Problems without complaint. The entire grant amounted to only ten thousand rubles, of which sum you received your due. So why write a lie?"

They kept silent. I realized they would not admit to denouncing me, though they could not disown the denunciation.

I have always disliked intrigue, but at that time I wished I liked it, because I clearly had to go to the counteroffensive. When I asked Dr. Gennadi Troyanski, the first secretary of the school's Party Committee, to investigate the matter and rein in my enemies, he replied, "There are several of them and all are Party members. Try to win over one of them. Without this the Party Committee would not be able to help you. A group of communists is always a powerful force. We cannot fire communists. But if they break their unity and start scheming against one another, it will be an entirely different matter. Then an intra-Party scandal will arise and the Party Committee will be in a position to step in and reestablish order."

It was distasteful to try to convert an enemy into a friend. However, I braced myself and had a talk with Dr. Kosmatov, whose thesis for a scientific degree I had written practically from scratch and who owed me his position of assistant professor.

We sat alone in a small square. "What surprises me most is that you agreed to sign that missive," I said, "you who had spared no words to express your gratitude to me for all I've done for you."

"I'm still grateful to you," he said uneasily.

"Then why did you sign that letter?"

"I couldn't turn down a request from my fellow communists. Had I refused to sign, it would have been tantamount to a betrayal of my Party duty."

"What duty?" I exclaimed indignantly. "Does your duty consist of squealing on your benefactor?"

"My duty is to be on the side of the communists all the time," he replied stubbornly.

It is beyond my power to combat this warped psychology! I cut short all efforts to flirt with them. It was vital that I counterattack, but I did not feel I could rise to the task. With their malicious perseverance and single-minded hatred, they were stronger than the soft intellectual slug that I was. Still I cast about in search of ways to save myself and my position. I sought out Irina and other people close to me for advice. My health deteriorated. All the denunciations, discussions, and mental torment were destroying me.

Irina watched my condition grow progressively worse; I slept poorly, lost weight, and relied increasingly on Valium and other tranquilizers. Yet I stepped up the intensity of my work. At last Irina decided to plead my case personally with Dr. Kornienko, also a secretary of the school's Party Committee. From prior experience he knew full well that wives would come to him either to complain or to seek aid. He received Irina very coldly.

"Your husband should seek accommodation with these people," he told her. "If he's innocent, why should he worry?"

"But they're persecuting him with their denunciations," Irina insisted.

"A letter from a group of communists is not a denunciation, but an expression of legitimate concern of responsible people taking a principled stand on a matter of state importance. Even if they're not one hundred percent right, I don't see any harm; anybody can make mistakes."

Irina was provoked into an ill-advised outburst: "If those slimy scoundrels don't stop hounding my husband, I'll find a way to get in touch with Western correspondents and the whole world will learn about this story on the Voice of America."

He cast her a vicious glance.

Needless to say, we had no connections with Western journalists, nor was I a dissident. But from time to time we did hear stories in Voice of America broadcasts about Soviet scientists being persecuted for anti-Semitic or political reasons. But we had no intention of seeking protection through publicity in the West.

In the meantime, an umpteenth attempt was made to investigate me: a special auditor appeared, an old Party hag notorious for maliciousness and sternness, known to have destroyed many Jewish physicians during open anti-Semitic drives. My enemies had composed yet another denunciation and sent it to the prosecutor's office, where a secret investigation was launched on its basis.

Finally I appealed for aid to my patient Colonel Alexei Musyachenko, an executive at the Economic Crime Unit. One night I went to see him at his office, which was in an old building without an identifying plaque on Sadovaya Street. My steps echoed dully down the empty, cold corridor. "My footfalls will sound exactly the same in prison," I thought involuntarily.

Colonel Musyachenko was a typical Russian peasant, very shrewd and wily. With a lifetime of experience with forgers, embezzlers, and thieves behind him, he was an expert on economic crimes and the psychology of people committing them. I did not fit into any of the criminal categories he knew.

"The malice of your enemies is really surprising!" he said after hearing my story. "And what's their goal? I suppose they want to undermine your career, but what do they stand to gain from it? I'm at a loss. You know, there was a similar case at the Botkin Hospital: malefactors started to hound a Dr. Ratner with denunciations. They hounded him so tenaciously that one day he applied for permission to emigrate to Israel. He left, and the hospital lost an excellent X-ray specialist. I was among the victims, because Dr. Ratner had treated me for a stomach ailment, but now I have no reliable physician to turn to."

I had not heard that story, but the colonel in effect pointed out to me that there was a way to save myself from slander: leave Russia. So the idea grew stronger.

Within six months, my enemies had blown my alleged sins to such proportions that many unflattering rumors started circulating in Moscow's medical world, tarnishing my reputation. True to form, the rumors distorted even the lies that constituted the substance of the charges invented by Dr. Mikhailenko.

In spite of the lies, I tried to remain cool. Our struggle became a test of nerves. For a while neither side could claim victory. Their charges were unsubstantiated through numerous investigations. My opponents turned into nervous wrecks. Dr. Mikhailenko was particularly unhappy.

"I can't last much longer," he once openly confided in me. "I can't sleep nights. If it goes on like this, I'll leave my job."

However stupid and ludicrous his naive complaint to—of all

people—me, I replied with a smile: "There's a cure for your condition: stop writing slanderous letters and you'll feel better immediately. Just relax."

"I can't," he replied. "My Party conscience doesn't allow me to relax."

One night I was visited at home by Party Committee Secretary Dr. Kornienko. He was a notorious KGB stooge, well-known in our medical school as a man to be distrusted, a kind of resident spy. I was aware of his activities, but was not in the least alarmed by his visit. He always took pains to show me he was on my side. Undoubtedly he knew that I counted many important generals among my patients and assumed that I had powerful support in high places.

He looked the picture of a revolutionary sailor of the 1920s —the way they are depicted in Soviet movies. With his rolling gait, legs spread far apart, all he lacked was bandoliers across his chest.

I offered him a drink and opened the bar of my Finnish wall unit. The bar was beautiful and I watched furtively for his reaction.

"Why, look at your bar! What a supply of booze and all of it foreign," he said admiringly. "But how about our Russian vodka?"

"No problem, it's in here." I poured vodka in glasses.

"To you," he said smiling.

"Thanks, and to you."

"Fine vodka," he grunted. "Tell me, did you really have an affair with Lena?"

"Lena who?"

"Well, that coed of yours, Lena Shalaeva . . ."

I was so surprised I almost choked on my drink. "Why are you asking?"

"You tell me first, did you or didn't you?"

"No, of course not."

"Hmm, yet she wrote a letter to the Party Committee testifying that you did."

"Lies! What exactly did she say?"

"I haven't seen the letter and can't even say who has it. But I decided to warn you as a friend. Surely you know that an affair with a coed is a very serious misdeed, a sure way to get yourself fired. But since you're saying it didn't happen, you have nothing to worry about. So much the better. Well, here's to you!"

"And to you!"

Clearly, it was a provocation. To begin with, I had to tell Irina to spare her an unpleasant surprise. Fortunately, I had once told her how Lena had tried to seduce me. Still, wives who can hear such stories repeated without at least a touch of mistrust and jealousy are few.

I could not read Irina's mind, but after my story she turned perceptibly gloomier. However, we tried to present a brave front in public.

For several weeks gossip-mongers had a field day with the letter, though nobody had seen it. Although the charge of my romantic involvement with a coed was not confirmed, people delighted in savoring and passing along the gossip. In itself the rumor did my reputation a lot of damage. But I was more intrigued as to how and why that slur had surfaced right in the midst of the overall campaign against me.

Dr. Georgadze by sheer accident met young Dr. Lena at Hospital #40, where she was undergoing treatment for asthma.

"What do you have against Golyakhovsky?" he asked.

"Nothing."

"Then why have you denounced him in writing?"

She told him. I had denied her surgical internship in my department, and she had wept behind the door of my office while my assistants tried to soothe her and prove to her that I was right. In a short while, her anguish subsided. She went through an internship in internal medicine, was quite content with her life, and contemplated marriage. Then one night, Dr. Mikhailenko suddenly called her and requested a meeting. Although they had never associated socially, she could not turn down her former teacher. He went to her apartment accompanied by two other assistants of mine, Dr. Pechenkin and Dr. Valentsev. Those three highly placed men, in their forties, pleaded with a young woman to lodge a written complaint against me with the Party Committee. She told them she had no score to settle and that she was even grateful to me for what I had done for her. But they told her I was spreading rumors about my conquest of her and that I had refused to admit her to the internship program because there was another pretender to the position, a young woman with whom I was romantically involved.

She weakened under the psychological onslaught, and they

stepped up their attack, insisting that it was her duty to unmask me. At long last, Lena told them: "My relationship with Golyakhovsky is my own business, but I'll sleep on your suggestion." Then Mikhailenko exclaimed: "Why wait? We've drafted your letter; all you have to do is read and sign it."

After that they spread a rumor that Lena was about to come to the Party Committee with a letter spelling my doom. But the letter failed to materialize. Did the letter exist or not?

I was never to find out. But when I imagined the scene of how they were trying to talk her into slandering me, I shook with fury and impotence. They were so single-mindedly bent on destroying me that morality lost all relevance. And to think that I had tried to fight them fairly! Fool. Incorrigible softy!

Yet another commission appeared to check my work and arbitrate the conflict. It consisted of three men: Party Secretary V. Kornienko, Professor S. Babichev, and Professor V. Rodionov. The latter two until recently had held high positions in the medical administrative hierarchy, but lost internicine fights and had been demoted. Despite losing their battles, both were past masters in the art of intrigue and demagoguery. Thanks to their connections, after their downfall they were able to cling to relatively high positions—those of heads of chairs of surgery. But they were not satisfied and boiled with fury and spite. Neither could be called a surgeon by any stretch of the imagination. Dr. Babichev was known among his colleagues as "an iron without a handle," an accurate representation of his prowess in the operating room. As for Dr. Rodionov's lectures on surgery, here is what my students, Victor and Igor, told me, mixing indignation with derision:

"He reads standard textbook material on surgery copied word for word on a sheet of paper. We took the trouble of bringing the textbook into class and checking his lecture by it—not a word of his own. What a waste of time! How on earth could such a man become a professor of surgery?!"

I knew the commission had been selected for the express purpose of doing a hatchet job on me. How could they form an informed opinion of my work when none of them was an orthopedist?

They were monsters destroying everything in their path. To

counterattack, I conspicuously displayed all my patent certificates and samples of inventions; the special diploma awarded to me by the Committee of Inventions and Discoveries as the outstanding inventor of the year; and reprints of all my articles and those written by my assistants. But the commission did not deign to have even a cursory glance at the evidence. Taking seats in my office, the commission members launched into a litany of accusations:

"What have you done!" Dr. Babichev said.

"Yes, a nasty business, a very nasty business," Dr. Rodionov confirmed.

"What do you mean?" I asked.

"What we mean is that you made fools of us in front of our students, that's what!"

"It must be a mistake," I said. "I'd never allow myself such an indiscretion. . . ."

"Yes, you did; you did!"

"But I've never even mentioned your names to my students."

"I should think not! But you did discuss the operation performed by the American surgeon Dr. DeBakey on Comrade Keldysh, did you not?"

"Yes, I did. I answered the students' questions about the operation. But I told them that I had not been present in the operating room. And I never said a word of you."

Of course, I understood perfectly well what they meant: my story of DeBakey's operation was true, while both of them had lied to the students. I continued to feign astonishment and pretended not to understand.

"Ideological education should be prominent in the training of a physician," Dr. Rodionov said didactically, in the tone of a former Party boss.

"Right!" Dr. Babichev confirmed. "We knew, of course, that the government had invited the American to perform surgery on Comrade Keldysh."

"But it was an exception to the rule and our students needn't know about it," Rodionov continued.

I had an acute impression that they had rehearsed their lines like a circus routine; it was impossible to watch and hear them without laughter. Even Dr. Kornienko, who listened in silence, could not help inwardly smiling, as his eyes mutely testified.

"So you had no call to tell them about it," Babichev continued. "We all know our surgeons can perform such operations just as well as the Americans."

There was no use arguing. I was utterly disgusted by their vicious glances, their lowbrow mindset, even their uncouth speech. I could only think: "My God, will it ever end?"

At that instant Party Secretary Kornienko entered the conversation:

"A rumor has been circulated among the students that our esteemed professors Rodionov and Babichev were not exactly telling the truth," he said.

"Exactly: the students call us liars," Rodionov said.

"We know it from reliable sources," Kornienko added. In other words, somebody had ratted to the Party Committee.

What was I supposed to say to that? Frankly, the students were right. But I had not mentioned the names of the two professors. It was clear I was charged with the crime of not supporting them in their lies. And in point of fact they were right: I really was against them. I was not strong enough to endure in such a posture all my life.

"Show us the texts of your lectures," Rodionov said sternly.

I handed to him a few sheets of paper stapled together. They contained figures, several quotations from famous surgeons, dates and outlines of lectures. And that was all. Rodionov took the thin sheaf, weighed it on his palm, shook his head, and asked with a derisive smile: "Is this all you read to your students?"

"It's only the gist of my lectures."

"And where are the lectures proper?"

"In my head. I don't deliver lectures from a written text. Each time I introduce something new, modify the material, improvise. The students have their textbooks with standard material, so I try to give them additional material, live examples, to stimulate their interest."

The professors stared at each other and their expressions clearly said what they thought: "Look at this idiot!"

"In other words, you can't prove with documentary evidence exactly what you tell your students in the course of those improvisations?"

"Sure I can. I have no text, but I can tell you any portion of the material of your choosing right here, if you wish. As I said, I keep all the material in my head."

"It should be on p-a-p-e-r, on p-a-p-e-r!" Rodionov almost squeaked in indignation.

I grew indifferent to everything. I shrugged: "Each man uses his own method."

"No, no, don't say that!" Babichev interjected. "The method of teaching is uniform throughout the whole country. Like I said . . ."

They spent the whole day in my office, systematically trying to prove to me that I was guilty of deviations and errors. They called in my assistant/slanderers and I had to leave the office while they interrogated my enemies. In the corridor two groups of physicians awaited the outcome—my supporters and adversaries. Each time I exited, my supporters surrounded me and tried to cheer me up, while the enemies stood aside, eyeing me sullenly.

In late afternoon, Dr. Babichev asked me: "Is it true that you dislike operating with our Russian instruments?"

"If the instruments are good, I use them with pleasure."

"Then how does it happen you have foreign instruments?"

"I received them as a gift from my Czech counterparts. They were presented at an official ceremony."

"Maybe you got them officially, but you must surely know that many so-called intellectuals in that country wanted to defect to the capitalist camp."

"So now we're talking politics," I responded, not sure what Czech surgical instruments had to do with defections.

"Yes, we're talking about politics," Rodionov said sternly. "None of us should shy away from politics. That concerns you, too, if you are still on our side."

I glanced at him sharply; things were taking a nasty turn. An accusation of being apolitical was a serious charge.

"You should know how it used to be: one thing led to another; at first foreign instruments, then foreign pals," Babichev interjected. "That's how it happened in the case of the late surgeon Sergei Yudin. Like I said, one is better off using our Russian instruments. . . ."

Finally they got up to go. There was one last question. "What's your opinion of student Egalevich?" Radionov asked.

"In my view he's a very good student, active and intelligent, one of the best."

"Ahem," he muttered, "I wouldn't characterize him in such glowing terms. In my subject he gets only poor grades. But you are known in general to be biased toward . . . you know . . ."

It was a relatively mild but unmistakable allusion to my Jewishness. And I understood that the student Egalevich story had also been added to my indictment.

The commission departed, smiling, the job well done. My enemies surrounded the commission and broke into smiles as well. Dr. Mikhailenko, like a boisterous puppy, scampered around and all but squealed with delight.

I followed the commission out of my office, exhausted. Apparently my expression was so eloquent, my back and shoulders drooping, that after a single glance at me, the group of my supporters dispersed without questions or comments.

50

What had happened to me? Once a confident, calm, and strong-willed man, now I was a neurotic, suspicious to the point of paranoia. I had not had a good night's sleep in six months and was addicted to Valium. Frequently and anxiously waking up in the night, I would think about my endless troubles, putting myself through the torture again and again. The only way to calm down and forget it all was to press myself against Irina. Warmed by her body and lulled by her measured breathing, I would drift into sleep—but only for a short while. I was so exhausted that my sexual drive was receding. But not even this was of concern to me. I felt I was plunging into an abyss, my self-esteem disintegrating, my personality falling apart. The trouble was I could no longer analyze the situation objectively. The blow to my morale was too painful.

I requested an audience with Dr. Kapiton Lakin, dean of the medical school. I expected nothing pleasant from our forthcoming talk. I was forced to wait in the anteroom for a good two hours. Many people, most of whom I knew, entered and left the dean's office and said hello to me; but my attention was riveted on a stranger sitting next to me, a smiling young man of about thirty who looked like a typical chauffeur. From time to time he glanced at me, smiling slightly. I did not like his smile; it seemed ominous to me. And then it occurred to me that he was a KGB agent assigned to shadow me. In my mind's eye I saw myself being arrested exiting from the office or the school. I tried hard to shake off the obsessive picture, but it would not go away. I understood there were no grounds for suspecting that man, but I could not help it. I was going crazy.

Over nearly three decades of friendship, there was hardly a topic the dean and I had not discussed. But this time he did not want to talk to me one-on-one and invited a host of witnesses: the secretary of the Party Committee, his deputy, the president of the trade-union committee, the vice-dean, some other people. I felt ill at ease in front of that unexpected sea of faces and could not speak coherently. My tongue betrayed me.

The conversation was brief, polite but indifferent, with an obvious undercurrent of hostility toward me. The people in the room evinced their enmity through ice-cold stares. The dean expressed his displeasure at the fact that powerful people outside of our institute or the medical profession in general had gotten involved in the case on my behalf. I replied, without much assurance: "I wish I could do without them, but I'm even less eager to fall victim to slander. If the Party organization of the school can't put an end to the rampage of its members, I feel I have the right to defend myself with all means at my disposal."

"Including the Voice of America?" Dr. Kornienko asked slyly, referring to Irina's threat.

"It was my wife who said it, not I. But you should appreciate her feelings; she suffers on my account and tries as best she can to shield me." I knew this was no defense against the Voice of America charge.

"The latest commission to check your record gave you low marks for ideology and teaching methods," the dean added dryly. "The commission could not so much as find the texts of your lectures. I realize one does not have to read lectures from a prepared text, but on the other hand there exists a uniform work rules directive for all medical schools and we cannot tolerate deviations from standard practice."

I did not argue. I had neither the stamina nor desire to protest my innocence again; the outcome would not have been affected anyway.

"The circumstances do not favor you, Professor Golyakhovsky," the dean said dryly.

It was a direct threat. I knew that by law they could not fire me because my position could only be filled through a contest. Even upon expiration of the five-year term I was entitled to yet another year of employment. I kept silent, and the dean went on:

"Nobody faults you for your performance on the job. But you are guilty of failing to create a normal working atmosphere in your department. You are handicapped by the fact that you do not belong to the Party."

Actually, that was the bottom line—my position vis-à-vis the Party. For over two decades I had managed to steer round the rock of Party membership and still move ahead. But this time it lay squarely in my path and I could not push it aside. I understood that my position was hopeless. Yet I was dying to tell them: "And you are handicapped by your Party membership." I made an extraordinary effort to refrain from shouting it in their faces. But what use would it be?—an open revolt of a helpless lone spirit. All of us understood that if I stayed outside the Party it could only mean one thing—my distaste for the Party.

We had nothing more to talk about. I left the office followed by the silent stares of the Party bosses. The young man in the anteroom, whom I had suspected of being a KGB agent, was no longer there. He was indeed a chauffeur and I had seen him driving his boss away. I was relieved, but still I felt bad. I had to make a decision. Again . . .

I drove my car down Leningradsky Prospect in the right lane, hugging the curb. My heart ached and I feared that in case of a heart attack I would not able to handle the car in traffic. Somehow I managed to get home. Irina and our son were there. She looked at me anxiously, but my son ignored me. All children are self-centered and give little attention to their parents. I had been that way, too.

Exhausted, I slumped on the bed. Irina sat down at my feet

and I started telling her about my conversation with the dean. We were interrupted by our son, who entered the room and butted in unceremoniously, preoccupied by his own concerns.

"Hey, listen," he said. "You promised to get me a release from the stint on the collective farm. How about keeping your promise?"

To keep it, I had to plead with one of those who a short while ago sat in the dean's office, gazing at me with animosity.

"I can't," I said impatiently.

"But you gave your word," he insisted.

All of a sudden I flew into a rage: "What do you want from me?" I yelled. "There was a time I could do anything, I succeeded in everything I undertook, but no more! Now I'm a total failure, impotent. Do you hear me?"

I grabbed at the first thing at hand—it happened to be my glasses. I viciously broke them and threw the fragments on the floor. Blood oozed from cuts in my hands. Frightened, Irina rushed to wipe my hands with her handkerchief. But I didn't care if I hurt my hands; I was on the point of a breakdown. And then I intercepted my son's glance; he was looking at me with a mixture of understanding and compassion; I saw pity in his eyes.

Twenty-four years ago I had looked at my father with just that measure of compassion and pity when he was waiting for arrest by the KGB. I had been following in my father's footsteps: I was successful and now I was on the verge of losing everything, just as he had been that time in 1952.

I called my disciple and friend Dr. Algis in the Lithuanian city of Kaunas, and asked him to arrange a short vacation for me and Irina in his country. He found a place for us in the the tiny township of Zarasas, population just 6,700, and on a rainy day, July 13, 1976, we set out on our journey. Two days later we arrived at the destination, the house of one of Dr. Algis' patients. The owner's wife, a Lithuanian peasant woman, led us to our makeshift quarters. It was a tiny wooden barn in the depth of an overgrown garden on the shore of Lake Zarasas. The barn contained just one small room accommodating two beds and not much else. At the sight of it, deep gloom enveloped me: so that was my lot now instead of the government palaces where I had lived in luxury not so long ago!

From the start we found out that the high standard of living the Baltic people had once enjoyed was gone. Meat, chicken, and even eggs were unavailable; dairy products were in very short supply. With her usual energy, Irina reconnoitered all neighborhood stores and found out where and when provisions could be procured. Speed was important because the shelves were emptied very fast the same day supplies were brought in. Well, we'd manage somehow.

Every morning, I went to the well in the garden and fetched water in pails. It took fifty pails to water the garden—excellent physical exercise. I turned the well handle, mulling over one question and one question only: what was I to do with my devastated life? I could not stay on my job, that much was clear. It was out of the question to try to brave it out in such a poisoned atmosphere. Having lost my position I could hardly entertain hopes of regaining it. At the least it would take years to accomplish such a feat, and I was in poor physical and mental condition.

"I think maybe the only right solution is emigration," Irina had once told me. And I had replied: "Are you crazy? It can't be the only answer!"

But, however long I turned the well handle, no matter how many pails of water I lifted and carried about the vegetable garden, no other solution presented itself. I knew that whatever happened, I would always smart from my defeat. Not only was I bound to lose my job, but my human and professional position in society was to go down as well.

To distract ourselves, we drove around the area in search of beautiful sites. Once we chanced upon a unique monument of nature eight miles from Zarasas—the Stelmuzh Oak, the oldest tree in Europe. The trunk of the two-thousand-year-old tree was thirteen meters in circumference, its canopy twenty-three meters across. The ancient giant still bore beautiful green leaves, though its gnarled trunk was dotted with holes cemented over to preserve the tree.

I was struck by its longevity and vitality. Just think of the hardships it had endured over its incredible life! Roman legionnaires sought shade under its branches. It was older than Jesus Christ. And its environment was so severe; it had had to endure two thousand cold, snowy winters! Amazing!

I have always loved trees, the crowning achievement of creation. It is trees that set the stage for living beings. Through photosynthesis they supply us with oxygen. They burn in a fire to save us from the cold. They lend their trunks for construction; the first huts, boats, chairs, from the simplest to the most stylish, all are made of wood. Trees give refuge to beasts, birds, and insects, and people, too. They bear fruit. They never demand anything but always have something to offer—what a contrast to human nature!

Yes, I definitely prefer trees to people!

I sat under the oak canopy, thinking and thinking. I recalled my acquaintances undeservedly hurt by the communists the way I was. In my mind's eye, I saw my professor, Dr. A. Geselevich, the "rootless cosmopolitan"; the surgeon S. Yudin; the composer Dmitri Shostakovich; the poet Boris Pasternack. And, of course, above all I thought of my father.

They all managed to survive, but they never overcame the damage to their morale. My father, too, stayed hurt. And how many people had not endured? No, I did not want to join their ranks. I made a resolution to survive physically and mentally. But how? The only way was to leave Russia.

I thought and thought, to the accompaniment of rustling leaves on the oak's branches. And I felt its wisdom seeping into my soul. My eyes opened and I could see now that everything that had befallen me was not an unfortunate accident, but an inevitable chain of events. I was wrong for Soviet Russia, too unpalatable to the communists. Since the day they had seized power, they had been systematically destroying all the best and most progressive things Russia had to offer. They had ploughed a bloody furrow of indiscriminate terror through the history of the country, imposing their designs on a mostly unwilling people. I was but a speck of dust in their path, but an alien speck—and so I was being wiped out like hundreds of thousands before me. To preserve my personality, I had no choice but to leave Russia. I was obliged to do it not only for my own sake but also for the sake of my son.

51

Irina and I returned home unrested and preoccupied with new concerns. The first order of business was to have a talk with our son and parents about problem number one: emigration.

I sat with my son in the kitchen and started the conversation: "Your mother and I decided that we would all be better off leaving Russia for good."

He did not seem perturbed. "Where to?"

"America."

"Gee, swell!" he exclaimed with boyish exuberance.

"Yes, swell, but I'm not sure I'll be allowed to emigrate. If I'm denied permission and you stay with me, you might well be the one who'll suffer the most."

"Why me?"

"Because mother and I have the better part of our lives behind us. But your life is ahead of you. They can be counted on to start making life miserable for you the very instant we apply for exit visas. You'll be at their mercy, defenseless. Worse still, I won't be able to protect you."

He was flushed with a sudden surge of resentment at the prospect. "Why?" he asked.

"Because the minute you apply for emigration you'll join the ranks of enemies of the regime. You might be targeted to 'flunk' any exam, be kicked out of school and drafted into the army, where you'd be marked for such special treatment you'll cry bloody tears. Think about it."

He dropped his head and fell silent. Then he said: "We should give it a try."

I was ecstatic. In a crisis, he proved to be really my son, as recalcitrant as I ever was.

I decided to relegate the task of talking to father to my mother; she had the best chance of making him understand. In order to be able to talk to her out of father's earshot, I invited her to accompany me to the premiere of a new ballet, *Icarus,* at the Bolshoi. Mother was delighted to go to the theater with me and dressed up for the occasion.

During the intermissions we discussed the matter and came to an agreement. What a beautiful and sweet disposition Mother had! No sooner had I started: "Mother, I want to leave for America and take all of you with me. . . ." than she interjected excitedly: "To America? Oh, how wonderful! When do we leave?"

"That's the trouble. I'm not sure yet whether they'll let me go. First, we have to apply. I wanted to discuss all the angles with you in advance. And you'll have to talk to Father; you know better than anybody the way he's been."

"Yes, he's changed for the worse. But don't worry; he'll do what I tell him. We'll go with you and everything will be just fine. What about your family, will they go?"

"Of course."

"And the boy [that's what she called her grandson], isn't he afraid of the radical change?"

"No, he's a real mensch."

"Splendid! We will go to America and see the world. I'll get to see Rodin's *Hell's Gate.*"

"It's in Paris."

"So what? I'll just have to go to Paris then. If we go to America, we'll be able to travel wherever we please, won't we?"

"It's a big 'if'. . . ."

"Don't worry, we'll get there."

Having dealt with those crucial problems, I told Irina to have a talk with her mother while I went to the medical school to see the dean and discuss my resignation. I had to resign for two reasons: first, it was unthinkable for me to apply for emigration while staying on as head of a chair and lecturer; second, word of my intention would undoubtedly have encouraged my enemies to double their efforts, which in turn could have an impact on the KGB decision. So once the decision to emigrate was made, I had to quit. But not before I found a job where I could stick it out to the very last day.

Our medical school was abuzz with excitement. Two events had shaken it. One was the death of Professor V. Shelekhov, a physiologist roughly my age. A competent specialist and a nice man, he had just been promoted to head of a chair, with the proviso that he should join the Party. Dr. Shelekhov was in poor health; at the age of forty-five he had suffered a stroke. He was reluctant to join the Party, but they forced him. The ordeal was too much for him;

no sooner had he emerged from the admission procedure meeting at the Party Committee than he dropped dead.

His death shook even the Party Committee stalwarts. One of them was actually heard to say, "We shouldn't have twisted his arm. There was no need to force him to join, maybe if we hadn't he'd still be alive."

I was sorry for my colleague and friend; we were on good terms and our sons were schoolmates. But at the same time I could not help congratulating myself on having resisted the pressure.

The other event also involved a death, this time a murder. Zhanna L., the forty-year-old secretary at the dean's office, was found stabbed in the elevator of her state-owned apartment house the day the admission list was posted at the school. Zhanna's husband, an important functionary at the Central Committee of the Party, raised hell at the Criminal Investigation Department and prodded the detective into action to hunt for the killer(s). He would have been better off, though, to sit tight, because the investigation opened a can of worms: it transpired that his wife had been killed in connection with bribes she and several professors had extorted from college entrants.

Two young Georgians, who had applied for admission but flunked, were arrested. Under questioning, both admitted paying Zhanna 5,000 rubles each. After that, criminal investigators and those from the Economic Crime Unit became fixtures at our school, interrogating all employees and checking every single scrap of paper at the admission office. I was also interrogated, but I had been on vacation when the secretary was murdered, and besides I had never had anything to do with admissions. Naturally, there was not a single word either of the murder or the bribery in the press.

Dean Dr. K. Lakin could think of little else than his troubles. Like all members of the Party Committee he was under investigation not only by the law, but also by a commission sent by the District Party Committee, which was even worse. The dean feared reprisals if their practices became known. We all knew that corruption was rampant at the school, so I was not surprised when the dean groaned at the prospect of speaking to me. My case was yet another drop into his bitter cup. I derived some satisfaction from knowing I had company in my ordeal.

Under the circumstances I could engineer things in such a

way as to have directors of our school, and not myself, lose their jobs. All I had to do was to sing to the investigators. But it would have meant another round of infighting and I was too exhausted for that. I was sick and tired of all and everything. I was sick and tired of my country. I did not want to start a new intrigue. I could not care less who devoured whom, who would be expelled, who would be demoted. I had my own goal: to part with them as quietly and put as much distance between us as possible.

I handed the dean an application requesting a discharge within a month's time. I planned to use that month to land a new job. In my mouth I felt a bitter taste of defeat. My plans notwithstanding, the application was a renunciation of everything I had pursued for many years and achieved at such a high price.

"We go back a long way together," I told the dean, "almost thirty years. So for old time's sake will you do me one last favor concerning my son? Promise that no one will harm him when I'm gone."

The dean glanced at me with a trace of friendliness. "I promise."

"Whatever may be?"

"Whatever may be." The friendliness left his eyes. "Well, now that it's over you must realize you have no one to blame except yourself. You were given ample warning not to touch Party members. . . ."

All right, I knew it. I had been warned on many occasions: by Katya in bed in Czechoslovakia; by the drunk Belousov receiving my gifts; by Party Secretary Kornienko. What had happened was dictated by my personality. But now all that was over; all I cared about was my son's security.

I found out that the Vishnevsky Institute of Surgery, where my father had once worked, was looking for a senior researcher for its purulent wounds department. The position was two notches below my status and payed 150 rubles less, but the job suited me. I went to see Dr. Kostyuchonok, head of the department.

"The job's yours if you want it," he told me. "But remember it involves classified research and therefore requires a category two security clearance. Do you have any security rating at all?"

"No."

"That complicates matters. It takes several months to get a clearance."

Of course, I did not tell him I was going to emigrate.

At the mention of the clearance, I immediately realized that I had to turn the job down even if it was crammed down my throat. No one holding a security clearance of any kind was allowed to leave Russia at least until several years after expiration of the period covered by the clearance. I thanked him and left.

Irina was waiting for the news of my new job.

"Nothing doing," I told her. "They need a security clearance, while we need nothing of the sort. I'll have to look for something else. Did you talk to your mother; did she approve?"

Tears welled in Irina's eyes.

"What's happened?" I asked. "She doesn't want to go?"

"No. My stepfather doesn't want to leave Russia. But that's not the problem. She doesn't want to go. She told me she had a dream in which my father appeared and pitied her being abandoned by her daughter. And many other things, so obscure I didn't understand them. Everything she said was full of spite and self-pity. I wept for two hours afterward. I swear to God I've never thought of it, but now for the first time I'd like to go to Father's grave and complain to him about Mother. I don't want to talk to her again, ever."

I had no trouble recognizing my mother-in-law's nasty temper in Irina's incoherent story. But what a difference between the two mothers! And how sorry I felt for my wife!

I had a friend of long standing, an eminent professor of immunology, Alexander I. A Jew roughly my age, he had several years ago decided to emigrate to Israel, and so quit his job; but he held a class 3 security clearance that gave him access to scientific material not printed by the official press, and he and his wife were denied permission to leave Russia. My friend tried to find some other research position to get by, however meagerly, until the ban was lifted. But no one hired him. During the year he spent job hunting he became thoroughly steeped in the technology of emigration and supplied me with a great deal of useful information.

"Your best bet is to become a consultant at a commercial outpatient department," he told me. "There are no employment restrictions there. It's sort of a halfway house between a permanent job and emigration. Scores of doctors have left Russia and all of them were able to work practically to the last day at commercial clinics. And the pay's not bad either: three rubles per hour."

I followed his advice and went to seek employment at Commercial Clinic #6, on Petrovka Street. The system of commercial outpatient departments clearly contradicted the law on free medical care, but it existed with official blessings. Patients were charged for the full range of services—from an examination to analyses to X rays to treatment. The rates were relatively cheap, but expenses had a way of piling up and each patient had to pay an average of 25 rubles. Commercial clinics were very popular and always filled to overflowing with patients from all over the country. The clinics were staffed by fairly experienced physicians, many of whom charged patients additionally. For doctors it was a good source of outside income.

Clinic #6 was housed in the depth of a small and dirty yard. It was a rickety wooden building, reconstructed many times. Lack of space was depressing; patients stood for hours in long lines to register, to pay, and to be seen by the physicians. The head doctor was my old acquaintance, Dr. Mikhail Khutorenko, a one-time head doctor of the Kremlin Hospital. In 1960, he had taken Dr. Yazykov and myself to Khrushchev's dacha. Now he was retired on pension, but boredom made him look for something to occupy his time and he came to this hospital. He didn't remember me, and I decided against reminding him that we had once known each other; prudence dictated that when the time came to apply for permission to emigrate the less people knew about me the better. The clinic needed an orthopedist and we struck a deal. I returned to my entry-level income, but I was not concerned, for I did not plan to work for more than a year; besides, we had enough savings not to have financial worries for some time.

The work was not exciting, but any change of job is interesting because one meets new people and new working conditions. The surgeon of the clinic was Dr. V. Sanyuk, a tall Jew past fifty. He made a favorable impression on me and was invariably courteous and attentive in a conversation. I did not disclose my plans to him, merely telling him that I was going to work at the clinic temporarily because I was busy organizing a new research laboratory, where eventually

I meant to work full time. I don't know if he believed me, but he did not ask questions. Soon afterward I found out that he was Party secretary at the clinic and he commended me on my reticence.

Once we sat together, reminiscing about the times past. "The Jewish question is my heartache," he told me. "If only you knew how close to my heart I take everything associated with the Jews!"

We became friends. He invited Irina and me to dinner and his wife Bronya treated us to delicious gefilte fish. Everything in his home was associated with the Jewish heritage. He had an enormous collection of Jewish records and took particular pleasure in listening to Israeli songs:

"We are coming out at dawn / The wind is blowing out of the Sinai / Raising clouds of dust to the skies / Before me lie the Sinai sands / Behind me lies my Motherland / Across my chest is my machine-gun."

While the record was playing, Dr. Sanyuk sang and danced along. The rousing music stirred up deep emotions in all of us, particularly in my Irina. She fell in love with that song and constantly hummed to herself: "Across my chest is my machine-gun."

Sitting in a cozy Moscow apartment, we almost felt like soldiers of the Israeli armed forces. And I thought: "My God, what tortuous paths we follow! Only three years ago I spoke at an imbecilic anti-Semitic meeting and mumbled incoherently something about Israeli aggressiveness to save my skin. And now I enjoy myself by singing along with a cheerful military song of Israel."

My new friend was very knowledgeable about Zionism. He was born and raised in Kiev, where Jewish traditions have always been much stronger than in Moscow. But how and why did he become a communist? He told me had joined the Party during World War Two, where he saw action as a much-decorated lieutenant in a reconnaissance unit. He did it out of hatred for the Nazis, particularly after learning about Babi-Yar. Those were the years of acute patriotism and hardship. What might not happen when one is just eighteen?

Under his influence, for the first time I developed a strong interest in the history and traditions of the Jews. I did not become religious, but on Yom Kippur in 1977, I fasted to share the Jewish experience. And for the first time I yearned to go to Moscow's sole synagogue to be able to immerse myself in a Jewish environment. But

I was afraid: uniformed police and KGB plainclothesmen kept vigil at the synagogue, photographing many, if not all, of the people who came there. I did not want to give the KGB any material that could be used against me and delay my departure, so I did not go.

An important advantage of my new job was that it occupied little of my time, so I was able to take care of my private affairs. And I was grateful to Alexander I. for having led me to such a convenient job. But he himself, try as he might, could not find employment; he was turned down because he was Jewish and because he had applied to leave Russia. What was he to do? Under the law, he could be officially branded a *tuneyadets* (social parasite), subject to banishment from Moscow. He had almost nothing left to live on.

After a year of ordeal he finally got a job as a night watchman at the Journalists' Club, for a night watchman could be of any ethnic identity. Once every three nights he went to work, for which he was paid 60 rubles per month.

"Never in my life have I held such a nice job!" he said cheerfully. "First of all, it's the only place where nobody asks about my nationality. Secondly, I work absolutely alone and thus don't have to suffer the company of imbeciles or attend their idiotic meetings. And above all, I've lots of free time to study at the library and write scientific papers on my own. Of course, I'm a little hungry, but somehow I get enough nutrition to cerebrate. And I've never felt so free!"

I introduced the professor–night watchman to the communist-Zionist. They liked each other. In general all would-be emigrants became friends easily, for we shared a lot of things. The professor–night watchman loved to listen to Jewish songs at the communist-Zionist's, while the communist-Zionist liked to listen to the stories the professor–night watchman told about refuseniks— Jews denied emigration permits. I, too, was enraptured by the stories. Gradually, my circle of friends changed. Now all my aspirations were directed toward emigration and I grew totally indifferent to what had once been the essence of my life: achievements, career, success.

I withdrew from Valium, I slept well, my "heart fatigue" was gone, and I no longer felt a burden in my chest. Now at night I embraced my Irina with youthful vigor as if I had been rejuvenated.

Yes, everything was changing within me and around me. I

looked into the future without apprehension and anxiety, but in anticipation of new and exciting things to come. I did not expect an easy life, but I did not seek one; I sought a *different* life.

And, like the professor–night watchman, I felt free, as never before.

52

We could only learn how to go about implementing our emigration plans from the grapevine, the sole source of information available to Russian citizens. The authorities told us nothing, although by 1977, emigration had been in progress for eight years, and 150,000 Jews, almost 5 percent of the Russian Jewish community, had left the country. Never in her thousand-year history has Russia experienced such an exodus. After the 1917 Revolution, emigration had been banned outright. And now it had reached massive proportions. Emigration was all Jews could talk about: some of them had already left; others were about to leave; still others were bracing themselves for the decisive plunge; yet others knew people who had left. But of course, all conversations were conducted in secret, and only among Jews; with rare exceptions, Russians were excluded.

The idea of emigration was so pervasive among the Jews that it even gave rise to this joke: A Jew approaches a group of three other Jews engaged in a heated debate and says, "I don't know what you're talking about, but, of course, the answer is, emigrate."

I and my friends, the professor–night watchman and the communist-Zionist, had amassed a mountain of useful information: what to do and in what sequence at all stages of the emigration process from filing a visa application in Russia to arriving in the United States or Israel. Our ears, attuned to rumors through a lifetime of habit, were now veritable radars. Experience guided us through the maze of rumors and helped us to pluck grains of wisdom from the chaff.

I was faced with several main tasks:

1. Before applying for emigration, to research how the authorities might conceivably treat would-be emigrants my son's age after they applied for visas; anticipate all possible moves and plan against any kind of contingency.

2. To obtain invitations from Israel for all five of us, including my parents.

3. To plan the sale of most of my property and try to smuggle at least a fraction of my wealth in any form out of the country.

4. To study English and cram for the forthcoming American exam to confirm my physician's credentials.

5. To try to smuggle out my diaries, manuscripts, and all our documents in the original; emigrants were not allowed to take with them anything on that list.

For Irina and myself, naturally enough, our son's well-being was the overriding concern. Already, Irina was nervous in advance and spent sleepless nights pondering what would happen to him if we were denied permission to emigrate and he were expelled from the medical school. In order to have at least a remote idea of what awaited teenage boys applying to leave Russia, Irina and I went to Riga, the foremost emigration gate for Russian Jews, where we hoped to have our questions answered.

As a member of the Managing Council of the Writers' Union Literary Fund, I approached the fund director, V. Voronin, with a request for two passes to a writers' sanatorium near Riga. Voronin was a newcomer to the Literary Fund. He had been an official at the Russian Trade Mission in London and was expelled from Britain in a group of 150 Russian spies. Back in Moscow, he was given a pension as a KGB colonel and a cushy job as a reward for past services. He issued me two passes to a deluxe suite at the writers' sanatorium.

For the last time I vacationed on privileged terms, for I intended to leave the Writers' Union very shortly; to improve our chances of getting exit visas, I planned to cut off all threads that tied me to any kinds of privileges and perks. Once in Riga, we found our old Jewish friends, many of whose acquaintances had already left for Israel or the United States. We spent nights with them, going over the case histories of all teenagers who had left Russia. By and large, it seemed, no special obstacles had been put in their way. But there were no guarantees, either, for several boys had been denied permission to emigrate and were drafted into the army. My friends also suggested that I invest my money in jewelry, provided I had a way to smuggle it abroad. The idea was tempting because I had more money than I could legally spend. But there was no way valuables and antiques could be officially taken through the customs. We had to devise a way to get our wealth out of Russia and get it back once we were safely beyond the Soviet borders.

At the sanatorium I took up English studies under Irina's guidance. Every day, my first teacher of English patiently taught me new words and the correct way to pronounce them. I was rather a dumb student.

When we returned to Moscow, I went to see a psychiatrist friend of mine, a Jew in whom I had complete confidence. I told him about my plans.

"If worse comes to worst," I asked, "and they attempt to draft my son into the army, can we make a medical document certifying him as a serious psychiatric case?"

"No problem," my friend replied without a moment's hesitation. "I'll register him as an outpatient, suffering from schizophrenia. Under the law, he's not obligated to inform anyone of his condition unless and until he has a need to. If they draft him, I'll send a transcript of his case history to the military commissariat and they'll have to waive your son under a special article of the Conscription Act."

"But what if they don't believe the diagnosis and decide to examine him themselves?"

"Then I'll set up your son for a consultation with Dr. Snezhnevsky, chief psychiatrist of the Ministry of Public Health. He's an incontestable authority. No one would dare dispute his opinion."

"But will Snezhnevsky say that my son is sick when he's not?"

"Don't worry, he will," my friend said confidently. "He has his own pet theory of expanded boundaries of schizophrenia. I'll coach your son in how to behave, and I'll write up his phony case history in such a way that Snezhnevsky will have no difficulty diagnosing schizophrenia."

I knew that Snezhnevsky had earned adverse publicity in the worldwide community of psychiatrists because he had expanded the boundaries of psychiatric diseases and diagnosed perfectly healthy dissidents as schizophrenics. But I also knew that no one in Russia would think of disputing his diagnosis. So I readily agreed with my friend's plan. But how terrible to have to pass off my healthy boy as a schizophrenic!

My father's cousin, Zina Churchin, seventy, lived in Antwerp, Belgium. I had never seen her because she had left Russia with her family immediately after the Revolution. For several years now we had been conducting intermittent correspondence. She had even invited us to visit her in Belgium in 1968, but our applications were turned down. I wrote Zina a letter hinting about our decision to emigrate. The hints were couched in cautious and vague terms in the hope that Zina would understand them while the Soviet censors would not. Zina did understand and came to Moscow together with my cousin Raimond for a three-day tourist trip—her first in sixty years.

We worked out a plan: Zina agreed to contact our distant relatives in Israel and prevail upon them to send us officially registered invitations. It was the only way to get permission to leave Russia. Later Zina told the whole story to my aunt Lyuba in New York, who expressed a desire to come to Moscow once again to discuss all the particulars about our coming to America.

Thus, bit by bit, I worked to ease our departure. But how could we smuggle out my documents and valuables? My friend from Holland, Lev Sinitsky, came again. I decided to discuss my problem with him:

"Will you agree to take my personal documents, diary, and manuscripts?" I asked. "I won't be angry if you say no, because I realize the risk you'll be taking."

He pondered for several minutes. "What's in your diary?" he asked.

"Nothing except my personal entires."

"Any sensitive stuff?"

"Absolutely none. But a lot of criticism about Russia."

"Usually I carry a lot of company documentation and I've never been checked by customs," he said. "I think I'll be able to take out your papers."

"Thank you." My relief and gratitude were boundless. "And one more thing: can you smuggle out a few jewels and gold articles for me?"

"Easily. I'll put them in my wallet, in the change compartment. So far they've never searched my pockets."

His agreement gave me a precious opportunity to smuggle out of Russia at least part of what we had saved. Even if I sold the smuggled valuables at half or even a third of the price, it would be better than nothing.

He also agreed to take out one sample each of my shoulder-joint, elbow-joint, and wrist-joint prostheses. I was overjoyed: now I would be in a position to show my artificial joints to new colleagues in America and continue work to improve on their design.

Over the last few years I had saved some 20,000 rubles, a substantial sum by our standards. I kept my money at the savings bank paying the highest available interest rate—3 percent. My father also had money in the bank, 14,000 rubles. Though he had worked twice as long as I had, he had saved less. I think that the reason for the disparity is simply that I had not yet passed along to my son as much as my father had passed along to me.

My cooperative apartment, car, and my berth at the cooperative garage, if sold, could bring another 20,000 rubles. We decided to pool all our financial resources and invest them as best we could with the goal of taking with us at least part of our fortune in gold and jewelry. I made my mother-in-law heir to 5,000 rubles in cash, our new furniture, and absolutely everything else we owned.

Now I had to find and buy jewelry. Private transactions in diamonds are prohibited in Russia on pain of being charged with currency speculation—a grave offense carrying severe punishment. But the state is the biggest speculator of all: it officially buys jewelry from the populace at low prices and resells it at an exorbitant markup. Therefore people prefer to sell their valuables privately on the sly. But quality diamonds were rare. I was given a few addresses and Irina and I spent several nights traveling to the sellers and examining their wares. All the jewels offered contained major defects, all were priced very high while their potential value in the West, where diamonds were a thousand times more valuable, was negligible. Obviously, the offers we received were losing propositions. I became very tired of the diamond chase: I was not a connoisseur of precious stones by any measure and I did not know the going prices, but it was up to me to make decisions. Irina's expertise was as meager as mine; all her life she was rather indifferent to precious stones and had very little jewelry in her possession.

Finally my mother came up with a good idea:

"Why don't you go to Chistopol and see our old friends, the Samovs. They had excellent old jewelry and gold coins. They won't be afraid of you and might gladly sell."

So early in December I set out for Chistopol, the town where I had spent my childhood. I took the train to Kazan, from whence I had to go either by bus or taxi to my destination, a distance of one hundred miles. The crowd waiting for the bus was too great. A taxi driver warned that he would not be able to take me all the way to Chistopol: the Kama River, about two miles wide, was in the way, bridges were unavailable, while the ice cover on the river was too weak to support the weight of the car. I decided to take the risk and persuaded three other passengers from the bus line, two Tatar men past middle age and a Tatar woman, to share the taxi with me and split the fare four ways. We came to the end of the highway where it reached the Kama River. Strong gusts of wind whipped snow over the ice sheet covering the wide river. Thick snow was falling, obscuring the view of the opposite bank. We were unsure what to do next. No official information about the ice condition was available. We could test our luck and walk across, but only at the risk of falling into the water and going under. It was getting dark; a strong wind was blowing; we were cold and miserably aware of being cast adrift.

Suddenly we heard the sound of a motorcycle and headlamp beams appeared, moving toward us from the opposite bank. Soon we saw a motorcycle with a sidecar, with a driver and two passengers. We all rushed down to meet the newcomers, whose arrival signified that the crossing was passable. The motorcycle driver agreed to take us across the river, charging five rubles per person. I had to position myself on the sidecar fender. Lest I be thrown off along the bumpy road ahead, the driver tied me down to the sidecar with thick rope. I retrieved my sharp tourist knife from a trouser pocket and kept it in my fist in the pocket of my fur coat. If the ice cracked and we started sinking, at least I would be able to cut myself free in a single swing. The motorcycle dashed off up the ice into the blinding snowstorm. Visibility was close to zero, but we had to drive fast so as to rush across weak ice spots. After a quarter of an hour of fear and hope we dashed up the steep bank. The driver unraveled my bonds and I started to flap my numb arms.

After the tiring journey it was a pleasure to warm myself in the house where I had spent my childhood. The house was crumbling away with age; the owners were even more frail than their home. I did not tell them that I was going to leave Russia; the news might have scared them. I simply said that I had saved some money and wanted to invest it in jewelry and gold. They kept their valuables at the bottom of a huge steamer trunk of the kind that can only be found in the homes of old merchant families, and agreed to sell me the lot for 15,000 rubles.

The next day was a Sunday, and I took my last stroll through the town, retracing the routes of my childhood. I came to my old high school and stood at the entrance for awhile, trying to evoke in my memory the episodes and faces of days long past. Beyond the school was a tall fence surrounding the two-story building of the city prison. I recalled that I had always been afraid of that building. The prison was old and dismal; its sight imbued me with a feeling of foreboding. The small windows were boarded over, the wood darkened by time and rain. I could see the figure of a sentry in a sheepskin coat with a rifle hulking on the tower at the corner of the fence. I turned and walked away.

On the way home I wandered into an open-air market. Trade was sluggish, the counters half-empty, the prices high. A long line stretched along one of the counters. People stood pressing tightly against one another. They were waiting for something; the counter was bare.

"What are you standing for?" I asked one woman in the line.

"Just waiting," she replied indifferently. "Maybe meat will be brought in, who knows? . . ."

The walk filled me with sadness. No, I was not sorry to leave this Russia. The thought pumped adrenalin into my blood and I hurried back.

The old lady sewed up the jewelry and gold in my trouser pocket, so the only way I could lose my fortune was together with the trousers. I took a taxi to the river. There were no vehicles, but many people were crossing the ice on foot. I joined them. It was quite a chore to walk on the slippery surface against a strong, biting wind. It took me almost two hours to get to the opposite bank.

By nightfall I reached Kazan, took a passing train, and by next morning got home. Irina cut open my sewn-up pocket, and the gold coins and jewels cascaded onto the floor.

53

Irina handed in her resignation. According to our plan, she was to quit before we applied for emigration in order to avoid any reference to her place of employment in our applications. The Institute of Microbiology and Epidemiology was a semi-secret institution where bacteriological weapons were developed, and though Irina had nothing to do with sensitive research we decided it wisest for her to quit in advance. Institute Director Dr. O. Baroyan, an old spy, could not divine the true reason for Irina's resignation and tried to keep her with promises of promotion and a pay raise. But she told him she had already found a better job.

I found it amusing that we were able to dupe the sly Armenian fox. But it was not so easy to fool her Jewish colleagues, many of whom sensed the reason Irina was quitting. Dr. Ida Uchitel, an intelligent and charming woman, asked Irina softly so nobody could hear: "You've made an important decision, haven't you?"

Without a word Irina nodded. Then Dr. Uchitel invited us to her home for dinner. When we came she pelted us with questions, and we spent the whole night discussing the problem of the Jewish exodus. It was pleasant to discuss the subject with a sympathetic person, although our hostess did not intend to emigrate and was consequently somewhat restrained.

She asked me: "Do you hope to become head of an orthopedic department in America?"

"Not at all."

"What *do* you hope for then?"

"To be able to start from scratch and step by step win the right to be a doctor again."

"But it'll be difficult and, pardon me, humiliating for you."

"I'm prepared for anything, even humiliation. Maybe I idealize America, but it seems to me it would never have achieved its successes unless its people could grow commensurate with their talents. I believe in success because I believe in America."

"Maybe you're right," she said thoughtfully. "Still, if I had the courage to leave, I think I'd go to Israel."

My aunt Lyuba came to stay for a month with us. This time customs officials went through her two suitcases with particular zeal and finally decided on a duty payment of 200 rubles. Naturally, Lyuba had no Russian money, while I had just 150 rubles on me.

"I don't have the two hundred; all I have is a hundred and fifty," I told the official.

"Okay," he waved his arm. "A hundred and fifty will do."

God knows what rules those Russian customs officials follow!

Lyuba and I discussed our forthcoming journey. HIAS, a Jewish agency, was to support us from Vienna to the United States, so we needed no help. But Lyuba gave us a lot of useful information on what to take and what to leave behind, making the packing much easier for us.

Soon after Lyuba's departure, Israeli invitations for us and my parents came through the mail. They were from Assya Berlovich. I had never heard that name before, but it made no difference. In her officially registered and stamped letter, she appealed to the Russian government to allow her kin—meaning all of us—to emigrate to Israel so that our families could, at long last, reunite.

Now we had to come out into the open. Our son went to see the dean of his medical school with an application that said that in view of his forthcoming departure for Israel he requested a document certifying his status as a medical student. Irina and I anxiously awaited the outcome of his mission: maybe Valdimir Junior would be instantly expelled from school; maybe the dean would refuse to sign the certificate. The dean had given me his word not to harm my son before we had declared our intention to leave for Israel. Each person applying for emigration automatically becomes an outcast, and all previous obligations are considered to be null and void; a distinct boundary line is drawn between the before and the after.

"They may try to talk you out of emigration," I told my son before he left on his mission, "lecture you on morals, insist that you think of your future and stand fast against outside influences. Respond like this: 'My parents have decided to go and I have to accompany them.' Lay all the blame on us and pretend you're a pawn in our evil hands."

The boy returned home at night beaming with satisfaction: the dean had signed the certificate and refrained from moralizing. There had also been a Jewish coed in the dean's office who had come with a similar request. The youngsters kept silent in the dean's presence, but once they left the office they burst out laughing with relief.

I went to see the head doctor of my clinic to have him sign my emigration papers. Knowing that he held a colonel's rank with the KGB, I steeled myself for a nasty dialogue. But to my utter astonishment, he glanced at my application and without a word signed it. My friend, the communist-Zionist, told me that later in the day Khutorenko had said to him, "You know, Professor Golyakhovsky came to me with an application for emigration to Israel."

"You don't say." My friend feigned indignant surprise; as the Party secretary of the clinic he was duty bound to disapprove of such a "crime."

"I signed his papers," the head doctor went on. "After all, it's up to him if he wishes to go. One is sometimes apt to be up to one's ears in trouble just to move from one apartment to another, while to emigrate . . . No, let him go, it's his own business."

"Right," said the Party secretary, who planned to follow in my footsteps shortly.

I filled out the necessary forms and took them to the OVIR office. Police Lieutenant Marina Duravko, who knew me, greeted me with a smile; she remembered that during my fight for a vacation in Yugoslavia important people had helped me. But when she read "To Israel" on the form, her thin eyebrows slid up in astonishment:

"Well, well, well, Doctor, you're really getting around, first to Yugoslavia, now to Israel. . . . "

"Well, you know how such things happen," I replied noncommittally.

The smile left her face. And I went out into the street with a new feeling: The die has been cast, the Rubicon has been crossed! Now there was no turning back.

The obligatory six months of waiting for the answer dragged on interminably; what would it be: permission or refusal? Before applying for emigration nobody, except our closest friends, had been told of our plans, but now there was no point in hiding anymore. I mailed my membership card back to the Writers' Union Secretariat and enclosed this note: "In view of my intention to move for permanent residence to Israel, I request dismissal from the Writers' Union." Several days later, Felix Kuznetsov, secretary of the union's ruling board, called on the phone.

"Did you write the application yourself?" he asked.

"Sure I have; haven't you seen my signature?"

"Oh, I saw your signature all right, but it crossed my mind that perhaps you feel victim to a provocation. . . . "

"No, it's my application."

"Well, that's different then," and he hung up.

That same day rumors started circulating about me among the writers. Since we lived in a writers' building, all our neighbors immediately got wind of the "event." The writer Vasily Aksenov alone was supportive, while the rest of them took to keeping away from me and stopped saying hello. I had anticipated just such a reaction; but what I was not prepared for was that my closest friends, those who had stood by me all my life, would try to avoid me. With each passing day we received fewer and fewer calls until one day our telephone line was almost totally dead. I was angry and sad: they had been with me all our lives; I had helped them all; I had treated their relatives; I had been their friend—and now they were trying to erase all memory of me!

How deep is the chasm of slavery in the Russian soil! I was certain they had not fallen out of love with me; they were just afraid of keeping in touch with the "leper" and, in case my telephone was bugged, of having their voices taped. Occasionally they did call from a public phone, always speaking briefly and in hushed tones. Such calls stressed my status as outcast and I disliked them. Sometimes one or another of them dared visit me, but invariably late at night, sneaking to my house under cover of darkness.

My ties snapped one after another. I had ceased sending articles to journals and no longer attended the sessions of scientific councils on which I still sat officially. I stopped seeing patients at the Ministry of Internal Affairs Outpatient Clinic and gave up contact with General Igor Karpets. Once another friend of mine, General Josef Cincar, military attaché of Czechoslovakia, paid a visit to my home, but the reason for our meeting was sad: our mutual friend, Dr. Miloš Janeček, had passed away.

Remote acquaintances, with whom we had not been close, behaved differently. Upon meeting us and learning that we were going to emigrate, almost all of them exclaimed in excitement, "Hey, it's great! If only we could leave as well!"

One such distant acquaintance, Irina's ex-colleague and the wife of a TASS correspondent in Austria, spread a rumor that I was being sent by the KGB on a spying mission.

"Don't you doubt it," she assured other people we knew, "believe me, people of his kind don't just up and go. He is going on a secret mission, masquerading as a Jewish refugee."

Having spent a good deal of time with her husband abroad, apparently her viewpoint was shaped by precedents.

The wait was frustrating. Our son still attended classes at his medical school and I continued to work at the commercial outpatient hospital. No attempts were made to expel or bother either of us. I learned that KGB officials had turned up at the medical school and rifled through my file to see if I had ever had access to sensitive material. I had not, although a security clearance went automatically with my rank. I was afraid that they would dig up my contacts with the cosmonauts and my project to provide spaceships with magnetic-field insulation. Everything associated with space exploration was considered sensitive material.

In the fall, our son was drafted for semiannual labor duty to pick potatoes on a state farm. It is a form of labor conscription compulsory for all students. This time our son had to spend a full month on the farm under particularly trying conditions. Once, Irina and I decided to visit him and drove sixty miles to the northeast of Moscow. There, near the town of Dmitrov, was a small village, Olyevidovo, the seat of the collective farm. The weather was gray and damp, the dirt road mired in mud; our tiny car slipped and skidded. The farm consisted of several one-story dingy log barracks behind a common fence. Outwardly it looked like a Gulag camp and the medical students inside were the picture of the Gulag inmates described by Solzhenitsyn. Everything was dirty, miserable, and desolate. Our son looked unhappy and lonesome. He was a member of some sort of "shock team" and "overfulfilled" his quota. Besides, as a "man on duty" he was responsible for keeping the barracks clean and his superiors satisfied. His position was unenviable, no question about it, but he had no other choice but to endure. To the rest of them he was a stranger.

I went inside the barracks to see how the students lived. The oppressive, foul air all but forced me outside. Irina and I were distressed. We put our son and a friend of his in our car, drove some distance away from the farm, and let the boys gorge themselves on chocolate and other delicacies. They were very hungry. We returned a short while later to find their commander, a stern-faced army captain, waiting impatiently. A veritable Gulag!

Soon afterward I sold my car and garage berth for 10,000 rubles, sewed up the money in a pocket, and again set out to buy jewelry.

Once a month I called the OVIR to ask Lieutenant Duravko where we were, but each time I got a standard reply: "No decision on your case has been handed down yet."

From the numerous rumors that swept the Jewish community I knew that 80 to 85 percent of the applications were given permission to leave the country. Still, that left 15 to 20 percent whose applications were turned down, and in each individual case the response was totally unpredictable.

I spent nights, sometimes till dawn, in my library, worrying. Earlier I had sat at that desk, writing treatises or poems or drawing sketches of my new inventions, but now I was doing nothing—just speculating on one subject and one subject alone: would they let us go or not? Sometimes Irina, who could not sleep either, joined me. She would sit in an armchair, tucking her legs underneath her, and we would silently ponder the nagging question.

I weighed and assessed all logical probabilities, although I was aware that *they* were not constrained by the rules of logic. But what could I base my predictions on? My current status of a lowly consulting physician at an ordinary outpatient clinic certainly favored our emigration prospects. On the other hand, almost all my previous career militated against leniency and provided the authorities with a host of pretexts to keep us in Russia. I cursed my hyperactivity. Why in hell had I fought to become head of a chair and director of a medical school department?

Another alternative was possible: I would be kept back while the rest of my family would be allowed to go. What was to be done then? I thought that Irina and our son had better go in any case, but my parents were sure to stay with me. Maybe I would be allowed to emigrate later, after a few years' hiatus! But how would Irina and our son do without me in a strange land? And suppose I would never be allowed to join them?

In those months I followed the Voice of America and BBC broadcasts particularly avidly. The Madrid Conference on the record of compliance with the Helsinki Accords had just begun. Almost every night I learned about the debates on the issue of emigration from Russia. Soviet media never mentioned a word of the Madrid meeting. It seemed to me I developed an ability to distill the foreign broadcasts and evaluate my chances for an exit visa from the general tenor of the diplomatic skirmishes in Madrid. Of course, it was merely a figment of my imagination, born of constant nervous tension.

I pondered another problem: if I was not allowed to go, what would I do with my active self? I had always detested mute obedience. So far the authorities had not touched me directly, and consequently I had refrained from raising my voice against them. But denied my right to emigrate, I would certainly pick a fight. In my mind I was getting ready to become an active dissident. I even thought it likely that in the long run I would be jailed or shipped to a concentration camp. The prospect did not dismay or sway me: if such a turn of events happened, it meant that such was my destiny. I recalled the old prison in Chistopol, with its boarded-up windows and dismal gray facade behind the tall fence. That might be my final home!

Irina had her own worries: how would we start anew in America? What awaited our son? Would we be able to find jobs? How would we survive the inevitable hardship before we gained our footing again? Irina was forty-five, and it was easy to understand the worries of a middle-aged woman faced with the prospect of a major upheaval.

Strange as it may be, I was not overly worried about our future in America. I knew that we would all find life difficult there, and I harder than the others because I knew almost no English and would have to take a difficult doctor's exam. But I planned as follows: it would take me three years to overcome the language barrier and pass the exam. All that time Irina would have to work to support the family, while I would try to sell our jewelry to tide us over. Our son would have to enter college and fall backward three years in his education if he was to eventually enroll in medical school. I knew that my parents would receive modest pensions and subsidized housing. No matter, we'd muddle through! If worse came to worst, I was ready to take any kind of job. The prospect of working as a nurse's aide did not in the least seem humiliating. I knew that a typical American biography followed this sequence: an errand boy—an ordinary clerk—a millionaire. Of course, it was too late for me to *start*, but I was prepared to do just that if I had to.

I was not in the least scared by anything *after* we left Russia. I was going to America with an open heart: I loved her and hoped she would reciprocate my feelings.

In the middle of December 1977, Lieutenant Duravko told me, "Call me on December thirtieth."

Her statement instilled terror and hope in us and we waited impatiently for the day. On the morning of December 30, 1977, I called the OVIR and heard Lieutenant Duravko say:

"You've been allowed to leave, together with your whole family."

Victory!

Our son called from school and, hearing the good news, quit immediately; as a would-be emigrant he found it hard to breathe in the animosity-filled atmosphere. The news came just in time: our son was shortly to be seen by Dr. Snezhnevsky, the psychiatrist. Now he was spared the ordeal of trying to pass himself off as a lunatic. I rushed to my parents to tell them the news. Mother wept with happiness, but Father was still nervous: what lay ahead for all of us? I went to see my mother-in-law and her husband. Since learning about our intention to emigrate, she had not spoken to Irina. I had to make them conclude a peace treaty before we were gone. Irina's mother went into hysterics; she wept and complained, picking on Irina in particular. I listened patiently; after all, I had put up with her all my life, so I could afford to endure just a while longer.

The next day we celebrated the New Year, 1978, at home, knowing that in the coming year we would leave Russia and go to America. Never had we been so happy.

In the frosty night beyond the window a bright star glimmered in the sky. It was the star of our happiness.

54

We had to wait a few more weeks for the exit visas. The waiting was agony. From time to time I called Lieutenant Duravko only to hear a standard polite reply: "Your visas are not ready yet."

I strained my ears, trying to interpret her inflection. Sometimes it seemed to me that she accompanied her reply with a smile as if to comfort me: "Don't worry, everything will be okay." At other times I had the impression that she coldly rapped out each word as if implying that my fate still hung in the balance. I oscillated between joy and despair; only an infatuated lover could examine a woman's voice with such zeal. Finally a day came when she told me sweetly: "You may come tomorrow to pick up your visas. Bring the money to pay for them."

"Thank you, thank you!"

Each one of us had to pay 500 rubles for the privilege of renouncing our citizenship.

"Suppose I wished to get my Soviet citizenship back," I asked a teller at a savings bank. "How much would it cost me?"

She looked at me as if I were crazy and handed me a citizenship petition form. "It says here," she said, "the assumption of citizenship costs fifty kopecks."

One-thousandth the price of giving citizenship up! I felt like laughing out loud.

With the visas in my pocket, I grabbed a cab and rushed to the Aeroflot International Box Office on Frunze Quay. The first order of business was to buy tickets for Vienna. All Jews with Israeli visas departed for Vienna first. From there on private Jewish philanthropies and societies financed by the Israeli and United States governments supported the emigrants. Each of us was allowed to convert into dollars just 90 rubles ($135); and for all practical purposes we crossed the border as paupers.

In the meantime I decided to buy first-class seats on a TU-134 airliner. Let us become paupers *there,* but I wanted to leave *this* country in style, as an ancient Russian tradition dictated. "Let the air hostesses serve us with the cognac and caviar due to first-class passengers," I thought. "Who knows when we'll be able to afford such luxuries again?"

The next morning, while it was still dark, I set out for the Dutch embassy, which represented Israeli interests in Russia, where I was to receive our entrance visas to Israel. Having ceased to be a Russian subject, I felt very strange in the streets of Moscow—I was beside myself with joy, with ecstasy. The thought that my pocket contained a permanent exit visa, not a Soviet passport, throbbed in my mind. I forgot all my achievements in life except this one: I had obtained a release from this country for my wife, my son, myself, and my parents! I was free!

I approached the ancient mansion housing the Dutch embassy. The sight of a policeman at the embassy door produced the customary reflex—a bout of inner timidity. Indeed, how could I *feel* free if my experience cried out that entering a foreign embassy was a grave crime in itself.

No sooner had I approached the door than the policeman spoke: "You've got the address right, but the reception starts at nine A.M. So you'll have to wait, but not here. Go where everybody's gone to wait." But where was everybody waiting, as he indicated?

I crossed the narrow street and looked around. At first I saw no one, but on second glance I noticed the doors of the adjacent buildings occasionally open and heads pop out, peering toward the embassy. People had come early and were killing the time in the lobbies of neighboring houses, protecting themselves against the January frost and the policeman's wrath.

Aha! So I, too, had to hide in a strange lobby? But the idea was not appealing. Better to stroll through the streets. After a good walk I returned to the embassy at five minutes to nine, feeling cold. I could see from a distance that the doors of the buildings in the street were open and knots of people stood in the doorways in fives and tens. All were staring transfixed at the embassy. A squad car stopped and disgorged two police lieutenants who then took up positions. The next instant the huge ancient door of the embassy swung open from inside, and, as if on cue, the waiting people surged forward. They ran across and along the street, exchanging shouts. An instant later, a line sprang up at the embassy door. The policeman set about bringing order to the chaos, working crisply and efficiently. I stepped up my pace, but to no avail; I found myself near the end of a long line of about three hundred men and women. The crowd irritated the policemen, who were apparently under orders to prevent congestion at the door lest passersby and foreign correspondents become unduly interested in the commotion. They tried to persuade the people to disband and come one after another, but the line responded by compressing even more tightly. The people behind me pressed forward and squashed me against the humanity in front of me. It felt like being in a subway during rush hour. But I did not want to surrender my place in the line either, and also pressed against my neighbors. Finally the policemen gave up and left us alone.

People from the line were allowed inside in small groups, ten or fifteen at a time. The policemen checked their visas, peering at the photographs and checking them against the faces of the bearers. Their paramount concern was to prevent any unauthorized persons from entering the sacred embassy grounds. The police knew that many would-be emigrants hoped to smuggle out their personal documents with the Dutch diplomatic pouch, and insisted that people leave their briefcases outside. However, the emigrants knew about that and secreted their papers in pockets or even behind trouser and skirt belts. In general I was amazed at how thoroughly informed and knowledgeable in all particulars of the emigration process my neighbors in the line were. I heard snatches of conversations around me: "Look, there are more people today than there were yesterday."

"There are many from Kiev who have come to have their invitations reissued. A lot of refusals there lately." "The cops today aren't as ferocious as they usually are." "It's because they haven't gotten angry yet. Just wait till they get hungry and tired."

At last I got inside, passed through another check, and as part of the crowd was led up to the second floor. From time to time a pretty woman emerged from an office with a stack of visas in her hands and started a roll call. She could not outshout the crowd, so people passed around the names she called. When the right person was found, his papers would be handed to him. Because of the bustle a simple procedure was transformed into a prolonged chaos. But it did nothing to dampen the general buoyance. At last the frustrated secretary stopped calling out names and fell silent, waiting for the people in the hall to calm down. Bit by bit, the crowd fell silent. Then she said in heavily accented Russian:

"Ladies and gentlemen, *gospoda*, I cannot outshout your chorus. Please be quieter."

A concerted outburst of laughter was her response. For the first time in our lives we were addressed as *gospoda* instead of the customary "comrades." Yes, indeed, life was changing!

Finally, I was cleared, all papers in hand. I had spent half a day among the Russian refugees. For me it was a sort of overture to what awaited us all in the months ahead. I saw that noise and hassle were to be my constant companions in the weeks and months to come.

I was done with one embassy. Now I had to visit another one —the Austrian embassy, to get a transit visa. But there the entire procedure took a mere half hour. Now everything was behind me, all my life in Russia. It was a life to which I no longer belonged.

55

During one of our last nights at home I sat down at my desk and wrote a farewell poem entitled "Fare Thee Well": "I will not rush into your arms / I will not take your ash with me, Russia / I am leaving you without regret / And I will never come back. / Neither your birch trees nor your wide expanse / Will lure me back, / Without gloom or heartache/I joyously say good-bye to you. / Nostalgia will not torment me / Nor will it force me to mope, / Everything in you, Russia, is alien to me / Everything cries to be forgotten."

Several days were left till our departure, and everything we were doing was *done for the last time.* Irina and I arranged a farewell party for seventeen of our friends, all of them Jewish, all of them either planning to leave, or thinking seriously about leaving, or at the very least supportive of the idea of emigration. We did not attempt to select our guests either by ethnic identity or by aspirations. Those who came to say good-bye were simply our remaining friends, the last few who had not betrayed us.

My friends and patients, the lawyer Keller and his wife, came. Their only daughter, Galya, had left for Israel in 1970.

"Do you remember how you tried to persuade me to leave six years ago?" I asked him. "Thanks a lot for sound advice."

"Better late than never," he said. We laughed.

Dr. Sanyuk, the communist–Zionist, brought a pile of Jewish records. None of us had ever heard so much Jewish music. The wonderful tunes made us merry; we wanted to laugh and dance.

My refusenik friend, the professor–night watchman, came wearing his work clothes because at midnight he was to go on shift. He was dressed in thick, warm trousers tucked into boots, an old military tunic, cowhide top boots, and a broad military belt. Even so, he merrily danced to Jewish songs, stamping his boots on the floor.

"I couldn't dance at my farewell party, so at least let me dance at yours," he shouted above the din. Irina circled him, waving a kerchief. They looked for all the world like Russian folk dancers, while the rest of us, clasping each other's shoulders, jumped and jumped in a Jewish Freilachs dance till we could hardly breathe.

Happy and drunk, I flashed our exit visas. Also hot with wine and revelry, the guests touched the visas reverently, as a sacrament. It was not difficult to understand their wistful glances: for them the documents meant freedom.

The professor–night watchman gave us this farewell speech:

"Swear to God you will be cautious till the very last moment. Remember, until you get off the Soviet plane you won't be free. But once your feet are firmly planted on Austrian soil, not before, then gather all the saliva in your mouth and spit toward the plane. And then spit again for me."

Twenty-four hours before departure we were required to bring all our baggage to the Sheremetyevo Airport and submit it to thorough customs inspection. I knew the procedure took several hours for each family and that some items, even though officially allowed to be taken out of the country, would be stopped. To be first in line, we came to the airport at 6:00 A.M. I was accompanied by my son, to help me lug the heavy suitcases, my father, and Irina. Although we indeed were at the head of the line, inspection of our baggage did not start until noon. We were all exhausted; Father, tended to by Irina, was in a particularly poor way. We had eight suitcases for the five of us. That was all. One suitcase contained my Russian-made and foreign-made typewriters, another my son's tape recorder, a third blankets. Minus these three, we had just a suitcase each for our personal belongings, as if we were going on a month-long vacation, not moving for good to another country. But Irina and I were against taking too many personal things: what good were they anyway? We were taking our wits with us and that was all that mattered. We would have plenty of time to acquire material possessions in the future.

Three customs officials examined all our belongings, down to the smallest trinket. They unscrewed the cover-plates of the typewriters and tape recorder and peeped inside to make sure no jewelry or other forbidden articles were secreted there. The silver spoons were carefully weighed and the two smallest ones were turned back —excess weight! Mother's family icon, which had faithfully blessed generations of newlyweds, was also barred from expatriation although it had little commercial value. My son's tapes were taken to a special room and checked for their contents—whether they really were music recordings or something else.

The officials' zeal reached its peak when they examined my father's seventeen combat decorations earned in World War Two. They checked the medals against their certificates, engaged in a debate, and then declared that we would have to leave the decorations behind. My poor father was so upset I was afraid he would have a heart attack. I tried to console him, all the while arguing with the officials. They repeated a barely intelligible jumble: "In general, of course, sometimes decorations can be allowed to go through, but only in special cases of personal agreement. . . ."

Clearly, what kind of personal agreement, except a personal bribe, could there be in a matter like this? I was aware that customs officials had a habit of milking the emigrants for huge sums. But to bribe them for the decorations for which my father had put his life on the line? Never! Under the law, the only way a person could be stripped of his combat decorations was by a special decree of the Presidium of the Supreme Soviet. I got on the phone to the customs administration and finally obtained permission for the medals. The officials yielded with undisguised but understandable reluctance—they had just lost a seemingly sure bet. The inspection took half a day, and there was a line behind us. Finally we returned home, all four of us, because my parents had already checked out of their apartment.

We had to spend one more night and one more morning in Russia. Vladimir Junior went to say good-bye to his girlfriend. I was afraid he might be beaten up as a parting rebuke by the authorities, so I let him go for just two hours with a warning to be careful. He came back in tears: ah, first love!

My mother-in-law and her husband spent the evening with us, she popping tranquilizer pills all the time. Although Irina and her mother had made up, there still was a residual trace of animosity between them. Irina's aunt came to pick up Irina's old shearling coat for her daughter. We gave away our possessions without regret. Only one thought swirled in our minds: let's go, and the faster the better! But those who were staying needed our things.

Early on the morning of February 8, 1978, we arrived for the last time at the airport. The weather was clear and bright—perfect flying conditions. The customs officials once again checked the contents of our handbags, pocketbooks, and wallets. Again we went over the allowable weight limit and I paid the duty with my last rubles. I knew it was within their power to do as they pleased, even to subject us to a body search. I had warned my family to be prepared for such an eventuality, that they should stay calm and refrain from expressing indignation. We were to avoid conflict with officialdom at all costs. Fortunately, everything went smoothly and we were not stripped or delayed. Only one barrier remained: a last passport check by the KGB before we could board the plane.

We heard the announcement of our plane over the PA system. It sounded like Beethoven's Ninth Symphony: "Attention, passengers. Passengers with tickets for flight Moscow-Vienna, Aeroflot TU-134, are requested to proceed for boarding to Gate Seven." The announcement was repeated in English, French, and German. Gate 7—seven is a lucky number!

We ascended the stairs to the second-floor border checkpoint in Indian file. I had planned our formation in advance: Vladimir Jr. was to be at the head of the column because, being the youngest of us, he was the likeliest target for last-minute harrassment (I had heard of such cases); next came Irina so that as soon as the boy crossed the border his mother would join him; she was followed by my parents—I did not expect them to have any difficulties. I brought up the rear to make sure all my family safely passed the checkpoint and were beyond the border. I distrusted the authorities till the very last moment and expected some act of treachery. If that happened, at least I would know my family was safe. My heart was pounding frantically.

The KGB officers took our visas, examined the photographs against the owners' faces, stamped the visas, and finally opened the turnstile in the passage to the border. I stood several feet to the rear, watching the proceedings intently, constantly alert for signs of trouble. The turnstile opened before my son and he crossed the border. Aha, now Irina followed him. At least they had each other if anything happened. My parents were waved through. Now my turn. I came to the booth and extended my visa to the officer inside, my hand trembling involuntarily. He looked at the photograph, turned his eyes to my face. His face was totally expressionless. He stamped the visa. . . . He handed it back to me. . . . The lock buzzed, I pushed the turnstile. . . . I crossed the Russian border. . . . I was walking as if in a dream.

Suddenly I woke up. The tension was gone and a wave of joy engulfed me. We started to kiss and smile, then we rushed to Gate 7. Of course, even now something could still happen, but once over the border, such a possibility was very small. We were taken to the plane in a bus. The stewardess smiled at us. Oho, not bad!

After takeoff the plane made a banked turn over the part of Moscow where we had lived. For the last time I had a bird's-eye view of the painfully familiar district. The flight to Vienna lasted two and a half hours. We had seats in the first-class section and enjoyed brandy with caviar and a delicious lunch. Marvelous! From time to time we nudged each other and exchanged smiling glances. Behind us, in the tourist section, were three KGB agents, whose presence was mandatory on all flights abroad. I spotted them easily, of course. They dozed in their seats, occasionally casting glances in our direction. All right, watch us to your hearts' content, I thought, use your powers over us to the hilt, for the hour of deliverance is near.

Vienna appeared in the distance. The airliner dipped its nose and started to descend. Any minute now we would leave the last piece of Russian territory. We landed. The plane taxied to the gate. I looked out of the window, then eyed the KGB agents. They stayed in their seats. The door opened and we left the plane. The air was cold, fresh, and fragrant.

We descended the stairway in the same order: our son first, followed by Irina, then my parents, and finally me. We stepped on Austrian land. A bus stood nearby—a Viennese bus, not a Russian one. I recalled my friend's request and, before climbing into the bus, spat toward the plane.

A charming young woman, representative of the Israeli Sohnuth, met us with a dazzling smile.

"Shalom." She sang the unaccustomed greeting melodiously. "Where are you going, to Israel or America?"

"Shalom! We are going to America."

Beyond the door we saw a welcoming committee: our Dutch friends Lev and Natasha Sinitsky, who brought our papers and valuables, and my father's cousins from Antwerp: Zina, who had made arrangements about our Israeli invitations, and Berta.

When we embraced, my aunts exclaimed: "Free, free at last!

Yes, it was true; for the first time in our lives we were free. Tears welled in my eyes. I looked at my family—Irina, my son, my parents, at our relatives and friends, at the new surroundings—and cried. Did it really happen? Was I dreaming?

We were taken in a car to a small hotel, the Donau, for Russian refugees. We were given just one room for all five of us, a large room but without a bathroom or a telephone. No matter, we would manage! The Jewish organizations paid all our expenses and we were grateful.

Irina and I went out into the snow-covered wide street. We went to the post office to call her mother in Moscow and tell her everything was all right. The surroundings were different from everything we had known in the past. While we walked, I suddenly experienced a strange, mystical feeling: as if I were inside a long and narrow pipe. A dim light glimmered at its end. I felt distinctly that something had left me and was slowly floating along the pipe toward the distant light. What was it? It seemed to me I had less difficulty breathing now. I stopped. Irina looked at me with surprise and concern. I told her:

"You know, my past life has just flown away."